Men'sHealth®

TOTAL-BODY HEALTH & FITNESS GUIDE

2010

RODALE®

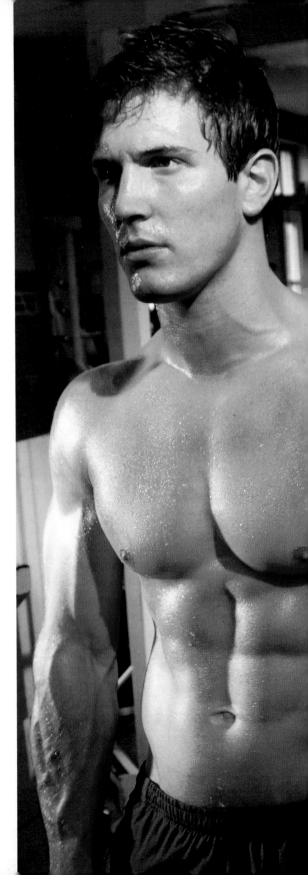

© 2010 by Rodale Inc.

All rights reserved.
No part of this publication may be reproduced or transmitted in any form or by any means, electronic or mechanical, including photocopying, recording, or any other information storage and retrieval system, without the written permission of the publisher.

Men's Health is a registered trademark of Rodale Inc.

Rodale books may be purchased
for business or promotional use or for special sales.
For information, please write to:
Special Markets Department, Rodale, Inc.,
733 Third Avenue, New York, NY 10017

Printed in the United States of America

Rodale Inc. makes every effort to use acid-free ∞,
recycled paper ♻

ISBN 13: 978-1-60529-721-7

Book design by John Dixon and Elizabeth Neal

Cover photographs: © Alan Cresto (left);
© Image Source (center left); © Claire Artman/Corbis
(center right); Scott McDermott (right)

2 4 6 8 10 9 7 5 3 1 hardcover

RODALE
LIVE YOUR WHOLE LIFE™

We inspire and enable people to improve their lives and the world around them
For more of our products visit rodalestore.com or call 800-848-4735

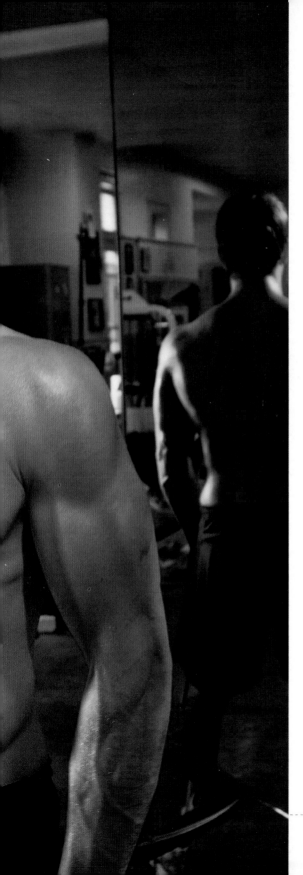

CONTENTS

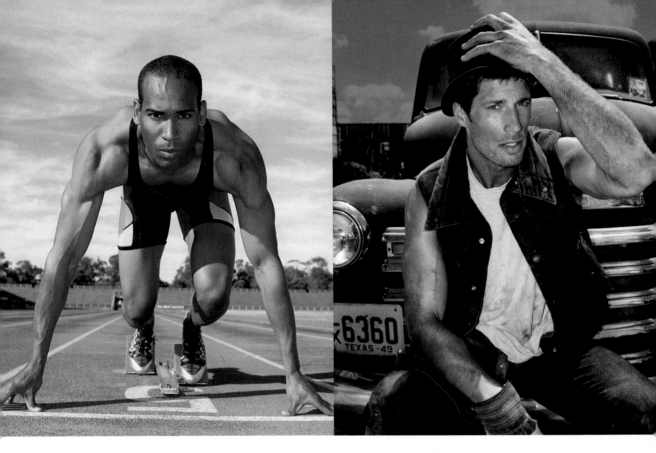

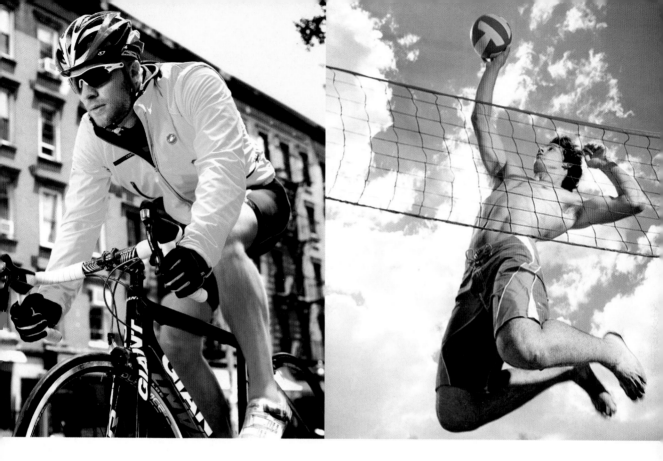

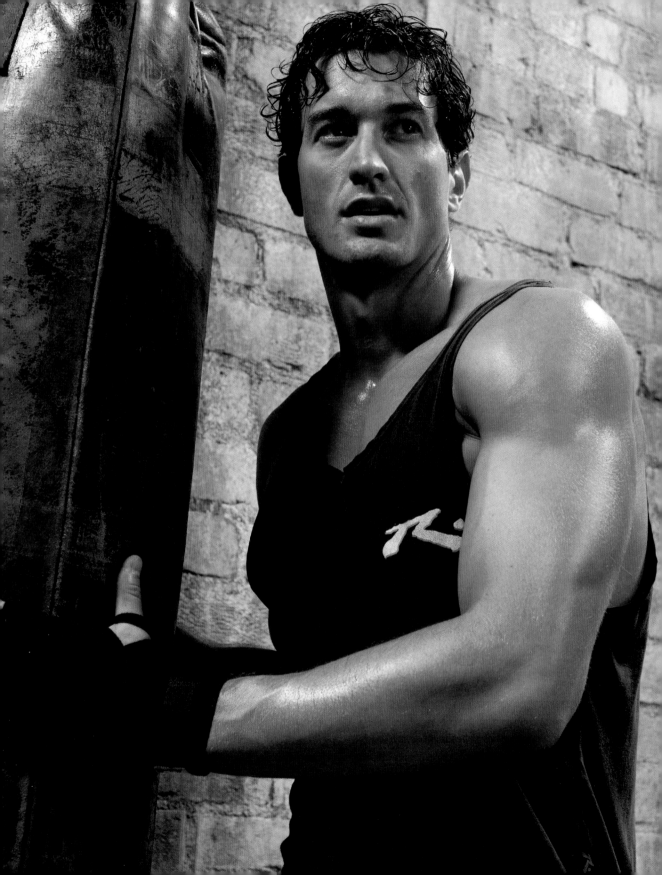

According to a Johns Hopkins study, by 2048 every single American adult could be over-weight. Scientists estimate that within 21 years, 1 out of every 6 health-care dollars will be attributable to the obesity epidemic.

We are slowly eating ourselves to death. And the risks of obesity are, well, enormous. According to the Centers for Disease Control and Prevention, obesity increases the risk of the following diseases and health conditions.

CORONARY HEART DISEASE

TYPE 2 DIABETES

CANCERS, SUCH AS OF THE COLON

HIGH BLOOD PRESSURE

HIGH TOTAL CHOLESTEROL OR HIGH LEVELS OF TRIGLYCERIDES

STROKE

LIVER DISEASE

GALLBLADDER DISEASE

SLEEP APNEA

RESPIRATORY PROBLEMS

OSTEOARTHRITIS

With this book, we aim to help you to help yourself improve your health and your fitness. Weight loss is one major part of that. But there's lots more, too.

In **Part 1**, Lose Your Gut, you'll find our best fat-fighting tips. Change your body one meal at a time in "Eat This, Not That." "Outsmart Your Stomach" with seven ways to fill your gut and lose it, too. Then learn why kicking your soda habit might be the easiest way to lose the weight for good.

In **Part 2**, Flat Belly Foods, you'll discover how to best fuel your body. "Power Up Your Diet" with the new superfoods. Need a pick-me-up? Read "Wake Up, Already" for the latest information on energy drinks. If all else fails "Get an Edge" with the caffeine advantage.

Because you're busy, **Part 3** will help you to Muscle Up Fast. First things first, "Test Your Strength" with our 1-minute muscle test. "Sculpt a Gold Medal Physique" with the secrets of Romania's muscle building wizard. Finally use our best strategies to "Get into the Best Shape of Your Life."

Part 4 offers our best style tips so you'll Look Better Instantly. Learn the 19 essential rules of male style so you can "Dress to Impress." Turn back time without going under the knife. And put a halt to your receding hairline, but "Don't Get Scalped."

Part 5 helps get and keep you on the road to good health, Live Longer, Live Better. Steal rich-guy lifestyle moves to "Be as Healthy as the Wealthy." "Take Charge of Your Health" by asking your doctor to check some critical blood markers. And stop putting off your doctor's "Checkup—or Check Out."

Finally, in **Part 6**, you'll Strip Away Stress. "Burn Fat, Not Fuel" by cranking out your commute. Tap into your primal marksman and "Sink Every Free Throw." And do it all without hurting yourself and "Injury-Proof Your Workout."

Here's all of our best advice—to make you your best. ■

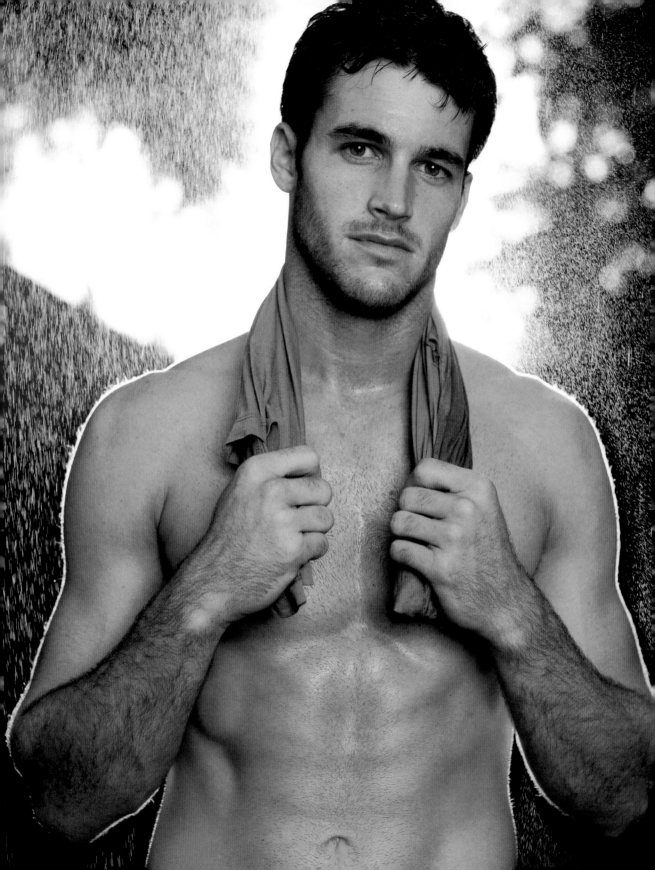

1

Lose Your Gut

Eat This, Not That

HERE ARE SIMPLE, SMART, FAST WAYS TO CHANGE YOUR BODY, ONE MEAL AT A TIME

Not all burgers are created equal. That's important, especially when you consider that the average guy will eat 100 of them this year.

Take America's two most famous burgers, the Whopper with Cheese and the Big Mac. A fair fight, right? Well, if you go for the Arch alternative, you'll save 220 calories over the BK behemoth. Use that strategy for every burger you eat this year, and you'll save 22,000 calories—the equivalent of 6 pounds of body fat.

See, the way you pick your favorite fixes—from burgers to banana splits—could help you make the transition from chubby to chiseled. In researching *Eat This, Not That!,* the best-selling book based on the popular column in *Men's Health* magazine, we found that the most effective weight-loss strategy doesn't require you to abandon the foods you love but simply to make better choices when selecting them. Do that, and you'll trade failed diets and wild weight fluctuations for healthy eating patterns and a lean, new you. Who wouldn't make that swap?

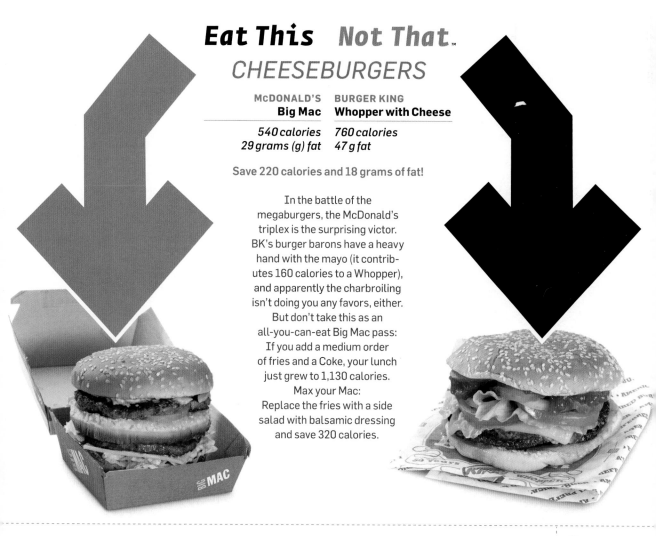

Eat This Not That.

CHEESEBURGERS

McDONALD'S Big Mac	BURGER KING Whopper with Cheese
540 calories	760 calories
29 grams (g) fat	47 g fat

Save 220 calories and 18 grams of fat!

In the battle of the megaburgers, the McDonald's triplex is the surprising victor. BK's burger barons have a heavy hand with the mayo (it contributes 160 calories to a Whopper), and apparently the charbroiling isn't doing you any favors, either. But don't take this as an all-you-can-eat Big Mac pass: If you add a medium order of fries and a Coke, your lunch just grew to 1,130 calories. Max your Mac: Replace the fries with a side salad with balsamic dressing and save 320 calories.

PIZZA

DOMINO'S
large cheese pizza with crunchy thin crust (2 slices)

360 calories
19 grams fat

PIZZA HUT
large cheese pizza with thin 'n' crispy crust (2 slices)

560 calories
24 grams fat

Save 200 calories and 5 grams of fat!

In the world of mass-produced pizza, nothing beats Domino's crunchy thin-crust pie. This is how Italians meant for pizza to be eaten—with a crackling crisp crust and balanced cheese and sauce. The average guy will consume 46 slices of pizza this year, so this one small change can save you nearly 5,000 calories—a down payment on a smaller waist size.

CHICKEN MEAL

BOSTON MARKET
Chicken
(1 thigh and 1 drumstick)

300 calories
17 grams fat

KFC
Original Recipe Chicken
(1 thigh and 1 drumstick)

460 calories
32 grams fat

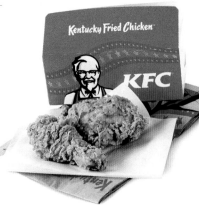

Save 160 calories and 15 grams of fat!

There's no secret recipe here, just a fryer full of bubbling oil and a breaded, grease-infused two-piece combo. Boston Market slow-roasts its birds on a spit, so they're naturally juicy (but not oil-saturated) with a great balance of fat and protein. Add sides of garlic-dill new potatoes and green-bean casserole for a meal you can savor now and not suffer from later. Sub in steer: Tired of chicken? Five ounces of sirloin will run you only 290 calories.

TURKEY SANDWICH

SUBWAY
6-inch Turkey Sub with provolone

330 calories
8.5 grams fat

PANERA
Sierra Turkey

840 calories
41 grams fat

Save 510 calories and 33 grams of fat!

Turkey, roast beef, and ham are all lean cuts. But Panera slathers its turkey with a thick layer of chipotle mayo and slides it into a heavy, oily wedge of focaccia, so this turkey is a porker. A Subway 6-incher not enough to quell your raging lunchtime hunger? Double up on the meat for just 50 calories more. Forget the focaccia: Panera's smoked turkey on sourdough has only 430 calories.

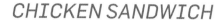

Eat This

Not That

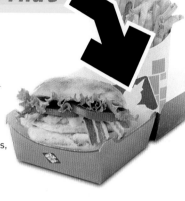

CHICKEN SANDWICH

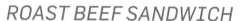

JACK IN THE BOX **Chicken Fajita Pita** (with side salad and salsa)	**JACK IN THE BOX** **Chipotle Chicken Ciabatta** (with natural-cut fries)
335 calories 12 grams fat	1,140 calories 51 grams fat

Save 805 calories and 39 grams of fat!

The chipotle chicken sandwich has more than double the calories, fat, and carbohydrates even before you factor in the fries.

ROAST BEEF SANDWICH

ARBY'S **Super Roast Beef Sandwich**	**ARBY'S** **Roast Beef and Swiss Market Fresh Sandwich**
398 calories 18 grams fat	777 calories 41 grams fat

Save 379 calories and 23 grams of fat!

Skip the seemingly healthy "Market Fresh" sandwich in favor of the classic Super Roast Beef, which has about half the calories.

BURRITO

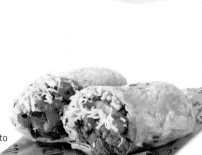

TACO BELL **Regular Style Steak Burrito Supreme**	**CHIPOTLE** **Steak Burrito**
390 calories 14 grams fat	1,033 calories 40 grams fat

Save 643 calories and 26 grams of fat!

Chipotle uses terrific fresh ingredients, but until the chain downsizes its football-size burritos, you have only two safe ways to quell your craving: Share half of your Chipotle burrito or swap in Taco Bell's leaner Burrito Supreme. (If you must, add a taco. You'll still save more than 450 calories.)

CAESAR SALAD

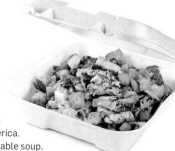

PANERA **Grilled Chicken Caesar Salad**	**CHILI'S** **Chicken Caesar Salad**
560 calories 34 grams fat	1,010 calories 76 grams fat

Save 450 calories and 42 grams of fat!

In the wrong hands, a Caesar salad can be murder. At Chili's, the innocent pile of romaine is swallowed up by a perfect storm of dressing, Parmesan cheese, and croutons, making this unnatural disaster one of the unhealthiest salads in America. Craft a combo: Round out your meal with a 90-calorie cup of Garden Vegetable soup.

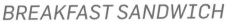

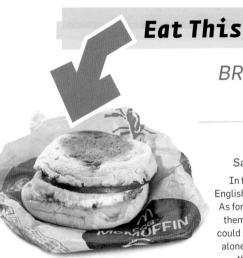

BREAKFAST SANDWICH

MCDONALD'S
Egg McMuffin

STARBUCKS
Classic Sausage, Egg & Aged Cheddar Breakfast Sandwich

300 calories
12 grams fat

460 calories
25 grams fat

Save 160 calories and 13 grams of fat!

In the nutritional hierarchy of breakfast breads, English muffins beat bagels and croissants every time. As for meats, bacon tops sausage, and ham trounces them both. Replace the sausage with ham, and you could save up to 500 calories a week from breakfasts alone. Case in point: Starbucks has a ham version of this sandwich that weighs in at 380 calories. Start strong: Eighteen grams of protein make this a surprisingly sound beginning to your day.

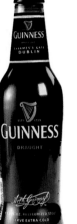

BEER

GUINNESS
Draught

SIERRA NEVADA
Pale Ale

126 calories
10 grams carbohydrates

175 calories
14 grams carbohydrates

Save 49 calories a beer!

Surprised? Most people think of Guinness as a beer milk shake: dark, thick, and rich enough to inspire guilt along with the intense pleasure. But a 12-ounce mug is as low in calories as many watery light beers, and it can save you up to 50 calories over other full-flavored brews, such as Sierra Nevada. Switch out a six-pack a week, and you'll save yourself more than 4 pounds this year. Brilliant! Sip smartly: Stick with this bottle because the Extra Stout version packs an extra 50 calories.

FRUIT SMOOTHIE

JAMBA JUICE
Power Mega Mango Smoothie

DUNKIN' DONUTS
Large Tropical Fruit Smoothie

420 calories
97 grams sugar

720 calories
142 grams sugar

Save 300 calories and 45 grams of sugar!

This sickeningly sweet concoction from Dunkin' has an ingredient list straight out of a chem lab and more sugar than seven Häagen-Dazs vanilla-and-almond ice-cream bars. So this tropical excursion will be bad for your equator. On the other hand, the Jamba version is 100 percent fruit, so there's a huge caloric discount and big antioxidant payload.

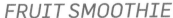

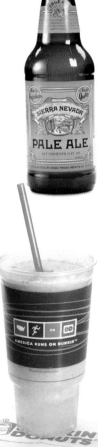

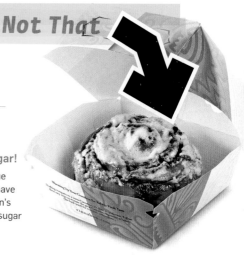

CINNAMON ROLL

AU BON PAIN | **CINNABON**
Cinnamon Roll | **Classic Cinnabon**

350 calories | 813 calories
21 grams sugar | 55 grams sugar

Save 463 calories and 34 grams of sugar!

Right. There's absolutely no nutritional value in a cinnamon roll. But when you just have to have one, take comfort in knowing that Au Bon Pain's sweet spiral more than halves the calories and sugar found in the Cinnabon catastrophe.

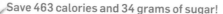

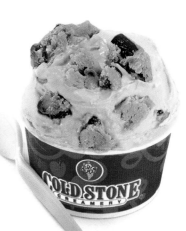

ICE CREAM

COLD STONE CREAMERY | **COLD STONE CREAMERY**
Cake Batter Light Ice Cream with Chocolate Shavings (Like It size) | **Cake Batter Ice Cream with Cookie Dough** (Like It size)

330 calories | 510 calories
11 grams fat | 26 grams fat

Save 180 calories and 15 grams of fat!

If you're going for a summer treat, stick with the light option. It has less than half the fat but all the flavor of the regular version.

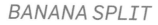

BANANA SPLIT

DAIRY QUEEN | **BASKIN-ROBBINS**
Banana Split | **Classic Banana Split**

530 calories | 1,030 calories
14 grams fat | 39 grams fat

Save 500 calories and 25 grams of fat!

Ever eat just half of an ice-cream sundae? Neither have we. So stay out of trouble: Ditch the Baskin-Robbins bomb in favor of the scaled-down version from Dairy Queen and spend the 500 calories you saved on another sundae (next week). Save energy: With more sugar than four Snickers bars, the Baskin-Robbins dish will make your energy level soar, then plummet. ■

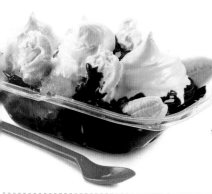

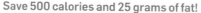

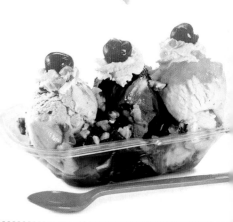

Know the Science

PROPONENTS OF THE GLYCEMIC INDEX SAY THE SECRET TO LOSING YOUR GUT IS TO EAT BY THEIR NUMBERS. BUT **WHAT HAPPENS WHEN THOSE NUMBERS LIE?**

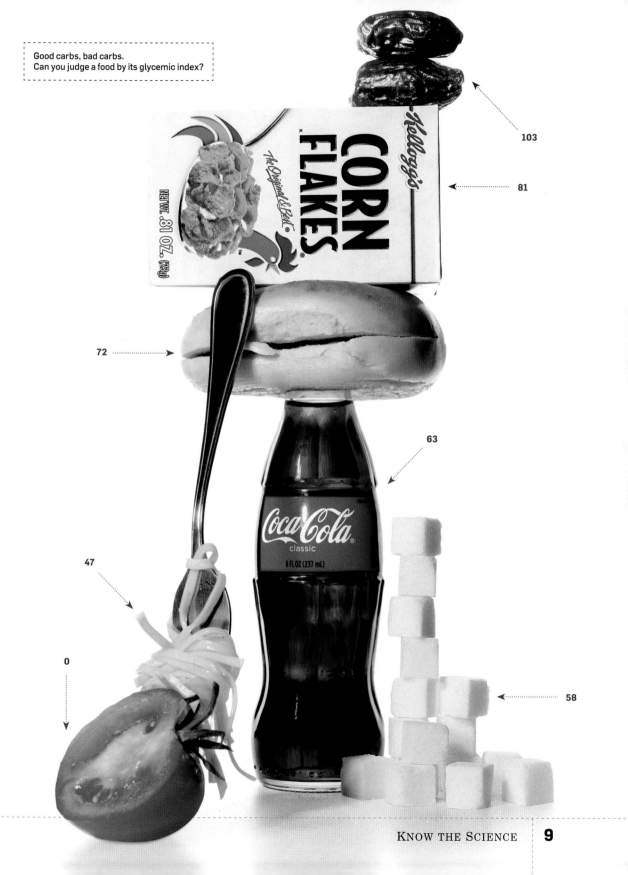

Good carbs, bad carbs.
Can you judge a food by its glycemic index?

103

81

72

63

47

0

58

Here's a riddle:
What do a Twix candy bar, a Pizza Hut supreme pizza, and a Betty Crocker chocolate cake have in common?

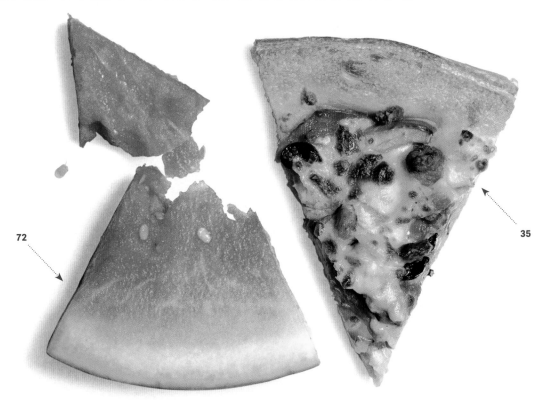

72

35

ANSWER: They're all "low glycemic" foods. And according to many nutrition experts, that qualifies them not only as healthy but also as great diet fare. For example, NutriSystem has pegged its marketing campaign on the science of the "glycemic advantage," which the company claims is the key to losing weight while allowing you to eat the foods you love.

What is all this glycemic science? A bit of background: The glycemic index (GI) ranks foods based on the impact they have on your blood sugar. So the higher a food's glycemic index, the higher it elevates the amount of glucose coursing through your veins.

The idea is that this overload of glucose leads to wild swings in blood sugar (it goes up, then comes crashing down), which ultimately causes you to crave more carbs. As a result, you overeat, or at the very least feel deprived from denying yourself, say promoters of the glycemic index. What's more, they argue that high blood sugar triggers the release of insulin, a hormone that helps lower blood-glucose levels, but that also signals your body to store fat.

This has led to the differentiation between good carbs and bad carbs. The good carbs are said to be low glycemic, meaning they break down slowly, which keeps blood sugar and insulin levels more stable and holds hunger at bay; the bad carbs are high glycemic and do the opposite.

All of which sounds smart, of course, but don't put Pizza Hut on your speed dial just yet. Turns out, the science of the glycemic index isn't that simple—and in fact, it's even a little sketchy.

THE FIRST FLAW

Let's say you decide to eat based on the glycemic index. So when given a choice, you'll choose the foods with the lowest GIs. Now consider the following GI facts.

- **Both pound cake and soda have a lower GI than watermelon.**
- **Chocolate ice cream has a lower GI than a parsnip.**
- **The GI of a Twix bar is lower than that of all the foods we just mentioned.**

According to this analysis, you should opt for a Twix over a slice of watermelon. A soda would be better, too. Intuitively, of course, that doesn't make sense. After all, per serving, the watermelon is lower in calories and higher in essential nutrients than the Twix. And, well, it's fruit—not junk.

What gives? It's simple: The glycemic index doesn't compare real-world portion sizes. You see, the GI of a food is determined by giving people an amount that provides 50 grams of digestible carbohydrates, which include starch and sugar but not fiber.

This is the amount of carbs in about three-quarters of a king-size Twix. However, you'd have to eat 5 cups of diced watermelon to match that number—not exactly an apples-to-apples comparison. So even though eating a lot of watermelon

According to the glycemic index, A SUPREME PIZZA IS HEALTHIER than watermelon.

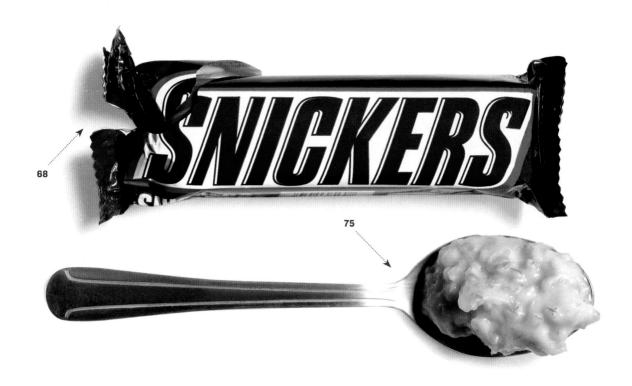

68

75

might raise blood sugar dramatically, a single serving of the fruit has significantly less sugar than a candy bar. (To see how GI researchers tried to remedy this problem, check out "Glycemic Load: A Better Number?" on page 14.)

Your takeaway: A food's ranking on the glycemic index doesn't necessarily indicate whether it's a good or bad choice. As a general rule of thumb, whole foods—such as produce—are superior to their processed counterparts, regardless of where the items fall on the glycemic index.

THE FITNESS FACTOR

Another surprise: The glycemic index of a food isn't a set number. University of Toronto scientists found that the value can vary by 23 to 54 percent from person to person. What's more, it can also differ within the same person. Scientists at Syracuse University discovered that a single weight-training session reduces the effect of a high-sugar drink on blood glucose by 15 percent for 12 hours after an intense workout.

Exercise uses the glucose stored in your

The best time to EAT FAST-ABSORBING CARBS is before, during, and after exercise.

Carbohydrates...Explained

SIMPLE CARBOHYDRATES

(a.k.a. sugar)
We eat many types of sugar, but the two main ones are glucose and fructose. They combine to create other sugars, such as sucrose.

GLUCOSE

Your body's main energy source, this is the "sugar" in blood sugar. Because it's already in the form your body needs, it's quickly absorbed into your blood.

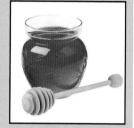

FRUCTOSE

To use fructose, your body must first send it to your liver, where it's converted to glucose or into fat and stored. This is why fructose doesn't spike blood-sugar levels.

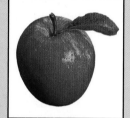

COMPLEX CARBOHYDRATES

The definition for these is simple: any carbohydrate that's composed of more than two sugar molecules.

STARCH

This is a bundle of glucose molecules held together by a weak chemical bond. As a result, it's broken down easily into pure glucose and absorbed quickly.

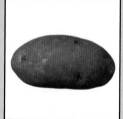

FIBER

Like starch, fiber is a bundle of sugar molecules. However, human digestive enzymes can't break the bonds that hold them together, preventing absorption.

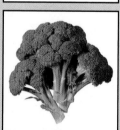

muscles. And to replenish those stores after a workout, your body starts shuttling more of the glucose from your bloodstream to your muscles, where it's packed away for future use. This helps reduce blood-glucose levels quickly, even after a high-sugar meal. Consider it another reason to lift weights: That extra muscle gives you a larger storage area for glucose.

Your takeaway: The more active you are and the more muscle you build, the less you need to worry about how foods affect your blood sugar. This is also why the best time to eat fast-absorbing carbs is just before, during, and right after your workout.

THE LOW-GLYCEMIC LOOPHOLES

Look on the back of a package of a king-size Twix and you'll find that it has 46 grams of sugar. How then, can it be a low-glycemic food? Three reasons.

1. Not all sugar causes spikes in blood glucose. Here's why: The nutrients you eat that have the greatest impact on your blood sugar are glucose and starch. (See "Carbohydrates . . . Explained" at left.) But most sweeteners, such as sucrose (table sugar) and high-fructose corn syrup, are only about half glucose. The rest is primarily fructose, a sugar that has just a tiny effect on blood sugar. So only a portion of the sweetener in a Twix bar is high glycemic.

Your takeaway: Don't be fooled into thinking low-glycemic junk food isn't still junk. Remember, eating highly sweetened snacks is an easy way to consume the excess calories that lead to a bulging belly.

GLYCEMIC LOAD:
A BETTER NUMBER?
EVEN EXPERTS WHO PROMOTE THE GLYCEMIC INDEX (GI) REALIZE IT'S NOT PERFECT. BUT IS THEIR SOLUTION REALLY AN IMPROVEMENT?

To address the flaws in the GI, Harvard University scientists came up with another number to base food choices on. It's called the glycemic load, and it takes into account a food's portion size as well as its GI. You can calculate a food's glycemic load by dividing its GI by 100 and then multiplying that by its grams of digestible carbohydrates (total carbs minus fiber).

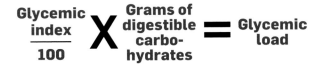

$$\frac{\text{Glycemic index}}{100} \quad X \quad \frac{\text{Grams of digestible carbo-}}{\text{hydrates}} \quad = \quad \text{Glycemic load}$$

TAKE MACARONI: It has a GI of 47, and 48 grams of digestible carbs. Do the math, and you'll find that its glycemic load is 23. A glycemic load of 20 or higher is considered high; 11 to 19 is medium; 10 or below is low.

$$\frac{47}{100} \text{ x } 48 = 23$$

There's little doubt that using the glycemic load is better than considering a food's GI alone. But here's a secret: If you're concerned about how a specific food affects your blood sugar, you don't need to figure out its glycemic load. All you must know is the number of digestible carbs it has. The higher the number, the higher your blood sugar will rise. Simply take the total number of carbohydrates listed on a product's label and subtract the number of grams of fiber. A rule of thumb: Any amount over 40 grams will likely send blood sugar soaring.

2. Fat lowers a food's GI. That's because it slows the absorption of glucose into your bloodstream (as does fiber). For instance, U.K. researchers found that adding full-fat Cheddar cheese to a baked potato reduced the meal's glycemic index. With a Twix bar, you're eating a combination of sugar and fat, which means that your blood sugar won't rise as high after you've finished it. Fiber also slows glucose absorption: That's why bread made from whole-grain flour has a lower glycemic index than the kind made from refined flour.

Your takeaway: Go ahead, have some fat. Adding a pat of butter to a slice of whole-wheat bread or tossing some nuts onto your cereal will ensure that your blood sugar rises at a more even rate after a meal—instead of all at once. Keep in mind, though, that this is not a license to overindulge. Total calories is the most important factor in managing your weight.

3. The glycemic index is relative. High-glycemic foods are those with GI values of 70 and up; medium-GI foods fall between 56 and 69 on the scale; low-GI foods are at 55 and below. However, within that low-glycemic category, for instance, there's broccoli, with a GI of 0, and macaroni, with a GI of 47. A serving of broccoli contains just 4 grams of digestible carbs and 31 calories, yet it shares the same classification with this pasta, which delivers 49 grams of carbs and 221 calories.

Your takeaway: Low glycemic doesn't necessarily mean low carb. The reality is that the most dominant factor affecting how much a food raises your blood sugar is the total amount of digestible carbs you eat.

Our recommendation: When you're trying to lose weight, limit higher amounts

You don't need the glycemic index to make wise choices. Just get the MAJORITY OF YOUR CALORIES from whole foods.

of carbohydrates—more than 40 grams—to the hours around your workout. The rest of the time, cap your carb intake at 40 grams per meal and 20 grams per snack.

THE FINAL WORD

Here's the bottom line on the GI.
Unless you're having just a soda, you're usually eating a mix of nutrients. That is, most meals with fast-absorbing carbs also include protein, fiber, and/or fat. (If yours don't, they should.) This makes the GI an unreliable tool, because fat and fiber both lower your blood-sugar response after you eat.

You don't need the glycemic index to make wise choices. Just get the majority of your calories from whole foods: meat, fish, fruit, vegetables, dairy, and whole grains. This automatically eliminates the junk and provides a filling diet rich in vitamins and minerals and other healthful nutrients.

Calories are king. If you don't overeat, you'll stay lean and healthy for life. So a diet that you find the easiest to maintain is probably the right one for you. ■

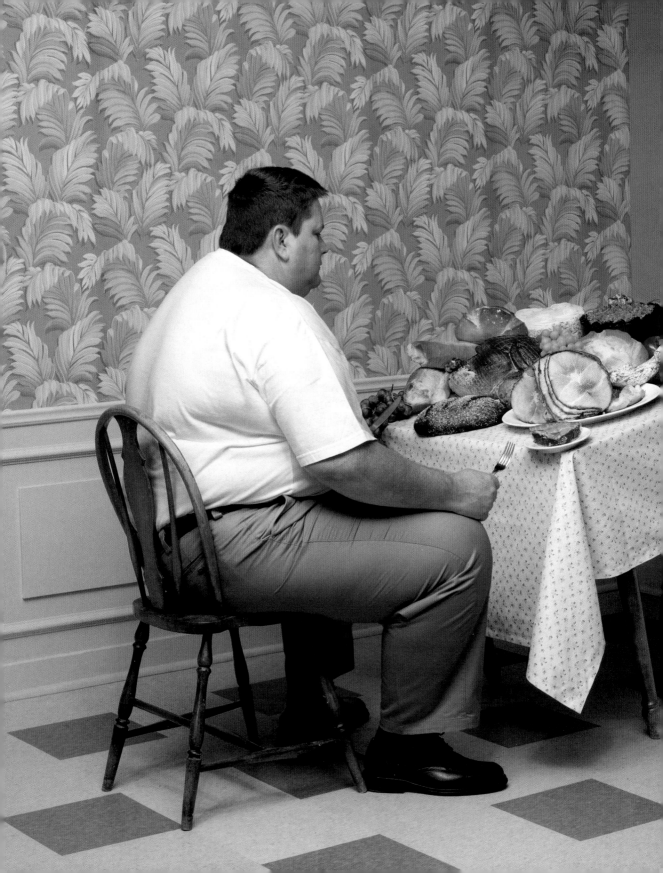

Outsmart Your Stomach

SEVEN WAYS TO FILL YOUR GUT—AND LOSE IT, TOO

Gut check. Are you really hungry or do you just think you are?

Recently, Cornell University researchers asked a group of people a simple question: "How do you know when you're through eating dinner?"

THE ANSWER MIGHT SEEM OBVIOUS. After all, doesn't everyone push the plate away when they feel full? Well, no. The leanest people do, according to the scientists, but people who are overweight rely more on what are known as "external cues." For example, guys packing a few extra pounds tend to stop eating when . . .

- **Their plates are clean.**
- **Everyone else in their group is finished.**
- **The TV show they're watching is over.**

Unfortunately, these cues have nothing to do with how they feel physically.

"People's brains are often out of touch with their bodies," says C. Peter Herman, PhD, a University of Toronto expert on appetite control. "And when eating becomes mindless, overeating becomes routine."

The key player in all of this appears to be a region of your brain called the left posterior amygdala, or LPA. This area monitors the volume of food in your stomach during a meal. Fill your gut to a comfortable level, and the LPA tells your brain to drop the fork. Trouble is, it delivers that information at dial-up speed in a DSL world.

"Many men consume calories faster than their bodies can say, 'Stop!'" explains Dr. Herman. "So they look to external cues to guide their consumption."

The bottom line is this: To shrink your gut, you need to start listening to it. We've scoured the science and tapped the top experts to help you learn how to do just that. Use the following seven simple strategies, and you'll fill up without filling out.

SIT DOWN TO SNACK

Turns out, the trappings of a formal meal make you think you're eating more than you actually are, and that may boost satiety levels. A 2006 Canadian study found that when people ate lunch while sitting at a set table, they consumed a third less at a later snack than those who ate their midday meals while standing at a counter. Think of it as the Zen of eating.

"If you treat every dining experience with greater respect, you'll be less likely to use your fork as a shovel," says sports nutritionist and behavioral psychotherapist Lisa Dorfman, MS, RD. "And that includes snacks as well as your three squares."

TURN OFF THE TUBE

University of Massachusetts researchers found that people who watched TV during a meal consumed 288 more calories on average than those who didn't. The reason: What you're seeing on television distracts you, which keeps your brain from recognizing that you're full.

SLOW DOWN AND SAVOR

"Pay close attention to those first three bites, which people usually wolf down due to excitement," says Jeffrey Greeson, PhD, a health psychologist at Duke Integrative Medicine. In fact, mimic a food critic.

"Examine the food's texture, savor the flavors in your mouth, and then pay attention and feel the swallow," he says. "Psychologically, this form of meditative eating boosts satiety and promotes a sense of satisfaction for the entire meal."

While you're at it, try spicing up relatively bland fare, such as scrambled eggs, with hot sauce or smoked paprika. "Hot, flavorful foods help trigger your brain to realize you're eating," says Dorfman.

TAKE A BITE, TAKE A BREATH

University of Rhode Island researchers discovered that consciously slowing down between bites decreases a person's calorie intake by 10 percent.

"Breathing helps you gauge how hungry you are, since it directs your mind toward your body," says Dr. Greeson. "It's also quite practical, since you can do it throughout a meal and not draw attention to yourself in a social situation."

DON'T SHARE YOUR FOOD

Researchers at the State University of New York at Buffalo observed that men

The leanest people PUSH THEIR PLATES AWAY when they feel full. Overweight people rely instead on external clues.

who ate with a group of buddies downed 60 percent more calories than when they ate with a spouse or girlfriend. That's because people often match their intake of food to that of their dining partners.

Of course, you shouldn't have to sit home on guys' night out. Choose one reasonable entrée for yourself, and skip the communal foods—bread, nachos, wings, and pizza, for example—which encourage you to take your eating cues from pals.

KEEP A FOOD JOURNAL

It's an effective way to remind yourself how much you're eating over the course of a day. But it doesn't need to be complicated: University of Pittsburgh scientists found that dieters who simply wrote down the size of each meal (S, M, L, XL) were just as successful at losing weight as those who tracked specific foods and calorie counts.

One useful addition: Detail the motivation behind your eating habits. "Were you really hungry or just blowing off steam before bedtime? Recognizing that you weren't feeling true hunger reinforces the idea of listening to your body," says Dorfman.

DON'T TRUST THE "HEALTHY" MENU

You're likely to underestimate your meal's calorie count by about 35 percent, according to a new study published in the *Journal of Consumer Research*. The best approach is to check the restaurant's nutrition guide before you order.

A University of Mississippi study found that people consumed 54 percent fewer calories when they used this simple strategy.

5 BELLY-FILLING FOODS

Silence a growling stomach with these satisfying options, courtesy of *Men's Health* nutrition advisor Jonny Bowden, PhD. Each offers a hunger-fighting dose of protein, along with fiber or fat, to help keep you full for hours after you've eaten.

1 ALMONDS

Along with 6 grams of protein, a handful (1 ounce) of almonds contains almost 9 grams of healthy monounsaturated fat.

2 OATMEAL

You can thank the 4 grams of fiber in a 1-cup serving for this breakfast staple's stick-to-your-ribs quality.

3 SALMON

A 3.5-ounce serving contains 22 grams of protein and is a top source of omega-3 fats.

4 QUINOA

Quinoa cooks up like any grain, but it contains the same type of muscle-building protein found in eggs and meat. For 10 ways to prepare quinoa, go to MensHealth.com/quinoa.

5 BLACK BEANS

All legumes provide a ton of nutrients, but black beans lead the pack with equal amounts of protein and fiber—15 grams in a cup. They're a great addition to almost any salad. ■

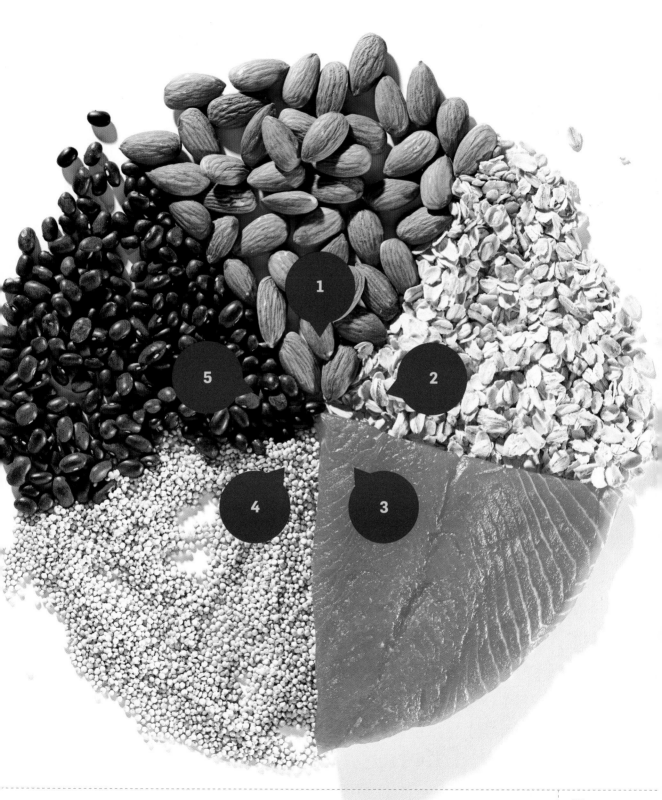

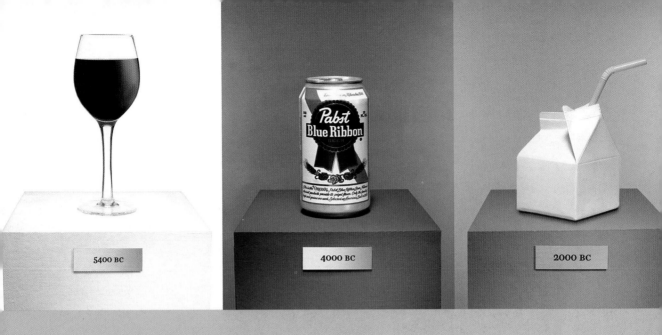

5400 BC   4000 BC   2000 BC

Think Before

KICKING YOUR LIQUID-SUGAR HABIT MAY BE

America has a serious drinking problem. But it's not the dirty martinis and shots of Patrón that we're hooked on. It's the soft stuff—regular soda, juice, and yes, the beloved grande mocha—that fuels our collective addiction.

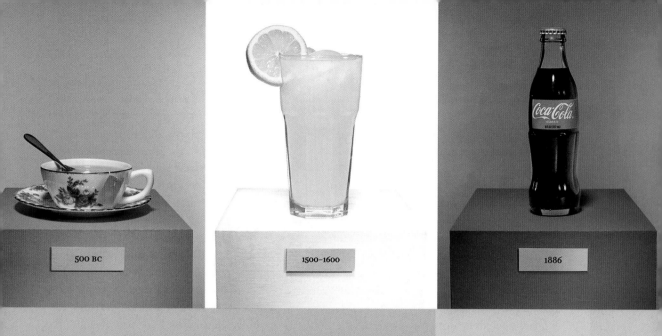

500 BC

1500–1600

1886

You Drink

THE EASIEST WAY TO LOSE YOUR GUT

AND PERHAPS MORE THAN ANYTHING else we swallow, these drinks are making us fat. "Our evolution over hundreds of thousands of years didn't prepare us to process liquid calories," says Barry Popkin, PhD, a distinguished professor of nutrition at the University of North Carolina. After all, he says, we drank only water for most of human history. For reference, you can figure that's a duration of, say, 200,000 years.

"High-sugar drinks didn't even exist until 150 years ago, and they weren't consumed in significant amounts until the past 50 years. This is just a blip on our evolutionary timeline," says Dr. Popkin.

The problem, it seems, is that beverages don't make us feel full. Dr. Popkin hypothesizes that we developed this way so that satisfying our thirst with water wouldn't also blunt our hunger for food.

Unfortunately, our bodies weren't reprogrammed for the 21st century, a time when more than 20 percent of our total calorie intake comes from beverages.

Perhaps all of this explains why our appetite for sugary drinks is seemingly insatiable: The drinks taste great but aren't filling.

When Purdue University researchers had people consume 450 calories a day from either jelly beans or soft drinks for 4 weeks, the candy eaters consumed no more total calories than usual. The soda swiggers, however, downed 17 percent more calories each day. So on a 2,500-calorie diet, for example, the pop drinkers would have taken in an extra 425 daily calories.

"People simply don't reduce their food intake when they drink their calories from soda and other beverages," says Dr. Popkin. Not surprisingly, the group that consumed the liquid calories gained weight during the study.

Now consider that the average person consumes 459 calories, most of which come from sugar, in the beverages he or she drinks each day. So by cutting back or even eliminating the kinds of drinks that contribute to those empty calories, you'll instantly kickstart weight loss. Where to begin? Start by slashing your consumption of regular soda, and focus on chugging more H_2O. (Reminder: Your muscles are almost 80 percent water, so don't be stingy with it.) Then use the following guide to fill out the rest of your drink list.

BEGINNING OF TIME

Our evolution over thousands of years DIDN'T PREPARE US TO PROCESS LIQUID CALORIES, such as those in soda.

DRINK OFTEN

Tea

After water, tea is the world's most popular beverage. But in the United States, regular soda rules. That's a shame, because tea contain antioxidants that might help protect against heart disease and fight cancer, and it's also calorie-free—that is, as long as you opt for the unsweetened kind.

Case in point: A bottle of Snapple original-flavor green tea contains 33 grams of added sugar—the equivalent of 14 sugar cubes. So check labels: You want beverages that provide little or no sugar. To make your own comparisons, remember that every 4 grams of the sweet stuff is the same as eating one sugar packet or sugar cube.

But what if the product label doesn't list nutrition information? That's good news, since it's an indicator that the calorie content is negligible. For instance, you typically won't find a nutrition label on tea bags, because they contain less than 1 gram of carbohydrates per serving, and thus, virtually no calories.

While green, black, and oolong bag teas are all great choices, there are many other types of tea that come in a variety of different flavors. Check out the following four, and experiment with as many as you can. You'll no doubt find several you enjoy, and you won't miss the sugar at all.

• **Mighty Leaf Bombay Chai:** Contains caffeine and bold flavors, making it ideal for kickstarting your day.

• **Adagio Roobios:** This South African herbal tea is caffeine-free, tastes naturally and subtly sweet, and comes in 13 flavors. For similar alternatives, try honeybush and chamomile teas.

• **Stash Peppermint:** A cup or two of this refreshing herbal tea is a great finish to any meal.

• **Tazo Sweet Cinnamon Spice:** It's spicy, but not overwhelmingly so, with a touch of sweetness. It makes for a soothing pre-slumber drink.

Coffee

Like tea, unsweetened coffee is filled with healthful compounds and almost no calories. But when was the last time you drank unsweetened coffee?

With the advent of Starbucks and similar establishments, calories from coffee are skyrocketing. In fact, gourmet-coffee drinkers consume, on average, 206 more calories a day than people who sip regular joe. But chances are, you might not be ready to kick your Starbucks habit entirely. So we scoured its menu for items that contain less than 20 calories. Here's what we found, all of which are good options.

• **Caffé Americano:** A grande (16 ounces) has just 15 calories.

• **Espresso:** One ounce—a Starbucks single-shot serving size—contains 5 calories.

• **Coffee of the week:** A grande has 5 calories.

• **Tazo Tea:** No, it's not coffee, but besides water, it's the only other drink on the Starbucks menu that has zero calories. Just make sure you order the plain version—not the syrup-spiked, juice-infused, or latte kinds, all of which contain added sugar and calories.

DON'T OVERDO IT

Milk

Like soda, milk doesn't make you feel full, says Dr. Popkin. However, other researchers disagree. And because milk contains bone-strengthening calcium and muscle-building protein, it's a worthy beverage to work into your daily calorie allotment. (Of course, you can also derive the same nutrients from solid dairy foods, such as cheese and yogurt.)

Still, some studies show that milk drinkers are leaner than those who skip the beverage—so unless you're downing it by the gallon, it's not likely to be the reason for your love handles. If you're trying to manage your weight, make it a policy to cap your intake at two glasses a day. Just make sure you opt for the unsweetened kind; flavored milk is loaded with added sugar. Interestingly, in an analysis of vending-machine sales in schools, flavored milk, such as chocolate and strawberry, outsold the regular kind nine to one. That just goes to show that our taste for sweet drinks isn't limited to sodas, coffee, and tea, and it probably starts at a young age.

Alcohol

The old saying, "You can get too much of a good thing," is right on the money. Moderate alcohol consumption—one to two drinks a day—has been shown to reduce your risk of heart disease. The downside, of course, is that alcohol contains liquid calories and might even boost your appetite. Plus, unlike fat, carbohydrates, and protein, the calories in alcohol can't be stored in your body—so they have to be used immediately. As a result, your body stops burning fat

until the alcohol is processed. This takes about an hour for every drink. So think about that at the next happy hour.

Juice

Here's the myth we've been sold for years: All juice is healthful because it comes from fruit. This has led many people to take a more-is-better approach to these beverages. The trouble is, many juices contain not only the natural sugar from the fruit, but also copious amounts of added sugars, so that they aren't as tart. Cranberry juice, in fact, is too sour to drink when it hasn't been sweetened.

Keep in mind, though, that a medium orange contains just 62 calories and 12

AMERICA'S 10 WORST DRINKS

Don't even think about it.

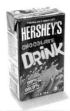 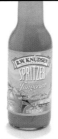 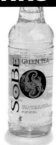 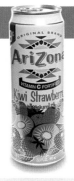 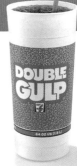

10	**9**	**8**	**7**	**6**	**5**
Worst milk beverage	**Worst soda**	**Worst spritzer**	**Worst bottled green tea**	**Worst juice drink**	**Worst fountain drink**
HERSHEY'S CHOCOLATE DRINK	**SUNKIST ORANGE**	**R.W. KNUDSEN FAMILY TANGERINE**	**SOBE GREEN TEA**	**ARIZONA KIWI STRAWBERRY**	**7-ELEVEN DOUBLE BIG GULP (filled with cola)**
Per 8-ounce carton: 130 calories, 20 grams (g) sugar	Per 12-ounce can: 190 calories, 52 g sugar	Per 12-ounce bottle: 200 calories, 46 g sugar	Per 20-ounce bottle: 250 calories, 63 g sugar	Per 23.5-ounce can: 352 calories, 82 g sugar	Per serving: 534 calories, 130 g sugar
Besides being loaded with sugar, it contains more water than actual milk.	More sugar per ounce than any other soda we found.	The label says, "No sugar added." Good thing.	To make regular tea this sweet, you'd have to add 16 packets of sugar.	You'd have to eat 11 cups of strawberries to consume this much sugar from the whole fruit.	This is 2 liters of soda.

grams of sugar, and it has 3 grams of belly-filling fiber. An 8-ounce glass of Minute Maid OJ has 110 calories, 24 grams of sugar, and no fiber. So the best approach is to eat the whole fruit, which also ensures that you get all the beneficial nutrients. (The skin of an apple is loaded with antioxidants.) And if you want juice, take it in smaller doses—2 to 3 ounces is a good rule of thumb. Another option: Go ahead and have the juice, but make sure you're monitoring your total calorie intake.

Diet Soda

Because diet drinks, such as diet sodas and Crystal Light, are artificially sweetened, they typically contain 5 calories max per serving. So they won't directly lead to weight gain. But guzzling these beverages all day long does lead to one potential problem: You drink less of everything else. So having one or two diet sodas a day is fine, but if you're downing five or six 12-ounce bottles, that means you're limiting your intake of healthful beverages, such as tea.

Also, emerging research suggests that consuming sugary-tasting beverages—even if they're artificially sweetened—might lead to a high preference for sweetness overall. And that might best explain why nobody takes their coffee black anymore. ■

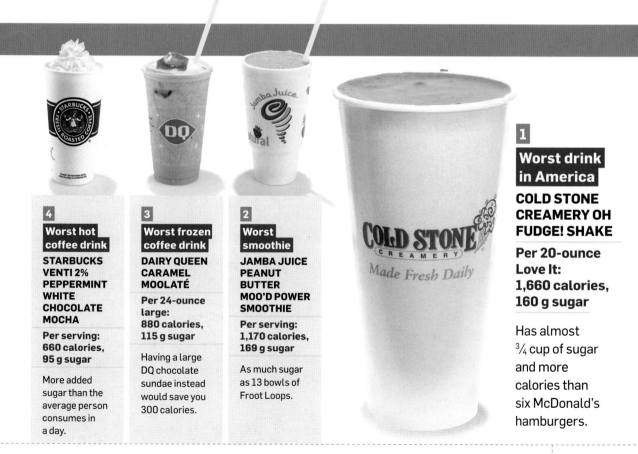

4

Worst hot coffee drink

STARBUCKS VENTI 2% PEPPERMINT WHITE CHOCOLATE MOCHA

Per serving: 660 calories, 95 g sugar

More added sugar than the average person consumes in a day.

3

Worst frozen coffee drink

DAIRY QUEEN CARAMEL MOOLATÉ

Per 24-ounce large: 880 calories, 115 g sugar

Having a large DQ chocolate sundae instead would save you 300 calories.

2

Worst smoothie

JAMBA JUICE PEANUT BUTTER MOO'D POWER SMOOTHIE

Per serving: 1,170 calories, 169 g sugar

As much sugar as 13 bowls of Froot Loops.

1

Worst drink in America

COLD STONE CREAMERY OH FUDGE! SHAKE

Per 20-ounce Love It: 1,660 calories, 160 g sugar

Has almost 3/4 cup of sugar and more calories than six McDonald's hamburgers.

Join the Belly Off! Club

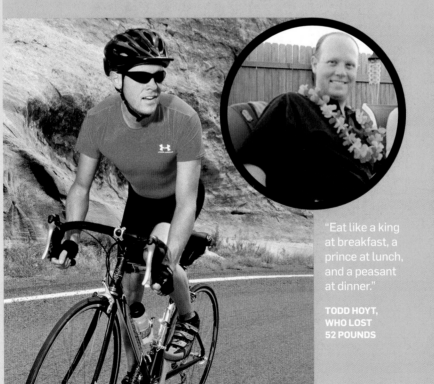

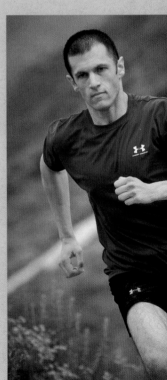

"Eat like a king at breakfast, a prince at lunch, and a peasant at dinner."

TODD HOYT, WHO LOST 52 POUNDS

TRANSFORM YOUR BODY—AND CHANGE YOUR LIFE—WITH **ADVICE FROM GUYS WHO HAVE LOST BIG,** AND WON

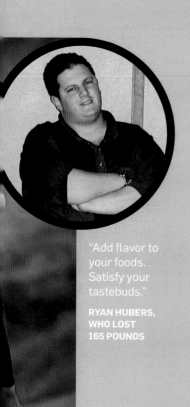

"Add flavor to your foods. Satisfy your tastebuds."

RYAN HUBERS, WHO LOST 165 POUNDS

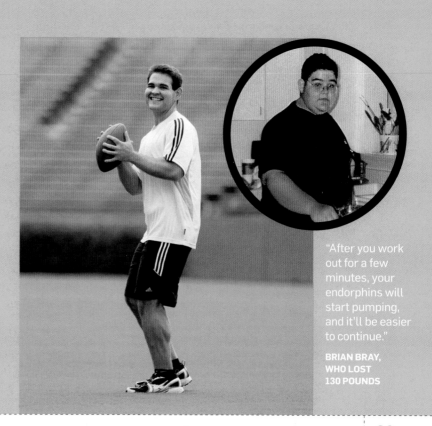

"After you work out for a few minutes, your endorphins will start pumping, and it'll be easier to continue."

BRIAN BRAY, WHO LOST 130 POUNDS

How do you lose nearly 2 million pounds?

WE WANTED TO KNOW, because that's the combined weight that members of the Men's Health Belly Off! Club—our online fat-loss community—have dropped since 2002. So we pored through their testimonials, searching for the common strategies that have helped more than 300,000 formerly fat men shrink their big guts. And we were surprised to find that many of our Belly Off! heroes cited the same simple weight-loss techniques, whether they'd lost 10, 60, 100, or even 150 pounds.

Those same real-world strategies, supported by scientific research, form the backbone of our new book, *The Belly Off! Diet*. What worked so well for so many men can work for you, too. *The Belly Off! Diet* is about real men eating real food and doing workouts designed to fit a hectic, real-world schedule. Consider it your no-fail, guy-tested weight-loss plan.

CUT OUT REFINED GRAINS AND SUGAR
Ninety-six percent of Belly Off! Club losers did this. This might be the simplest way to eliminate empty-calorie junk foods from your diet. The list of products to pass up includes white bread (and other baked goods), soda, candy, and potato chips.

These foods are full of fast-absorbing carbs that raise your blood sugar quickly. A sugar spike is typically followed by a crash, which can leave you feeling sluggish and hungry—a detrimental combination for any diet. So try to avoid products that contain sugar in any form (sucrose, high-fructose corn syrup, or cane syrup) and refined flour. (If it doesn't start with the word *whole*, as in *whole wheat*, cut it out.)

EAT MORE PROTEIN, HEALTHY FATS, PRODUCE, AND WHOLE GRAINS
Almost as many members, 93 percent, did that. This is the balanced diet you're looking for.

Protein fills you up while you're eating and provides the raw material to help you maintain and build muscle. Fat tastes good and keeps you satisfied for hours after a meal. And fiber, which is also filling, slows down the absorption of carbohydrates into your bloodstream, so you'll have energy all day long.

The final part of the picture is produce. Vegetables and fruits are low in calories, high in fiber, and packed with healthful antioxidants.

WEIGHT-TRAIN AT LEAST 3 DAYS A WEEK
That's what 90 percent of Belly Off! members do. Pumping iron vigorously burns calories, and it also can boost your metabolism for almost 2 days afterward, research shows.

The trouble is, heavy guys tend to be intimidated by gyms and their grunting clientele. That's why many Belly Off! Club members began their weight-loss journey by working out in the privacy of their garages and basements.

EAT BREAKFAST EVERY DAY
Three-quarters of the men in the Belly Off! Club start their day, every day, with breakfast.

EAT THIS, DROP FAT
YOUR GAME PLAN FOR A LOSING SEASON

Over the past 4 years, Ben Lewis gained 50 pounds. How? "I play on a rugby team, and we like to go out for a few beers," says the 28-year-old Chicago resident. "Eating hot dogs and deep-dish pizza at midnight won't do you any favors."

After ballooning from 183 to 233 pounds, Lewis finally decided he'd had enough. He checked out the Belly Off! Diet at the urging of a friend. To drop pounds with lightning speed, Lewis adopted our new plan. And now when he goes out with friends, he makes sure he eats some protein before he leaves home, so he can avoid the temptation of high-calorie snacks. Here's a typical day on the Belly Off! Diet.

BREAKFAST
"It all starts at breakfast. Make a good start and you're set for the rest of the day."
Two egg whites and one whole egg, whole-wheat toast or bowl of oatmeal, hot tea

SNACK
"I eat almonds half an hour before lunch so I'm not ravenous."
Two handfuls of raw almonds

LUNCH
"I try to bring my own lunch. That helps me control portions and carbs."
Strips of grilled chicken over a salad

SNACK
"Get out of the three-meals-a-day mindset. Snacks are what keep you going."
Apple or dried apricots or protein bar, water

DINNER
"Find new ways to cook good foods. If you enjoy them, you'll eat more of them."
Grilled salmon, broccoli , romaine-lettuce salad with vegetables and an olive oil/balsamic vinaigrette, unsweetened iced tea

For the complete diet and exercise weight-loss plan, order your copy of *The Belly-Off! Diet* by Jeff Csatari at **MensHealth.com/bellyoff.**

Post photos, track your progress, and lose weight with one of three exercise plans from our free, 8-week Belly Off! program at **MensHealth.com/bellyoff**.

In the morning, you have an entire day's worth of activity to fuel. After dinner, you lie motionless for 8 hours. You don't have to be a nutrition scientist to understand why you should eat big right after you rise.

In fact, researchers at Virginia Commonwealth University found that dieters who regularly ate a protein-rich, 610-calorie breakfast lost significantly more weight in 8 months than those who consumed only 290 calories and a quarter of the protein. Turns out, the big-breakfast eaters, who lost an average of 40 pounds each during the study, had an easier time sticking with the diet even though both groups took in similar daily calories.

DO CARDIO Eighty percent of our online community do cardio workouts. And perhaps the leanest use intervals.

A growing body of research suggests that intervals—short bursts of intense exertion interspersed with periods of slower activity—burn fat and improve fitness more quickly than long, moderate bouts of exercise. And intervals trigger an afterburn effect similar to strength training, keeping your body churning through calories long after you've hit the shower.

Consider this Canadian study from 2006: A group of people were asked to exercise on stationary bikes every other day for 2 weeks. They alternated 10 sets of 4-minute bursts of riding at 90 percent effort with 2-minute rest intervals of slow pedaling. The study participants who did intervals had more of a muscle enzyme that burns fat, and they used more fat for energy. So intense intervals turbocharged even easy-level exercise.

GET MOTIVATED One hundred percent of Belly Off! Club members are highly motivated. Call it the X factor: Strong motivation is what all big losers have in common. Without it, none of the techniques described above would have worked. ∎

Be a Big Loser

TAKE THE ADVICE OF STARS OF *THE BIGGEST LOSER* AND LOSE YOUR GUT FOR GOOD

This is a tale of two fat men and their quest to lose big.

Their journey began 8 months ago, when both were morbidly obese and at high risk of premature death.

That's when they became contestants on *The Biggest Loser*, the popular NBC reality show that challenges dangerously overweight people in a weight-loss competition.

Almost instantly, the men's waistlines—and lives—were dramatically transformed. In fact, after just a few weeks on the show, their combined weight loss totaled more than 160 pounds.

Do the math, and you might think losing that much fat, that fast, is impossible. But these guys are clear proof that it's not. So how'd they do it? You're about to find out.

CHICKEN-FRIED EVERYTHING

Ed Brantley, 31, is a laid-back southern chef from Raleigh, North Carolina. At his first-day weigh-in at the ranch, he tipped the scales at 335 pounds. (The ranch, if you're not familiar with the show, is the *Biggest Loser* campus, located about an hour north of Beverly Hills.)

You wouldn't be surprised at Brantley's weight if you saw him dive into a meal of fried chicken, macaroni and cheese, meat loaf with brown gravy, buttered biscuits, and sweet tea. That's what he cooks up every day as owner of a catering company. And before *Biggest Loser*, that's what he wolfed down after he untied his apron.

"I wouldn't eat until 2 or 3 in the afternoon, because I didn't think I deserved it. Not until my work was done," Brantley recalls. "When everybody was fed, okay, bring it on. I had earned it. And did I eat."

Brady Vilcan, 37, from Houma, Louisiana, is part Native American, from a small tribe called the Chitimacha. He weighed 341 pounds when he started on the show. How so?

"Well, in South Louisiana, anything that moves, you fry it," he laughs. "That's the food culture down there. All the cardiologists line up to study us. We're in the high-cholesterol capital of the world."

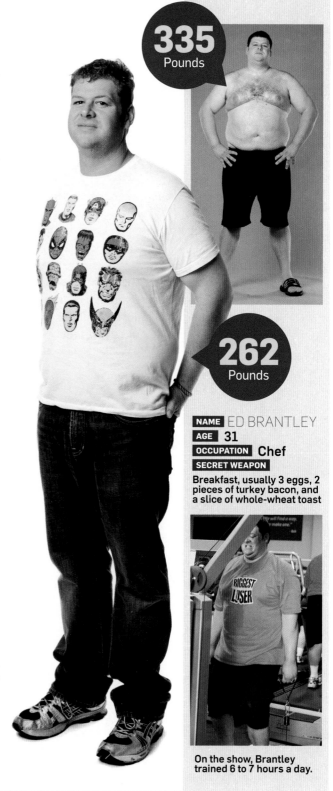

335 Pounds

262 Pounds

NAME	ED BRANTLEY
AGE	31
OCCUPATION	Chef

SECRET WEAPON
Breakfast, usually 3 eggs, 2 pieces of turkey bacon, and a slice of whole-wheat toast

On the show, Brantley trained 6 to 7 hours a day.

Then the men came to the ranch with their wives, Vicky Vilcan (246 pounds) and Heba Salama (294 pounds). And their lives turned upside down.

NO PICNIC AT THE RANCH

Double doors—one marked "Bob's Gym," the other "Jillian's Gym," referring to the two competing trainers, Bob Harper and Jillian Michaels—open to a facility that looks like the University of Florida Gators weight room. It's a musclehead's nirvana, jammed with free weights, benches, medicine balls, and banks of elliptical machines, stair-steppers, and treadmills.

The ranch routine doesn't vary much. Wake at 7. Eat breakfast. Hit the gym for weight training. Have a midmorning snack. Go for a run. Eat lunch. Get back into the gym. Break for a snack. Go for a hike. Dinner. Evening workout. Sleep. Start over.

"The workouts are hard, but I'll tell you what's harder," says Brantley. "The swarms of people around you all the time. I'm sick of these children [the show's producers] telling me where to be and what to do all the time. The mental side is the toughest."

The contestants undergo emotional lobotomies during the first week at the

"I was literally HOOKED ON THE EUPHORIA OF EATING," says *Biggest Loser* contestant Ed Brantley.

The sparkling new gym stands in stark contrast to the downtrodden dorms the contestants live in. The rugs are shabby. There's bad '70s art on the walls. It smells of college-dorm sweat on a hot September day. It's sticky and damp; empty yogurt cartons and no-cal iced tea bottles litter the floors. On this day, the kitchen stinks of bait because someone forgot to take out the trash and the remnants of last night's fish dinner.

As nasty as the place seems, nobody wants to leave. That's because this is where the big weight comes off. "You are working out 6, 7 hours a day," says Vilcan. "And you've got these trainers kicking your tail."

ranch. Not only do they find it difficult to get used to the cameras, lights, and mikes, there's no TV, phone, Internet access, or any other contact with the outside world. But worse, they're forced to examine why they got so fat.

"These people didn't get lazy and have too many margaritas on vacation in Cabo," says trainer Jillian Michaels. "You're dealing with people who are suiciding slowly. You've got to get to the bottom of what is psychologically motivating them to self-destruct."

Whether you're bordering on obesity or you would simply like to become fitter and trimmer, here are six strategies—both psychological and physical—from Brantley,

Bob Harper, who was a trainer for 20 years prior to joining *The Biggest Loser*, believes the brain is the most powerful muscle for weight loss. "I know that this struggle always has an emotional component," says Harper. "Losing the weight isn't all that hard; it's about understanding your relationship with food and taking control of your life." Here are his top tips.

ASK YOURSELF A QUESTION
"Are you ready to change your life? That's the first thing I ask my cli-

ents. They have to decide for themselves if they are serious about committing. They have to intellectualize it and see the path ahead of them as a long-term thing."

TREAT CALORIES LIKE COIN
"I'll limit a 400-pound guy to 2,200 calories a day. I tell him it's like you have a bank account with 2,200 calories in it. You can eat whatever you want; just don't go over the limit."

EAT TO PROGRAM YOUR BRAIN
"First thing I tell my people is that

they've got to eat to lose weight. Eat every 4 hours. They know they have to eat within the first 30 minutes of getting up in the morning to set their clock accordingly. And that first meal has to have a good balance of protein, carbs, and good fats."

LEARN TO COOK
"If you are cooking your own food, you know exactly what you're putting in your body and how proper fuel makes you feel," says Harper.

Vilcan, and the *Biggest Loser* training team that might inspire you to lose big.

FIND A GOOD REASON TO LOSE

It took some time, but Brantley finally realized he had a food addiction.

"The cravings would come and I would be like, 'Hey, let's get high,'" says Brantley. "I was literally hooked on the euphoria of eating." It didn't help that he and his wife, Heba, had a full social calendar with many an opportunity to wine and dine.

"If we want to have children, and we do, we knew we had to change our lifestyle and take control of this," he says.

Brady Vilcan took a hard look at his life and realized he was setting a poor example for his two kids. "We rarely got a lunch break at CVS," says Vilcan, a pharmacist. "I'd often go all day without touching food. If Vicky cooked, I might have three large servings. But mostly I'd pick up cheeseburgers or pizza."

He would also bring candy home from the pharmacy for the family. While watching TV, he might have two or three bowls of ice cream. "My grandfather was heavy. I remember going to Weight Watchers with my mom when I was a kid. Now my 4-year-old daughter, Lucy, outweighs my 7-year-old son, Chance. We've got to break this chain."

NEVER SKIP A CHEESE STICK

After six seasons with the show, nutritionist Cheryl Forberg, RD, says the two most common mistakes made by nearly all the contestants who've passed through the ranch are skipping meals, particularly breakfast, and not consuming enough calcium.

"They feel they don't have time to plan ahead, but skipping meals can lead to grabbing fast food and overeating because you're starving," she says.

To keep their metabolism revving high, Biggest Loser contestants are trained to

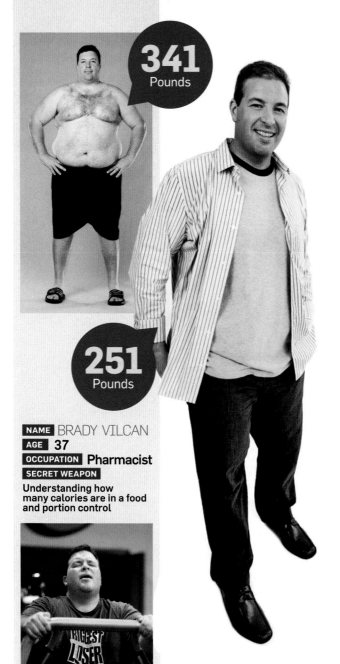

341 Pounds

251 Pounds

NAME	BRADY VILCAN
AGE	37
OCCUPATION	Pharmacist

SECRET WEAPON
Understanding how many calories are in a food and portion control

Vilcan burns blubber on a cardio machine

eat five or six times a day—breakfast, lunch, and dinner, small meals made up of high-water-volume vegetables and fruits, whole grains and lean protein, plus two or three snacks.

"Most people don't get enough dairy products in their diet," Forberg says. "Men need 1,000 milligrams of calcium. You can achieve that through three servings of milk, yogurt, and/or cheese a day. We encourage a low-fat cheese stick with a piece of fruit for between-meal snacks."

WEIGH YOUR FILET

The first thing Vilcan did when he returned home from the ranch was buy a food scale.

"Portion size can get away from you in a heartbeat," he says. "If you want to lose weight, you have to know what a serving is and how many calories are in it."

Do you really need to order that 16-ounce filet when the 8-ouncer will fill you up? Each *Biggest Loser* contestant's daily calorie limit is calculated using a formula that considers starting weight, body-fat percentage, activity level, and goal weight. For Vilcan, it's between 1,750 and 2,000 calories, depending on how much he's exercising.

"If you want to lose weight, YOU HAVE TO KNOW WHAT A SERVING IS," says Brady Vilcan.

"Realizing how much exercise it takes to expend the calories in food really puts things into perspective," he says. "I mean, look at these cheese fries from Outback Steakhouse. They're 2,900 calories. No friggin' way am I gonna eat that."

START WITH WEIGHTS, FINISH WITH CARDIO

Strength training with weights creates an afterburn effect that keeps your body churning through calories at a higher rate, even at rest. And it's widely known that muscle is more metabolically active than fat. So *Biggest Loser* contestants pump weights about 2 hours a day.

"In the beginning we focused a lot on weight lifting to build up the muscle," says Brantley. "Then we switched to more cardio to shed the pounds."

The key with cardio is to find something you enjoy doing to beat boredom.

"I hated the elliptical; it was too easy, I didn't feel like I was doing anything. Now the spinning cycle, that's fun, and it is a real workout. I'll do 2 hours a day on that."

PIG OUT ONCE A WEEK

One day a week at the *Biggest Loser* ranch is designated a high-calorie day, when contestants can go over their calorie limits.

"We do it to make the point that this isn't going to be a life of deprivation," explains Harper. "You can't sustain that. You want to develop healthy habits you can live with."

The contestants typically choose to order out for burritos. "The next day, they really feel the effects of all the sugar and sodium-filled food," says Harper. "They feel like crap. They learn very quickly that a healthy body that's been exercising and eating right doesn't want all that fat and processed junk."

BOOK COURT TIME FOR 2015

The biggest lesson *Biggest Loser* contestants learn is that their healthy lifestyles don't end when the cameras stop.

"There's no finish line. That's a big pill for people to swallow," says Harper. "Every single day for the rest of your life, you are going to have to make better food choices and move around a bit more."

Michaels calls it "composing a life." "You use fitness to re-create a different set of experiences and attitudes: You go from past experiences of 'I'm a loser, I'm fat, I'm worthless' to 'I'm capable, I'm strong, I'm confident.'" Once you've made that paradigm shift, Harper and Michaels say, you've won. ∎

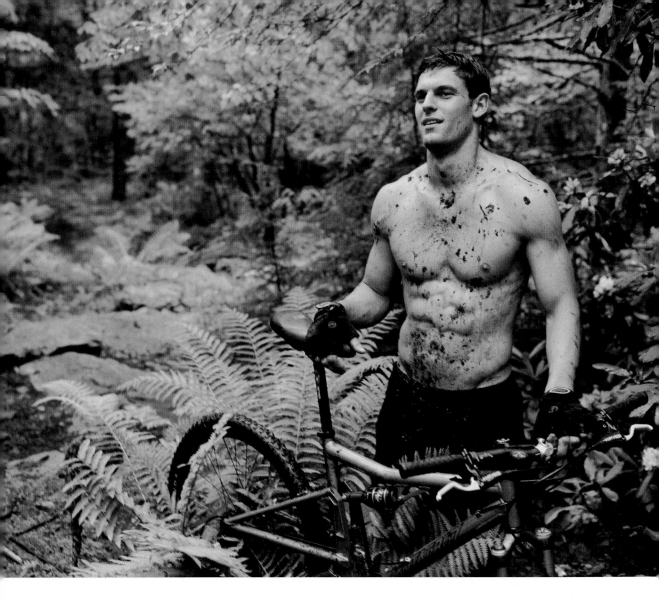

If you can't see your abs, don't assume it's because you're missing out on a magical abdominal exercise or secret supplement. Blame your mindset.

You see, losing belly flab is a boring process. It requires time, hard work, and most important, dedication. Take the right steps every single day and you'll ultimately carve out your six-pack. But if you stray from your plan even a few times a week—which most men do—you'll probably never see your abs.

Pick Up Your Six-Pack

NOW THAT YOU'VE FOUND YOUR MOTIVATION, USE THESE **SIX SECRET STRATEGIES** TO FINALLY REVEAL YOUR ABS

THE SOLUTION: six simple habits, which will help you strip away your lard for good. Think of these habits as daily goals designed to keep you on the fast track to a fit-looking physique. Individually they're not all that surprising, but together they become a powerful tool.

The effectiveness of this tool is even supported by science. At the University of Iowa, researchers determined that people are more likely to stick with their fat-loss plans when they concentrate on specific actions instead of the desired result. So rather than focusing on abs that show, follow our daily list of nutrition, exercise, and lifestyle strategies for achieving that rippled midsection. The result: automatic abs.

1.
WAKE UP TO WATER

Imagine not drinking all day at work—no coffee, no water, no diet soda. At the end of an 8-hour shift, you'd be pretty parched. This is precisely why you should start rehydrating immediately after a full night's slumber.

From now on, drink at least 16 ounces of chilled H_2O as soon as you rise in the morning. German scientists recently found that doing this boosts metabolism by 24 percent for 90 minutes afterward. (A smaller amount of water had no effect.) What's more, a previous study determined that muscle cells grow faster when they're well hydrated. A general rule of thumb: Guzzle at least a gallon of water over the course of a day.

2.
EAT BREAKFAST EVERY DAY

A University of Massachusetts study showed that men who skip their morning meal are 4½ times more likely to have bulging bellies than those who don't.

So within an hour of waking, have a meal or protein shake with at least 250 calories. British researchers found that breakfast size was inversely related to waist size. That is, the larger the morning meal, the leaner the midsection. But keep the meal's size within reason: A 1,480-calorie smoked-sausage scramble at Denny's is really two breakfasts, so cap your intake at more like 500 calories.

For a quick way to fuel up first thing, try this recipe: Prepare a package of instant oatmeal and mix in a scoop of whey protein powder and ½ cup of blueberries.

3.
AS YOU EAT, REVIEW YOUR GOALS

Don't worry, we're not going all Tony Robbins on you. But it's important that you stay aware of your mission.

MUSCLE CHOW
ALTERNATIVE WORKOUT FUEL

Tired of making protein shakes after your workout? Eat some eggs. Or try this tasty sandwich; it packs 19 grams of protein per serving.

Egg Salad Sandwich

2 hard-boiled eggs
4 hard-boiled egg whites
2 tablespoons fat-free sour cream
1 tablespoon chipotle mustard (We like Bookbinder's.)
2 tablespoons finely chopped onion
¼ teaspoon dried dill
  Dash of ground black pepper
4 slices whole-grain bread, toasted
1 box (1½ ounces) seedless raisins

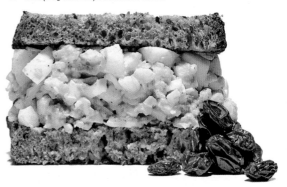

1. In a bowl, mash the eggs and egg whites into small pieces with a potato masher. Stir in the sour cream, mustard, and onion until well mixed. Add the dill and pepper.

2. Spread the mixture on two slices of toast and top each slice with another piece of toast.

3. Serve the raisins on the side.

Makes 2 servings

Per serving: 353 calories, 23 g protein, 53 g carbohydrate, 63 g fat, 1.7 g saturated fat, 213 mg cholesterol, 7 g fiber, 194 mg sodium

Men who skip breakfast are 4½ TIMES MORE LIKELY TO HAVE BIG BELLIES.

University of Iowa scientists found that people who monitored their diet and exercise goals most frequently were more likely to achieve them than were goal setters who rarely reviewed their objectives.

4.
PACK YOUR LUNCH

This habit should be as much a part of your morning ritual as showering. Here's what we recommend packing into your cooler.
- **An apple** (to eat as a morning snack)
- **Two slices of cheese** (to eat with the apple)
- **A 500- to 600-calorie portion of leftovers** (for your lunch)
- **A premixed protein shake or a pint of milk** (for your afternoon snack)

By using this approach, you'll keep your body well fed and satisfied throughout the day without overeating. You'll also provide your body with the nutrients it needs for your workout, no matter what time you exercise. Just as important, you'll be much less likely to be tempted by the office candy bowl.

You might want to adopt this simple rule: Don't eat anything that's not in the cooler.

5.
EXERCISE THE RIGHT WAY

Everyone has abs, even if people can't always see them because they're hidden under a layer of flab. That means you don't need to do endless crunches to carve out a six-pack. Instead, you should spend most of your gym time burning off blubber.

The most effective strategy is a one-two approach of weight-lifting and high-inten-sity interval training. According to a recent University of Southern Maine study, half an hour of pumping iron burns as many calories as running at a 6-minute-per-mile pace for the same duration. (And it has the added benefit of helping you build muscle.) What's more, unlike aerobic exercise, lifting has been shown to boost metabolism for as long as 39 hours after the last repetition. Similar findings have been noted for intervals, which are short, all-out sprints interspersed with periods of rest.

For the best results, do a total-body weight-training workout 3 days a week, resting at least a day between sessions. Then do an interval-training session on the days in between.

6.
SKIP THE LATE SHOWS

You need sleep to unveil your six-pack. That's because lack of shut-eye might disrupt the hormones that control your ability to burn fat. For instance, University of Chicago scientists recently found that just 3 nights of poor sleep might cause your muscle cells to become resistant to the hormone insulin. Over time, this leads to fat storage around your belly.

To achieve a better night's sleep, review your goals again 15 minutes before bedtime. And while you're at it, write down your plans for the next day's work schedule, as well as any personal chores you need to accomplish. This can help prevent you from lying awake worrying about tomorrow ("I have to remember to e-mail Johnson"), which can cut into quality snooze time. ■

Banish Fat for Good

STILL SEARCHING FOR YOUR SIX-PACK? HERE'S THE ULTIMATE WEIGHT-TRAINING AND CARDIO PLAN FOR ROCK-HARD ABS

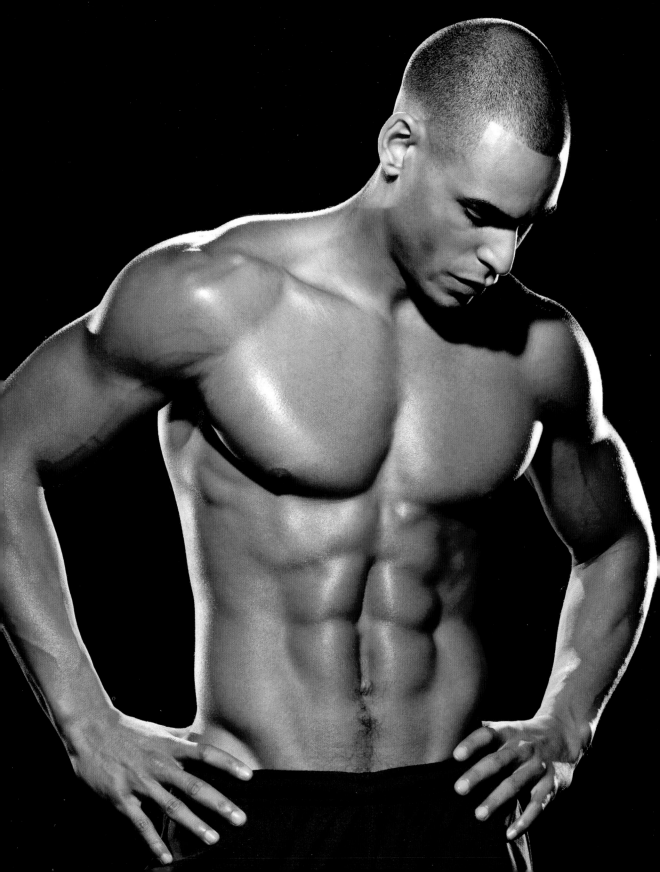

BUILD YOUR BEST BODY EVER

Yes, you have abs—they just need to be uncovered. And the most effective way to torch fat above your belt is by building more total-body muscle, which in turn will stoke your metabolism.

The compound exercises in this plan—squats and deadlifts—stimulate strength gains, and they also train your trunk muscles harder than many traditional core exercises do, according to researchers at Appalachian State University.

As a result, you'll build a leaner, stronger midsection, all without doing a single ab exercise. Not ready to give up your crunches? Set a timer for 5 minutes after you've completed all the exercises in this plan, and then finish your workout with your favorite ab moves.

1
Chinup

Hang from a chinup bar with an underhand grip, your hands spaced about shoulder-width apart and arms straight. Pull yourself up as you keep your elbows pointing down, and then slowly drop to the starting position.

2
Dumbbell Step-Up

Stand facing a bench as you hold heavy weights at your sides. Lift one foot, place it on the bench, and then press your heel into the bench to push your body up. Now raise your opposite knee until it's bent 90 degrees. Return to the starting position.

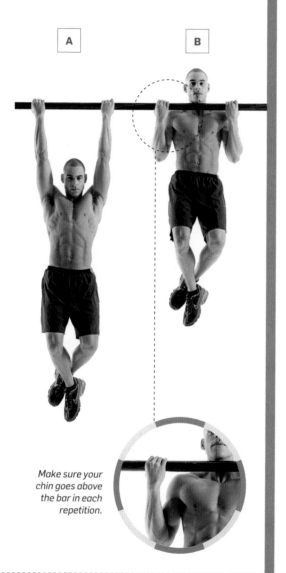

Make sure your chin goes above the bar in each repetition.

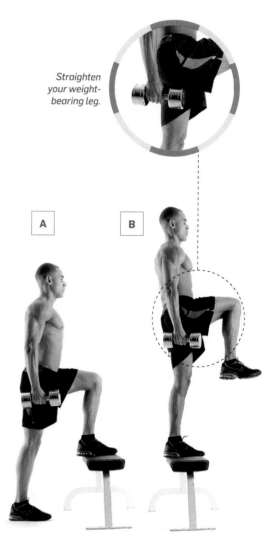

Straighten your weight-bearing leg.

3
Dumbbell Squat to Press

Stand holding dumbbells at your shoulders with your palms facing each other. Lower yourself into a squat until your thighs are at least parallel to the floor. Push back up and press the weights overhead. Return to the starting position.

4
Dumbbell Row

Stand holding a pair of dumbbells at your sides with a neutral grip (palms facing each other). Bend forward at the waist until your back is almost parallel to the floor. Pull the weights up to your rib cage, and then lower them back down.

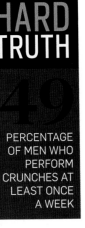

HARD TRUTH

49

PERCENTAGE OF MEN WHO PERFORM CRUNCHES AT LEAST ONCE A WEEK

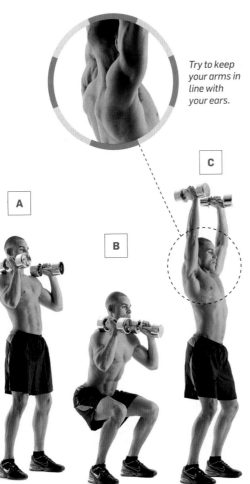

Try to keep your arms in line with your ears.

A

B

C

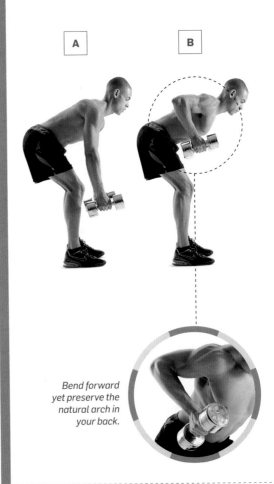

A

B

Bend forward yet preserve the natural arch in your back.

1
Barbell Front Squat

Stand holding a bar with an overhand grip. Bring your elbows forward so the bar rests across the front of your shoulders with your palms up and elbows high. Lower your body and then press back to a standing position.

2
Dumbbell Incline Bench Press

Lie faceup on an incline bench with your feet flat on the floor. Hold a pair of dumbbells above your chest with straight arms, palms facing each other. Slowly lower the weights to the sides of your chest. Pause and then push them back up.

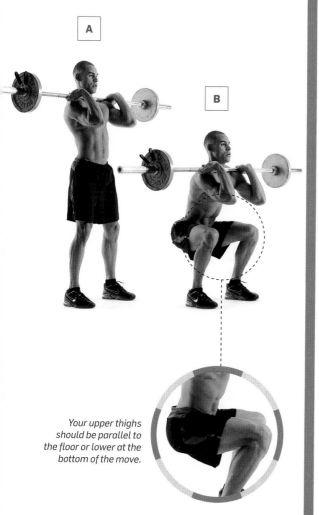

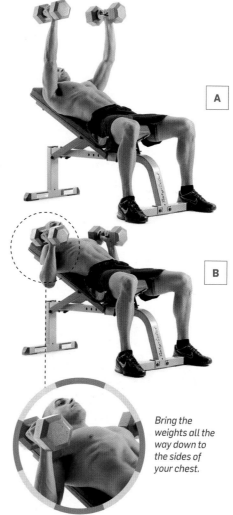

Your upper thighs should be parallel to the floor or lower at the bottom of the move.

Bring the weights all the way down to the sides of your chest.

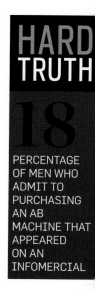

HARD TRUTH

18

PERCENTAGE OF MEN WHO ADMIT TO PURCHASING AN AB MACHINE THAT APPEARED ON AN INFOMERCIAL

3
Barbell Romanian Deadlift to Row

Stand holding a barbell in front of your thighs. Keeping your knees slightly bent and your back arched, push your hips back to lower the bar to your shins. At the bottom, draw it up toward your rib cage, lower it, and then return to the starting position.

4
Cable PNF

Stand to the left of a cable station. Grab a low-pulley cable handle with your left hand. Pull it up and across your body so that at the top of the move your palm faces forward. Reverse the path. Finish a set before repeating with your other arm.

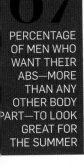

HARD TRUTH

67

PERCENTAGE OF MEN WHO WANT THEIR ABS—MORE THAN ANY OTHER BODY PART—TO LOOK GREAT FOR THE SUMMER

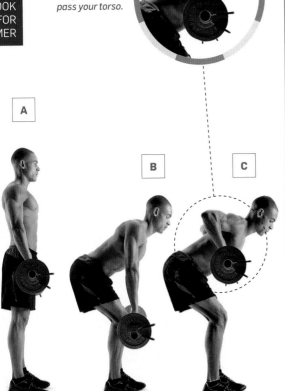

Pull the bar up until your elbows pass your torso.

A

B

C

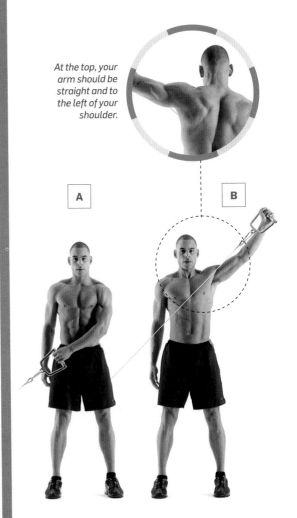

At the top, your arm should be straight and to the left of your shoulder.

A

B

The All-in-One Abs Workout

Lift weights 3 days a week, alternating between the two routines—Workout A and Workout B, and resting at least a day between sessions. For example, if you do Workout A on Monday and Friday and Workout B on Wednesday of this week, then next week schedule Workout B for Monday and Friday and Workout A for Wednesday.

WEEKS 1-3

Start with 5 sets of 5 repetitions of the first exercise—either the chinup or front squat. Rest 2 minutes between sets. Then do the next three movements in your routine as a circuit, completing just 1 set for each exercise before progressing to the next move. Do 8 to 10 reps of each movement in the circuit, resting 60 seconds between sets. Repeat for a total of 3 rounds.

WEEKS 4-6

In each workout, perform 6 sets of 3 reps for the first exercise, resting 2 to 3 minutes between sets. Then do the next three exercises as a circuit, just as you did during Weeks 1 to 3—except you'll be completing 10 to 12 reps of each exercise and resting 60 seconds between moves. Do a total of 4 rounds.

Accelerate for Abs

Run off extra pounds by following this interval-training plan twice a week. Run, rest, and repeat according to the schedule at right, preferably on days when you don't lift weights. You can also cycle, run stairs, or use the cardio machine of your choice.

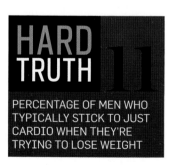

HARD TRUTH 11

PERCENTAGE OF MEN WHO TYPICALLY STICK TO JUST CARDIO WHEN THEY'RE TRYING TO LOSE WEIGHT

	MAX-EFFORT SPRINT (in seconds)	RECOVERY (in seconds)	REPS
Week 1 Day 1	60	180	3
Day 2	60	120	4
Week 2 Day 1	60	180	4
Day 2	60	120	5
Week 3 Day 1	60	180	5
Day 2	60	120	6
Week 4 Day 1	60	180	5
Day 2	60	120	3
Week 5 Day 1	60	180	6
Day 2	60	120	4
Week 6 Day 1	60	180	7
Day 2	60	120	5

EXERCISE SCIENCE

SAVE YOURSELF

If your pants feel tight, take action soon: A gain of just 13 pounds can harm your health, say German researchers. They determined that lean men who experienced small but significant weight increases developed resistance to the hormone insulin.

"Not only does this lead to both metabolic syndrome and diabetes, but the extra insulin in your blood signals your body to store more fat," says one study author, Johannes Erdmann, PhD.

Still not motivated? Consider the fat/cancer connection.

Excess heft accounts for one in seven cancer deaths in men, according to the *New England Journal of Medicine*. Here's how those pounds can kill.

1 Extra fat tissue causes your cells to become resistant to insulin.

2 The result is higher levels of insulin in your bloodstream.

3 Excess insulin spurs the growth of both healthy and cancerous cells.

4 Insulin also increases levels of the hormones that stop cell death.

5 Unchecked cell growth can develop into a tumor.

PRESERVE YOUR BICEPS

Warning: Shedding your gut might lead to smaller biceps. Scientists at Louisiana State University found that when overweight men cut 25 per-

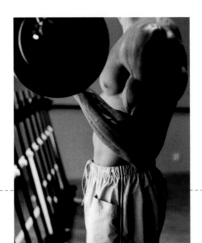

cent of their calories, a quarter of their weight loss came from muscle.

So what's a dieter to do? Protect your muscle by hitting the weights three times a week. In a West Virginia University study, this strategy prevented muscle loss even though men were taking in just 800 calories a day. (For a cutting-edge fat-loss plan, see our workout on page 45.)

MAKE WATER WORK

Thirst can masquerade as hunger, which is one reason dieters should stay hydrated. Now German researchers have found another reason: Water fuels your body's fat burners. For 90 minutes after drinking 16 ounces of chilled H_2O, adults saw their metabolisms rise by 24 percent over their average rates.

According to the study au-

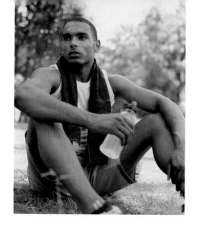

thor, Jens Jordan, MD, the mechanism is partly due to the energy your body generates to warm the water during digestion. For more H_2O benefits, check out "Work Out With Water" on page 179.

EAT TO LOSE

The right postworkout meal can speed fat loss, according to a British study. Men who ate a snack high in protein (43 grams) and low in carbs after an intense exercise session burned 21 percent more blubber than men who chugged a sugary drink.

You spend more energy processing protein than you do digesting carbohydrates, says the study author, Adam Cunliffe, PhD.

For a great meal after a workout, whisk 1 tablespoon each of peanut butter and sesame oil with 1 teaspoon soy sauce and the juice of a lime. Pour over 8 ounces diced, cooked chicken breast, then toss with salad.

UNDERSTAND WHY DIETS WORK

Even lots of exercise is no match for bad eating habits, say University of Missouri scientists. In the study, people lost their guts with a strict diet and a vigorous, 5-day-a-week workout. Then they were split into two groups: One did no exercise, and the other kept training. However, they all ate an average of 500 additional calories a day. The result? The belly fat returned—for everyone.

"If you take in more calories than you burn, fat will come back whether you exercise or not," says study coauthor Shana Warner, PhD.

SPEED UP YOUR WORKOUT

Lift fast to lose fast. Salisbury University scientists recently found that explosive weight training burns more calories than pumping iron slowly.

"Lifting quickly targets your fast-twitch muscle fibers,

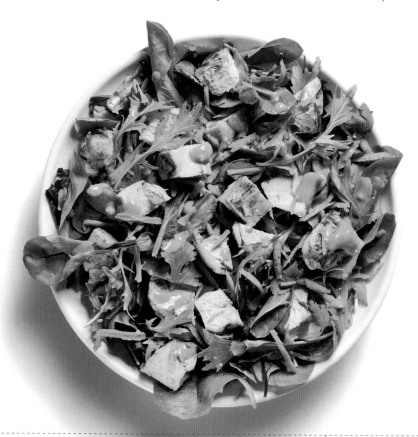

which have been shown to require more energy to contract than slow-twitch fibers," says study author Scott Mazzetti, PhD. In the study, the fast-lifting participants took 2 seconds to lower the weight and then pressed it back to the starting position as forcefully as possible.

For an explosive workout that burns fat, go to MensHealth.com/powertraining.

TRICK YOUR BODY THIN

It might be as easy as replacing your glass of apple juice with an apple. A small study published in the *International Journal of Obesity* reports

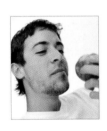

that people reduced their daily calorie intake by as much as 20 percent if they substituted a piece of fruit for fruit juice with their lunch.

The reason: Chewing stimulates satiety hormones better, say the study authors, while the whole food takes longer for your intestines to process, helping you stay full. The benefit was also observed when participants ate cheese instead of drinking milk.

LOSE FAT, BUILD MUSCLE

The best combination for chiseling your abs: dumbbells and a fork.

University of Connecticut researchers found that men who lifted weights and ate a low-carb diet lost 17 pounds of fat and gained 2 pounds of muscle in just 12 weeks. What's more, the low-carb dieters cut twice as much lard as lifters who followed a low-fat plan.

"Restricting carbohydrates forces your body to burn fat instead of sugar, while lifting spurs muscle growth," says study author Jeff Volek, PhD, RD.

Go to MensHealth.com/tnt to find the TNT Diet, a plan based on Dr. Volek's study.

SLOW DOWN TO LOSE FAST

Make sure you come up for air between bites: Fast eating might lead to diabetes and weight gain.

In a recent study, Japanese scientists found that peo-

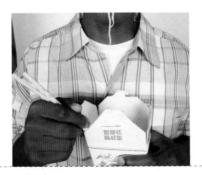

ple who wolfed down their food were more likely to be overweight and insulin resistant—both of which are early signs of future diabetes—than those who ate at a slower pace. The researchers are planning more studies to determine the connection.

Do you need to slow down at the dinner table? Be your own judge. The study participants were classified as fast or slow eaters based on how they rated their own eating speed.

Fifty-five percent of young men say they're "fast eaters," according to a University of Rhode Island survey.

LOSE BIG, STAY SMALL

If your goal is long-term success, perhaps the "best" diet is simply the one you can best stick to.

In another recent study, this one at Brown University, scientists tracked the diets of people who had dropped at least 30 pounds and maintained their new weight for 3 years. Contrary to popular opinion, the researchers discovered that low-carbohydrate dieters were just as successful at keeping weight off as dieters who followed a low-fat approach. This just goes to show that more than one weight-loss method can be effective.

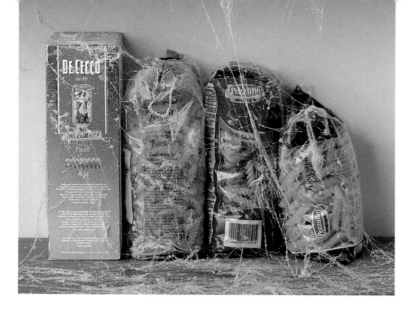

weight, even fast walking can damage your knees.

Researchers at the University of Colorado discovered that obese men had 51 percent more knee torque than their lean counterparts, increasing their risk of arthritis.

"Obese people walk with wider steps, which compounds the stress on their joints," says study author Ray Browning, PhD.

But there's no need to unplug your treadmill: The scientists determined that slowing to 2¼ miles per hour might keep knee strain within safe limits.

Compensate for the slowdown by using the incline function to ramp up intensity. A new A.T. Still University study found that walking 3 miles per hour on a treadmill set at an incline can be as challenging as running on a flat surface. ∎

Interestingly, the carb cutters—who didn't bother to count calories—reported feeling less deprived than their low-fat counterparts.

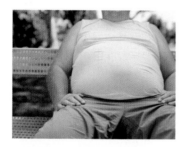

TARGET BELLY FAT

Switching to whole grains can melt away your gut. Penn State researchers compared two groups of overweight dieters: One group swapped white bread and pasta for whole-wheat products, while the other ate the same number of calories as the first group but didn't make the switch. Although all the dieters lost about 10 pounds in 3 months, the whole-grain eaters dropped twice as much abdominal fat.

The study authors credit the extra fiber and antioxidants in whole grains, which help control inflammation and insulin, which is a hormone that tells your body to store belly fat.

POSTPONE THE KNEE REPLACEMENT

It's no surprise that jogging with a big gut pounds your joints. But if you're a heavy-

HARD TRUTH 17,400
THE NUMBER OF ADDITIONAL CALORIES A MAN WHO DRINKS AN EXTRA 50 OUNCES OF COLD WATER DAILY WILL BURN ANNUALLY

TRAINING TIPS

Q: What's the ideal body-fat percentage for the 40something man?

A: Anything between 10 and 25 percent represents a healthy body composition, but if you can manage 15 percent, you'll look fit and toned. Above 25 percent, health risks start to climb, including those for type 2 diabetes and heart disease. But don't get carried away and grind yourself into the land of manorexia. Anything below 5 percent jeopardizes the immune system. Visit healthstatus.com to calculate your BMI, which is a good indication of body composition.

Q: How can I lose 10 pounds for a big event that's a month away?

A: It's entirely possible to lose that much in a month, but it's going to take increased visits to the gym and major discipline in your diet. To lose 10 pounds in 4 weeks, you'll need to create a calorie deficit of about 500 calories a day. That means reducing your food intake by 20 percent and burning off the rest with exercise. Here's your plan.

At the gym: Aim for three weekly exercise sessions, split between 20 minutes of strength training and 20 minutes of cardio. Your strength sessions should involve at least four exercises divided into supersets, which simply means running pairs of exercises back-to-back. Begin with dumbbell chest presses and body-weight split squats, doing 4 supersets of 8 reps per exercise with 1 minute's rest between supersets. Next, pair dumbbell rows with decline pushups. Same sets and reps as the previous superset. Finish off with a 20-minute interval workout of your favorite cardio exercise (e.g., running, cycling, rowing): a 5-minute warmup, 10 minutes of alternating between 30 seconds of intense effort and 90 seconds of active rest (at a cooldown pace), and a 5-minute cooldown. Short bursts of intense activity boost metabolism for up to 30 hours after you work out and increase the production of fat-burning hormones.

In the kitchen: Calculate how many calories you eat each day (use nutritiondata.com to add up the caloric value of what you eat) and then reduce that by 20 percent—probably about 400 to 500 calories. You won't starve. Just decrease your intake of processed foods, which tend to cause swings in blood sugar, triggering feelings of hunger, and bulk up on unprocessed foods such as eggs, spinach, oatmeal, and lean meat. The fiber in the produce and the protein in the meat will help keep you fuller longer.

Log your food and workouts at fitday.com, a free Web site that tracks your progress. For added insurance, challenge a buddy to lose 10 pounds, too. Research shows that the support and accountability provided by a training partner boost exercise adherence and weight-loss success.

Q: I sit on an exercise ball instead of a chair at my office. Will I lose weight?

A: Sitting on a ball might help strengthen your core, but it won't help you shed significant calories. The misconception comes, in part, from studies on nonexercise activity. Fidgeting, a common example, is often cited as a way to help burn extra calories. Mayo Clinic researchers found a significant increase in energy expenditure if you fidget while standing. But that effect is not as pronounced if you fidget while seated. So any difference between ball sitting and chair sitting is probably too small to have a real impact. So save the ball for the gym. Work is stressful enough without the extra task of balancing your way through it for minimal returns.

Q: If I work out after lunch, should I still eat afterward?

A: Yes. But you don't need to scarf something immediately, as you would if you'd skipped the preworkout lunch. The idea of a fast-acting recovery meal or shake as soon as possible after training is rooted in research on endurance athletes. One study focused on athletes who trained to glycogen depletion through a 2½-hour combination of intensive cycling and sprinting. On top of that, they were training after an overnight fast—and without a preworkout meal. Under those circumstances, a quickly absorbed meal or shake would be smart. But since your body isn't running on empty, try a meal that balances carbs and protein, like a meat-packed deli sandwich, within an hour after your workout.

Q: Can I use the same plan to lose both visceral and subcutaneous fat?

A: Yes, but visceral fat will take longer to shed. Unlike subcutaneous fat, which resides close to the skin's surface, visceral fat is located behind the abs in the spaces between organs. It's what potbellies are made of, and the best way to lose it is to alternate strength and cardio workouts.

Researchers in Korea found that performing each type of workout for 30 minutes three times a week resulted in 4 more pounds of weight loss and 11 percent more visceral fat loss than cardio alone. Lose 10 percent of your body weight, and you'll lose up to 40 percent of your visceral fat. ■

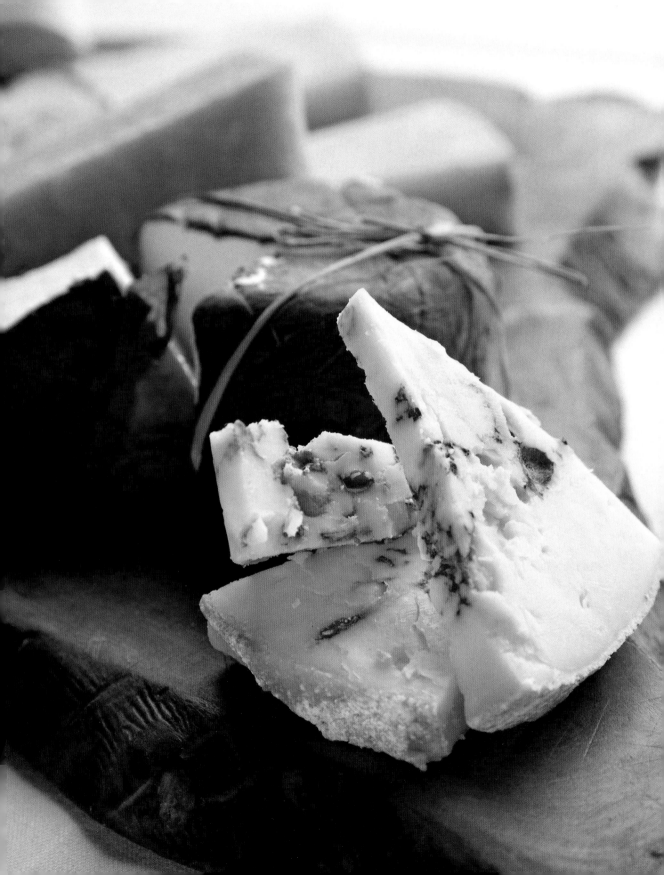

2

Flat Belly Foods

Upgrade Your Diet

YOU DON'T HAVE TO SACRIFICE FLAVOR TO EAT HEALTHIER. LET OUR ALL-STAR PANEL OF DOCTORS, NUTRITIONISTS, AND CHEFS SHOW YOU HOW

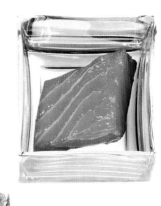
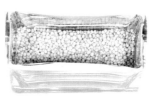
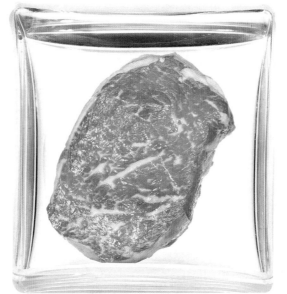
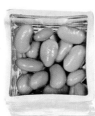
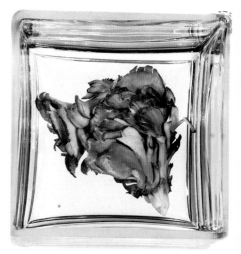
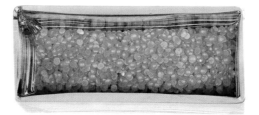

Men tend to eat the same foods over and over,

and so small changes in diet can have big effects. Try these tweaks to effect some major health improvements.

1. LOWER YOUR BLOOD PRESSURE AND CHOLESTEROL

HOW: EAT SHIITAKES AND MAITAKES INSTEAD OF BUTTON MUSHROOMS.

Nutritionally speaking, earthy-flavored shiitakes and maitakes are to button mushrooms as whole grain is to Wonder bread. A growing body of research links the Japanese fungi, which are packed with antioxidants and laced with selenium, to lower cholesterol and blood pressure, anti-tumor activity, and possibly better prostate health, says Donald Abrams, MD, director of clinical programs at the University of California at San Francisco's Osher Center for Integrative Medicine. Buttons, as well as creminis and portobellos (which are the same species), don't have these benefits.

The upgrade: Chad S. Luethje, executive chef at Red Mountain Spa, in St. George, Utah, has two favorite recipes.

The easiest—sautéed mushrooms with truffle oil—takes 5 minutes: Slice and cook 1 pound shiitakes and maitakes (also known as "hen of the woods") for a few minutes over medium heat with 1 tablespoon olive oil and ½ cup chopped chives. Add a splash of white truffle oil once it's hot; serve.

More ambitious, but still straightforward, is his 10-minute mushroom broth: Simmer 1 pint vegetable stock while you're sautéing 1 pound chopped mushrooms and ¼ cup diced leeks. Add the stock to the veggies when they're soft. Simmer for 5 minutes more, add a splash of white truffle oil, and serve.

2. SHRINK YOUR BELLY FAT

HOW: EAT GRASS-FED BEEF INSTEAD OF CORN-FED BEEF.

Now you can have your red meat and eat it, too. The fact that grass-fed beef is leaner and contains fewer hormones and antibiotics than regular beef is reason enough to upgrade. But what seals the deal is that grass-fed beef contains more conjugated linoleic acid (CLA), which has been shown to reduce abdominal fat while building lean muscle.

What's more, the ratio of detrimental omega-6 fatty acids to beneficial omega-3 fatty acids in grass-fed beef is about half that of corn-fed beef, says registered dietitian Susan Bowerman, assistant director of UCLA's Center for Human Nutrition. That's important because omega-6s can cause inflammation, increasing risk for heart disease and cancer.

The upgrade: Cook and slice a roast, and you will have leftovers you can keep in the freezer for quick sandwich fillers, says Laurie Erickson, wellness chef at coastal Georgia's Sea Island Spa.

"Put a slab of beef in a roasting pan, sprinkle it with salt and pepper, and cook at 350°F or 400°F until the meat thermometer reads 120°F for medium-rare," she says. "But be aware that there isn't a lot of fat in grass-fed beef, so it's going to become dry if you overcook it." Another option is to use ground grass-fed sirloin in your burgers or Bolognese sauce. If you can't find grass-fed beef in your supermarket, check out lacensebeef.com or americangrassfedbeef.com.

3. STAY TRIM AND WARD OFF DIABETES

HOW: EAT RED LENTILS INSTEAD OF MASHED POTATOES.

Despite their diminutive size, red lentils out-punch potatoes in three key nutritional ways: "They're packed with much more protein and fiber," says registered dietitian Stacy Kennedy, senior clinical nutritionist at Harvard's Dana Farber Cancer Center. That's important, but it's not their greatest strength. As men hit their forties, says Randy Horwitz, MD, PhD, medical director of the program in integrative medicine at the University of Arizona, they can develop metabolic syndrome: hypertension, obesity, and even diabetes. Eating high-glycemic carbohydrates, such as potatoes, can lead to this predicament. Lentils, however, are absorbed much more slowly and have less of an impact on blood sugar.

The upgrade: "I would take this in an Indian mash direction," says Lee Gross, formerly Gwyneth Paltrow's personal chef and now the executive chef at Los Angeles's macrobiotic M. Café de Chaya.

You can have your red meat and eat it, too. Go for grass-fed beef, which is LEANER AND CONTAINS FEWER HORMONES than regular beef.

Some liquids contain MORE ANTIOXIDANTS THAN THE FLESH OF THE FOOD from which they're derived.

"Heat a few tablespoons of olive oil in a saucepan. Throw in 1 teaspoon cumin seeds, 2 bay leaves, half a cinnamon stick, and ¼ teaspoon black mustard seeds. Fry the spices until they begin to pop. Add 3 tablespoons minced ginger and a few cloves of minced garlic, along with 1 teaspoon curry powder, then fry for 1 minute. Add 1 cup rinsed and dried red lentils. Then add 2 cups vegetable broth, chicken broth, or water. Bring it to a boil and simmer for 20 to 25 minutes until the lentils dissolve. You may substitute an Ethiopian berber spice blend of coriander, onion, chilis, ginger, and paprika."

Refrigerate the leftovers and eat as a dip the next day.

4. SUPERCHARGE YOUR VITAMIN INTAKE

HOW: DRINK POMEGRANATE JUICE INSTEAD OF ORANGE JUICE.

Nobody likes to criticize vitamin C–rich OJ. But the truth is, pomegranate juice has a greater disease-preventing capacity because of its off-the-charts antioxidant content.

"It also looks like pomegranates have the ability to reduce the risk of developing certain cancers, including prostate cancer," says Bowerman. Drinking 100 percent juice might actually be better than eating a pomegranate, she says, because the juice is squeezed from the whole fruit, so you get the nutrients from the seeds as well as from the peel, which is packed with phytochemicals.

The upgrade: "I like mixing 4 ounces 100 percent pomegranate juice concentrate with sparkling water," says Erickson. "Add a twist of lime for freshness." The concentrate has a lot less sugar than regular juice and more flavor, she says. Die-hard OJ lovers can mix pomegranate concentrate with their morning juice. You can also use pomegranate concentrate to deglaze sautéed chicken and pork dishes: Simply add 4 to 6 ounces to the pan after cooking and stir.

Concentrates are available online at health food sites like brownwoodacres.com and dynamichealth.com.

5. STIMULATE YOUR BRAIN

HOW: EAT WILD SALMON INSTEAD OF ALBACORE.

Wild sockeye or red salmon beats out albacore tuna for two reasons, both of which are related to what it eats: plankton, rather than other fish or cornmeal. It has 1.25 grams of omega-3s per 100 grams, which is 30 percent more than albacore, and it has 90 percent less mercury, according to the FDA. (To check the mercury count of other fish, go to gotmercury.org.)

Omega-3 fatty acids are a natural anti-inflammatory, which is beneficial for cholesterol levels, brain health, and reducing the risk of many chronic diseases. Sockeye cannot be farmed and is always wild. It's a good choice whether it's canned, fresh, frozen, or smoked, says Andrew Weil, MD.

The upgrade: "Green-tea-poached wild salmon is quick and easy," says Luethje. "For four servings, make 4½ cups of strong tea and use it as poaching liquid. Add the juice of 1½ lemons as well as the lemon zest.

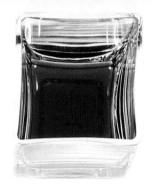

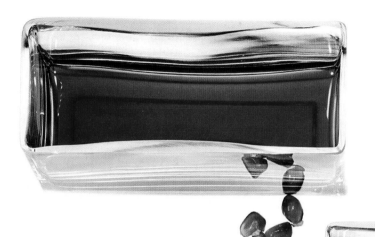

Put the liquid in a pan and submerge four 4-ounce fillets of fish. Poach for 7 minutes at just below a simmer. Then chill the salmon, and serve over sautéed kale."

Another upgrade is to use canned wild salmon in place of tuna. Combine a can of wild salmon with a dollop of Dijon mustard and some chopped dill and parsley in sandwiches; use it in a quickie whole-wheat pasta salad or mix it into whole-wheat mac and cheese.

6. PACK ON MORE MUSCLE

HOW: EAT QUINOA INSTEAD OF PASTA.

Pronounced "*KEE-nwah*," this Incan seed is the rare high-in-fiber whole grain that is easy to cook. Fiber's importance goes beyond regulating digestion: It also reduces the risk of heart disease and diabetes.

"Quinoa has significantly more fiber than pasta, plus it's rich in iron and protein," says Bowerman. "And it takes only 15 minutes to prepare." Its chemical content also intrigues nutritionists. "It's high in lysine and rich in methionine, amino acids that are in short supply in soy protein and vegetable protein," she says.

The upgrade: To cook quinoa, boil 1 cup quinoa to 2 cups water. It fluffs up when it's done. Maria Hines, chef and owner of Tilth, an acclaimed organic restaurant in Seattle, favors a simple herbed quinoa dish. Boil the quinoa. In a separate skillet, add 1 tablespoon olive oil and sauté 2 cloves chopped garlic, 2 shallots, the juice of half a lemon, ½ cup fresh chives, and ½ cup basil. When the garlic starts to brown, add the quinoa and stir for 2 minutes; serve. Quinoa is also a good base for salads, says Luethje. He combines 1 cup chilled quinoa (sometimes cooked in chicken broth to add flavor) with 1 cup grilled marinated vegetables or grilled chicken breast, and ¼ cup black beans or garbanzos. He tops it with ¼ cup Cotija cheese.

7. BOOST YOUR LIVER

HOW: EAT KALE INSTEAD OF GREEN BEANS.

Once relegated to ornamental status because of its brightly colored leaves, kale is enjoying a renaissance. A dark, leafy cruciferous vegetable in the same family as broccoli, kale is loaded with beta-carotene, vitamins C and E, calcium, and lutein, and it's extremely high in antioxidants.

"Green beans are rich in fiber, but kale has a much higher concentration of phytonutrients and cancer-fighting indole-3 carbinol compounds," says Kennedy. "And it keeps the liver healthy by providing a natural detoxification, helping to regulate liver enzymes that assist in the clearing of toxins."

Plus, kale has a high amount of folate, which is good for blood cells.

The upgrade: The knock on kale is its metallic taste when served British-style (i.e., boiled to a pulp). Lately, though, chefs are sautéing it and using baby kale leaves, which have a buttery taste. Hines keeps her kale simple, sautéing it with 2 cloves garlic, 2 shallots, and ½ cup white wine. Sauté it until the wine evaporates, and finish with a squeeze of lemon juice and a dash of red chili flakes.

Other chefs are using different kinds of kale. "Dinosaur or Tuscan kale, for instance, is delicious," says Gross, "but red Russian is my favorite." He uses it in a Thai peanut dish. Combine 3 tablespoons soy sauce, 2 tablespoons peanut butter, a few tablespoons of honey, 1 tablespoon minced ginger, 1 clove minced garlic, and 1 tablespoon crushed red chili flakes in a bowl. Mix it up, and use to dress the freshly blanched or steamed kale. Sprinkle chopped peanuts on top to serve.

8. ATTAIN A HEALTHIER, LONGER-LASTING CAFFEINE BUZZ

HOW: DRINK GREEN TEA INSTEAD OF COFFEE.

When it comes to a caffeine rush, green tea is the tortoise and coffee is the hare. Along with providing a gentler, more sustained buzz, green tea is easier on your heart (coffee can raise blood pressure) and stomach (coffee can cause an acid-reflux response), and it's loaded with antioxidants.

"Green tea is packed with the polyphenol EGCG, which helps prevent cancer," says Dr. Abrams. No wonder you can now find green tea even at Starbucks.

The upgrade: Traditionally, the Japanese drink green tea—either brewed in bags or made from a potent powder called matcha—straight with no milk or sugar. Good Earth (goodearthteas.com) makes a high-quality tea-bag blend. Recently, it has become popular to turn matcha into a hot latte or ice-blended latte.

"I steam soy milk—usually Vitasoy, because it makes a rich froth—and then I brew a strong shot of matcha powder and sweeten it with agave syrup," says Gross. O-Cha is considered the premier powdered green tea (o-cha.com). Do three parts milk to one part tea.

9. STRENGTHEN YOUR IMMUNE SYSTEM

HOW: EAT SOYBEANS INSTEAD OF POTATO CHIPS.

Immunity-boosting, heart-protecting, and superfilling, soybeans prove that "healthy snack food" is not an oxymoron. "Soybeans are rich in fiber, iron, protein, and omega-3s," says Kennedy. "And they give you not only standard protein, but also plant-based protein, which is the most healthy for your immune system. It's also a complete protein, meaning it gives you all the amino acids you need to build muscle without the less desirable aspects of red meat. What's more, soybean protein satiates you better than a carbohydrate snack, and your system absorbs the compounds slowly so you won't be susceptible to energy swings."

The upgrade: Steam these sweet and mildly nutty beans in a pot or in the microwave, and then salt lightly.

"For a bargain, purchase them frozen in the pod," says Erickson. "Add a few drops of water and microwave on high for 5 minutes." Soybeans can also be used in dips with crudités, she says. "Combine 1½ cups canned white beans with 1½ cups cooked edamame, 2½ tablespoons lemon juice, ¼ cup olive oil, 3 cloves garlic, and a dash of salt. Blend it in a food processor."

10. PROTECT YOUR HEART AND LOSE YOUR GUT

HOW: DRINK ORGANIC RED WINE INSTEAD OF BEER.

A variety of research has determined that red wine has heart-protecting qualities, but a new study shows that organic domestic red wine is the best. It has the highest levels of resveratrol, which improves cardiovascular health, and very high antioxidant activity, which can help prevent cancer.

"The red grapes from other countries have higher levels of pesticides," says Kennedy. "One negative aspect of pesticides is that they inhibit the plant from fully developing its own immune system, so the phytonutrients in the fruit are decreased."

Teetotalers can reap the benefits of organic red wine by drinking organic domestic grape juice instead.

The upgrade: Organic red wines do not age as well as conventional wines, so it is wise to drink them as soon as you can. Try merlots from northern California's Bonterra vineyard (bonterra.com) and pinot noirs from Oregon's Ponzi vineyard (ponziwines.com). To find other popular vineyards, visit the Organic Wine Company (ecowine.com).

HEALTH BONUS

Most Americans are turned off by fishy fish, but Spanish or Atlantic mackerel is becoming popular because it is so rich in omega-3s. It has close to double the amount of wild salmon.

"I cook mackerel in a Japanese fashion," says chef Lee Gross. "Season with coarse sea salt and cook over a very hot grill or grill pan until the skin is blistered and crisp and the flesh is cooked through. Transfer to a plate and drizzle with fresh lemon juice and a splash of good soy sauce or tamari. Eat the fish with a bit of grated daikon radish mixed with freshly grated ginger. The daikon and ginger help to cut the oiliness of the mackerel and temper its fishiness." ∎

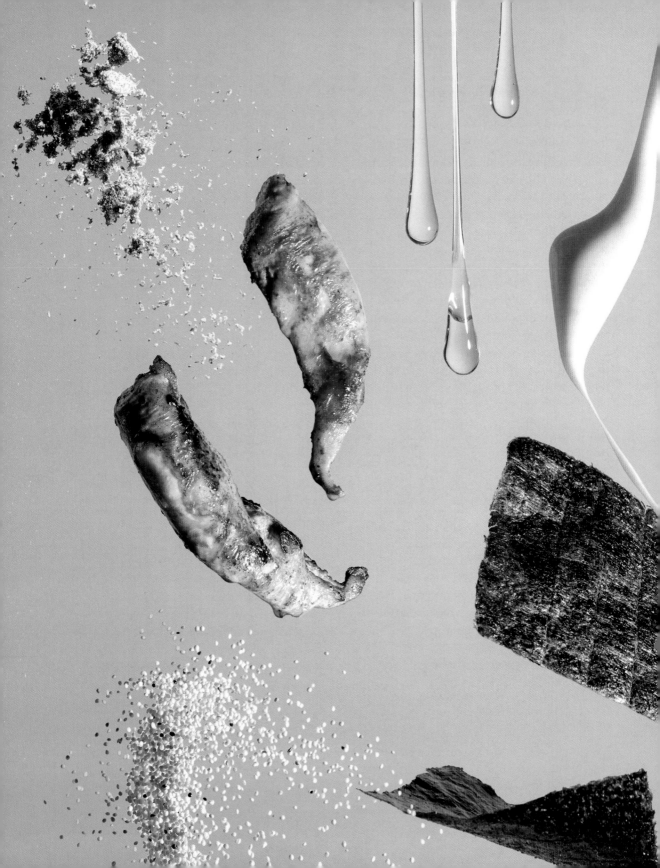

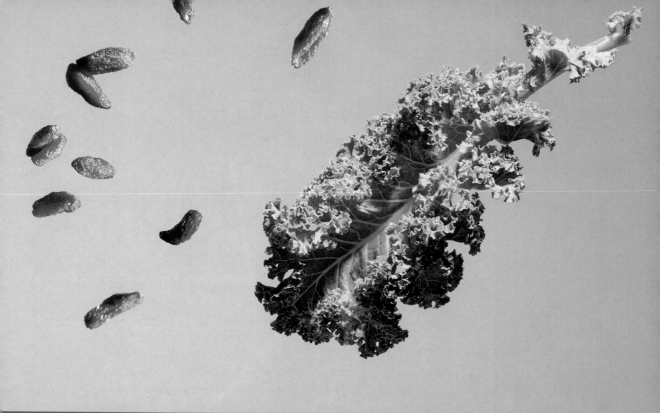

Power Up Your Meals

ONCE YOU'VE MADE SOME SIMPLE CHANGES TO YOUR DIET, TRY THESE NEW SUPERFOODS

A man can eat only so much salmon and spinach. Spike your diet with these grains, berries, meats, and beverages to stimulate your tastebuds, boost your immune system, strengthen your heart, sharpen your brain, and trim your waist.

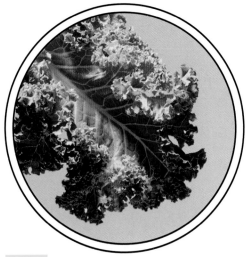

KALE

One irony of our nation's obesity epidemic is that kale is largely used to garnish buffets. Throughout the rest of the world, however, it's recognized as a body-boosting superfood that is rich in vitamins A and C, potassium, calcium, iron, and folate.

"It's also dense with carotenoids, such as beta-carotene and lutein, which studies have shown fight macular degeneration and several types of cancer, including that of the lungs and mouth," says Dave Grotto, author of *101 Foods That Could Save Your Life*.

Serving tip: When adding kale to salad, preserve its vitamin C content by not chopping or tearing it until you're ready to serve.

GOJI BERRIES

No need to pay $35 for 1 liter of goji juice. You can buy whole berries in many Asian markets for a fraction of the price. Although they're not especially rich in any one vitamin or mineral, the bittersweet berries are packed with the phytochemicals beta-carotene and zeaxanthin, which studies have shown reduce the risk of lung and bladder cancers.

"Goji berries are also unique among fruits for their ability to reduce LDL (bad) cholesterol and raise HDL (good) cholesterol," says Grotto.

Serving tip: Use dried goji berries like cranberries. Add them to your favorite trail mix or sprinkle them on top of cereals, stews, or baked goods.

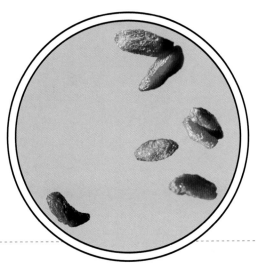

KEFIR

Created by culturing fresh milk with kefir grains (made from yeast and bacteria), this fermented beverage is an upgrade to yogurt.

"It has a different range of bacteria than yogurt, but similar benefits, such as the ability to lower cholesterol and boost immune function," says Susan M. Kleiner, PhD, RD, a nutritionist in Mercer Island,

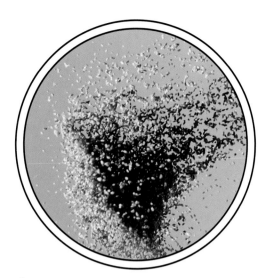

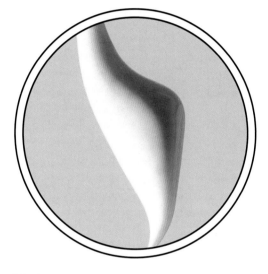

Washington. A recent study also found that it's more effective than fruit juice and other dairy beverages at curbing hunger.
Serving tip: Use in place of milk or yogurt in a morning or postworkout smoothie.

TEFF

In Amharic, the official language of Ethiopia, the word *teff* means "lost," which is exactly what will happen if you drop a seed.

"It's the world's smallest grain," says Grotto. "Even so, it packs more heart-healthy fiber than almost any other food on the planet." And unlike other grains, it's gluten-free, making it an excellent wheat

alternative for people with celiac disease.
Serving tip: Mix cooked teff with herbs, seeds, beans, garlic, and onions to make superhealthful veggie burgers.

ROOIBOS TEA

Think of rooibos as the new green tea, although it's red, made from a root, and packed with even more digestion-enhancing phytochemicals and disease-fighting antioxidants. A Japanese study found that it might even help prevent allergies and fight cancer.

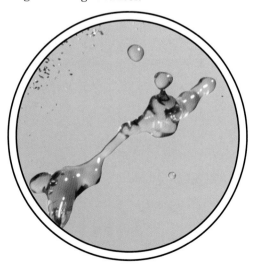

Serving tip: Look for Celestial Seasonings rooibos teas (we recommend Madagascar Vanilla Red), or order organic varieties on-line at adagio.com.

AGAVE

Most commonly served distilled with a side of lime, the nectar from the agave cactus is also a sweetener.

"The honeylike syrup has twice the sweetness and half the calories of sugar," says Grotto, "but it is digested slowly, so it won't cause swings in energy." Agave is also one of the only nondairy foods to contain digestion-enhancing bifidobacteria.

Serving tip: Drizzle on pancakes instead of maple syrup, or use in cocktails in place of simple syrup.

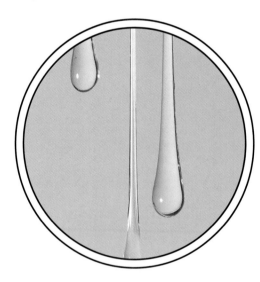

FLAXSEED MEAL

Unlike whole flaxseed, "flaxseed meal is easily digested and rich in lignans, prebiotic compounds that nourish bacterial cultures in the gut," says Dr. Kleiner.

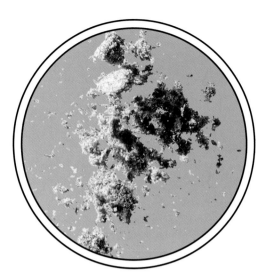

The result is healthier intestinal flora, and, in turn, enhanced immune function. Flaxseed oil does not offer the same benefits. In fact, studies have suggested that consuming the oil may increase one's risk of prostate cancer.

Serving tip: Buy ground flaxseed at your local health food store (or grind it yourself in a coffee grinder) and sprinkle it on top of cereal, yogurt, or fruit.

AMARANTH

The Aztecs mixed this nutty-flavored grain with human blood to build stamina and strength. You can reap similar benefits by

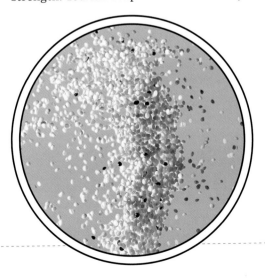

The Aztecs mixed amaranth with human blood to
BUILD STAMINA AND STRENGTH.

eating the cereal version (arrowheadmills.com) mixed with kefir.

"Amaranth is one of the few grains that is a 'complete protein,' meaning it has all eight essential amino acids," says Grotto. "It's also rich in the antioxidant squalene, which studies have shown to inhibit prostate cancer."

Korean researchers have also found that it's uniquely effective at reducing LDL (bad) cholesterol.

Serving tip: Boil and serve instead of rice, or toast and sprinkle on salads.

ALLIGATOR

High in protein and packed with omega-3s, the "other other white meat" is a savory, heart-healthy alternative to steak, says Dwain Johnson, PhD, a professor of meat science at the University of Florida.

The mild-flavored meat, which sits between chicken and rabbit on the taste

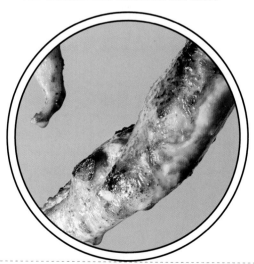

spectrum, is still a rarity in most supermarkets, but it can be ordered online at fossilfarms.com.

Serving tip: Tail meat is the most tender. Rub with blackening seasoning and then grill or pan-sear.

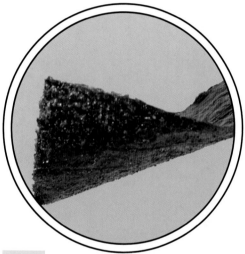

NORI

Best known as the dark outer wrapping on sushi rolls, this sea algae is particularly high in fiber, calcium, iron, and zinc.

"It's also rich in lignans, which recent studies have shown to help prevent tumor growth," says Dr. Kleiner. Look for it in the international section of your local supermarket or online at edenfoods.com.

Serving tip: Grind a sheet of nori in a coffee grinder and use the powder as a salt substitute to season food. ■

Be the Big Cheese

IF YOU ADD ONLY ONE FOOD TO YOUR IMPROVING DIET, MAKE IT CHEESE. FULL-FAT CHEESE IS LOADED WITH PROTEIN, CALCIUM, AND FLAVOR, AND THE FAT IT CONTAINS JUST MIGHT HELP YOU LOSE YOUR GUT FOR GOOD

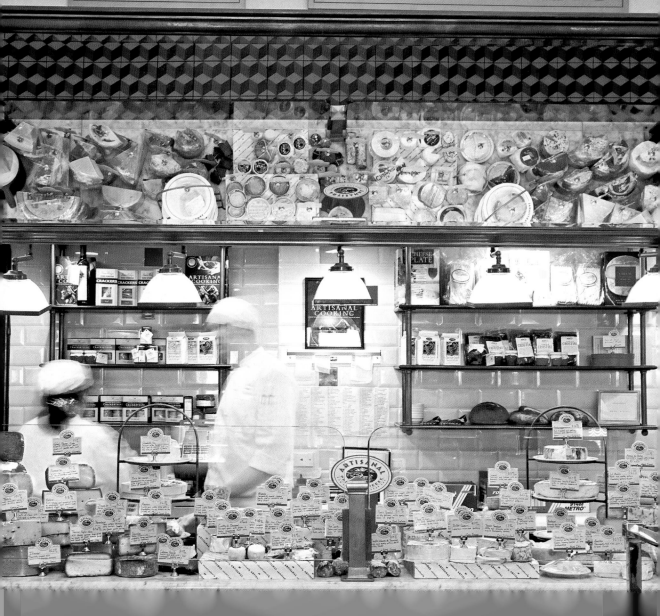

It's unavoidable advice:

If you're going to eat cheese, it should be the fat-free or low-fat kind. Trouble is, that usually limits your choices to mass-produced, vacuum-sealed cheeses that have had much of their flavor sucked out along with the fat. So it's hardly an appetizing proposition. And for what real benefit? Fewer calories and a lower risk of heart disease?

Not so fast.

"The combination of protein and fat in regular, full-fat cheese is very satiating," says Alan Aragon, a nutritionist in Westlake Village, California, and the *Men's Health* Weight-Loss Coach. "As a result, eating full-fat cheese holds your appetite at bay for hours, and I've found that it cuts down my clients' food intake at subsequent meals."

Aragon's advice: Enjoy snacks of full-fat cheese, especially if you're on a diet. "Just don't eat it mindlessly," he says.

And if you're worried about your cholesterol, chew on this: Danish scientists found that when men ate a whopping 10 daily 1-ounce servings of full-fat cheese for 3 weeks, their LDL (bad) cholesterol didn't budge. Which isn't to say you should live on the stuff—just that you don't need to fear it. Full-fat cheese can be a healthy snack and a great way to make a bland meal taste better.

"Cheese is the new wine," says Terrance Brennan, chef and owner of Artisanal Fromagerie, Bistro & Wine Bar and Picholine restaurant, both in New York City. "There are thousands of different aromas, textures, and flavor profiles."

So look beyond the singles and strings and into the gourmet cheese section of your supermarket (or shop online at artisanalcheese.com), and use our guide to discover the best cheeses you aren't eating.

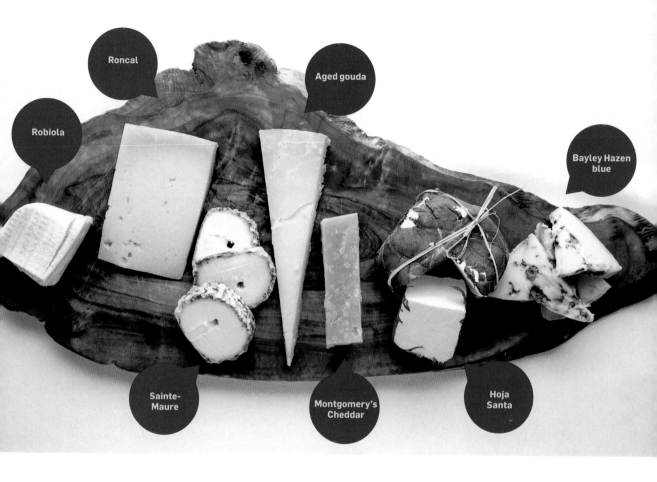

Roncal

Aged gouda

Robiola

Bayley Hazen blue

Sainte-Maure

Montgomery's Cheddar

Hoja Santa

THE SUPERSPREAD
ROBIOLA

Step away from the Cheez Whiz: Robiola is the best way to top a Triscuit. This Italian cheese is soft, like Brie, and it tastes as rich as butter. Spread it on a whole-grain cracker or baguette slice, and round out the snack with grapes or cantaloupe.

For another great spread, try Brillat-Savarin, which is so creamy it's been called the cheese equivalent of ice cream.

THE ANYTIME SNACK
RONCAL

A firm sheep's-milk cheese, Roncal's nutty flavor and chewy texture make it a fine stand-alone snack. Or, to add a touch of sweetness, you can give it a light glaze of cherry or raspberry preserves.

A delicious alternative is Comté, which is one of the most popular cheeses in France. Besides being a great snack, Comté can also be a tasty filling for a grilled-cheese sandwich.

THE SALAD ENHANCER
SAINTE-MAURE

This French goat cheese makes any salad taste better. But don't try to crumble Sainte-Maure like you would other kinds of goat cheese. It's too soft.

Instead, serve it on the side of a mixed-green salad. For the dressing, combine 2 tablespoons sherry vinegar, $1/3$ cup walnut oil, 1 tablespoon finely diced shallots, 1 teaspoon kosher salt, and some black pepper. Nab a bit of cheese with your fork, stab some lettuce, and bite down. The lemon and black-pepper flavors of the cheese blend perfectly with the earthy walnut oil.

THE FLAVOR KING
AGED GOUDA

Most cheeses can be aged for weeks to months, but a well-produced Gouda has spent 3 to 5 years in a cave.

"Cheese is aged to develop its flavors," says Scott A. Rankin, PhD, an associate professor of food science at the University of Wisconsin at Madison. The result is like a good Parmigiano-Reggiano, but with rich caramel flavors. Eat thin slices with a green apple or pear.

THE BEER BUDDY
MONTGOMERY'S CHEDDAR

When you chomp into this cheese, don't expect it to taste like the factory-formed orange bricks you find in your supermarket's dairy section. This is authentic Cheddar, from Manor Farm in Somerset, the county in England where the cheese originated. Its lingering flavors of buttermilk and horseradish balance well with any kind of beer and make American Cheddar seem bland.

"English farmhouse Cheddars from Somerset are the Cheddars of choice," says Steven Jenkins, the author of *Cheese Primer*.

STORAGE SECRETS

■ There are dozens of ways to store cheese, but the worst method may surprise you. It's cling wrap, says cheese expert Terrance Brennan. Wrapping cheese tightly in plastic, he says, keeps it from breathing, causing a stale, refrigerated flavor. Whether you're storing Gouda or Brie, here's how to keep your wedge tasting great.

Put it in the crisper

Your refrigerator's vegetable bin is the zone with the highest humidity, which keeps soft cheeses from turning into inedible rocks. Even better: A wine fridge keeps cheese at a near-perfect temp and humidity.

Wrap it right

Different cheeses call for different storage methods.

RIND CHEESES (such as Brie, Tomme de Savoie): Cover only the cut sides in light plastic wrap, but leave the rind exposed so the cheese can breathe.

BLUE CHEESE: Wrap tightly in foil, but change the wrapping frequently— once a day is ideal—so pools of moisture don't form.

SOFT CHEESES (such as Robiola, Sainte-Maure): Store these in a plastic container. If you see water droplets on the surface of the cheese, punch several small holes in the lid.

HARD AND SEMISOFT CHEESES (such as aged Gouda, Cheddar, Roncal): Cover these in two-layer cheese paper, like the kind made by Formaticum ($9 for 15 sheets, formaticum.com). Butcher paper or waxed paper also works.

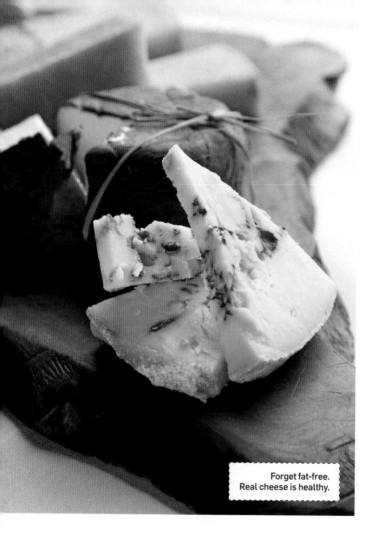

Forget fat-free.
Real cheese is healthy.

"Eating full-fat cheese HOLDS YOUR APPETITE AT BAY."

THE WINE COMPANION
HOJA SANTA

This creamy goat che ese from Texas is wrapped in leaves of hoja santa, which is an herb that imparts licorice and mint flavors. Serve it with a glass of Riesling or sauvignon blanc. White wine is usually a better complement to a cheese plate than red is, because its acidity balances the fat in most cheeses, says Brennan.

Another great cheese to eat with vino is Cypress Grove Chevre Purple Haze, which is a goat cheese from northern California.

THE DESSERT CHEESE
BAYLEY HAZEN BLUE

After biting into this Vermont-made blue cheese, many of our tasters exclaimed, "It tastes like chocolate." The fudgelike flavor even has a hint of apricot--quite a feat considering this is just moldy milk. Eat it alone, or drizzle a drop or two of honey on it for an even sweeter (but still healthy) treat. ■

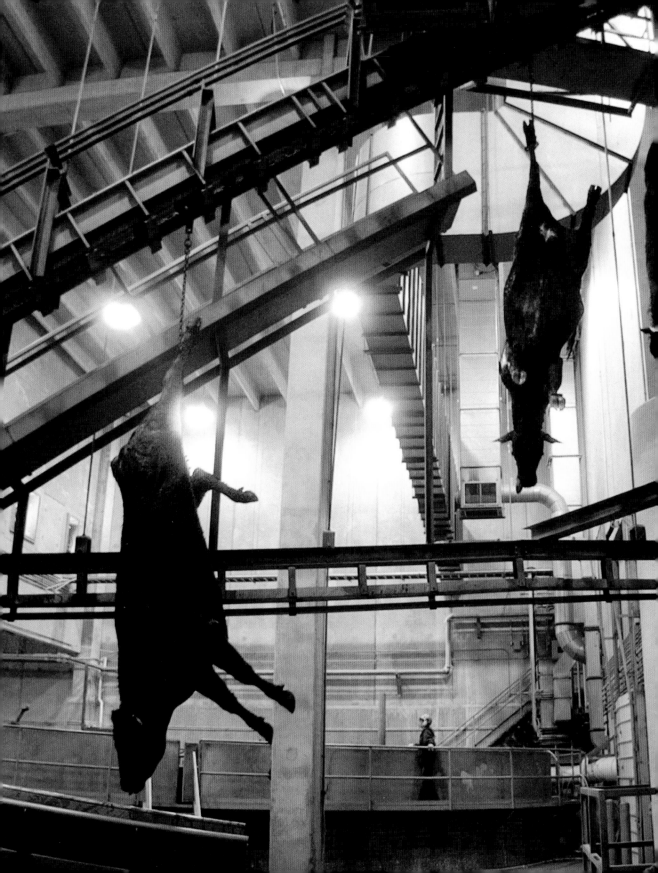

Think about What's Inside the Bun

WHILE YOU'RE OVERHAULING YOUR DIET, YOU MIGHT WANT TO PUT THAT BURGER BACK. THE AGENCY CHARGED WITH SAFEGUARDING OUR FOOD SUPPLY HAS A DIRTY LITTLE SECRET: IT TESTS JUST 0.05 PERCENT OF THE NATION'S GROUND BEEF FOR BACTERIA THAT COULD KILL YOU

Writer Tom Groneburg investigates: It's a Friday night in Missoula, Montana, when my buddy Eric and I walk into the Oxford Café. We make our way through the usual crowd of gamblers, players, and drinkers and take a seat against the far wall. The waitress looks weary, and we look like work to her. "What'll you have?" she asks. Eric orders a burger. I point at the menu and order eggs and brains, nicknamed **"He Needs 'Em."**

"IMPOSSIBLE," THE WAITRESS SAYS flatly. "Since mad cow disease, the USDA won't let us serve that."

"I don't know why you'd want to eat brains," Eric says. This from a guy who thinks nothing of gutting an elk.

I've eaten calf testicles and cow hearts and all sorts of things, but I'd never eaten brains before. I'd heard about the Oxford's fabled dish and figured this would be my chance to try something new, to taste something considered a delicacy in many parts of the world. It didn't seem particularly risky. In fact, no one in Missoula (or anywhere else in the United States) had ever been sickened from eating mad-cow-contaminated meat.

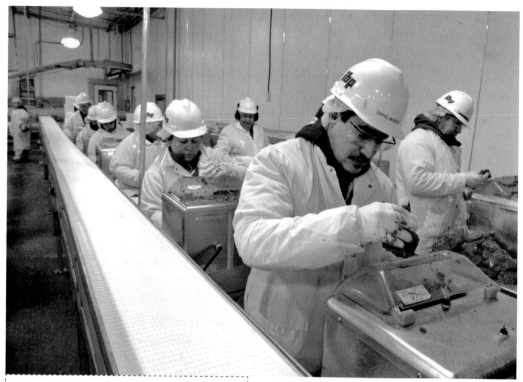

The top four meat-packing companies process more than 60,000 head of cattle a day.

"They'll let us sell pig brains," the waitress offers, "but who wants to eat those?"

I follow Eric's lead and order the state-sanctioned part of the cow, though if we're talking food safety, I really should pass. Turns out, the humble hamburger might be the most dangerous item on the menu.

YOU KNOW THERE'S TROUBLE WHEN your average American carnivore thinks twice about biting into a burger. The appetite-killer in question: *Escherichia coli*, a.k.a. E. coli, the bacteria behind the spate of recalls that recently hit the nation's beef supply. From June to September 2007 alone, ground beef contaminated with E. coli sickened 55 people while also shuttering one business and shaking up the USDA.

Not all E. coli are evil. There are actually hundreds of different strains, some of which are residing in your body right now, helping you absorb food and process waste. In fact, it's estimated that the average person excretes 10 billion *Escherichia coli* bacteria with every bowel movement.

One strain that definitely does not belong inside you is E. coli O157:H7. These bacteria normally live in the guts of cattle. However, if the slaughtering process is sloppy, feces or stomach contents can come into contact with meat and contaminate it with the bug. Next thing you know, you're weathering a weeklong bout of stomach cramps and bloody diarrhea. That is, unless your immune system isn't at full strength, in which case you're facing kidney failure or death.

Prior to 1982, little was known about E. coli O157:H7. That year, the strain was identified as a pathogen after a number of people were sickened by tainted hamburgers. A decade later, the bug popped up again, this time in burgers from the fast-food chain Jack in the Box. Hundreds were hospitalized, and four children died.

Still, it wasn't until 1994 that the USDA began testing for E. coli in samples of beef in packing plants. Five years after that, the agency added an extra safeguard by implementing a system known as Hazard Analysis and Critical Control Points (HACCP), which placed the main responsibility for testing in the hands of the major

slaughterhouses. Theoretically, if they detect a bad batch of beef, it won't be shipped to the smaller "down-line" processors, whose job it is to grind and package bulk beef for the public.

For a while, the system appeared to be working. On April 14, 2005, the USDA, FDA, and CDC released a joint report stating that the incidence of E. coli infections decreased 42 percent from 1996 to 2004. In the press release, then–USDA Secretary Mike Johanns proudly noted, "The continued reduction in illnesses from E. coli O157 is a tremendous success story, and we are committed to continuing this positive trend in the future."

So you have to wonder, what's going wrong now? In 2007, more than 30 million pounds of ground beef were recalled for possible contamination with E. coli.

Thirty million pounds.

How to Build a Burger, Hold the E. Coli

Choose nuked

Look for ground beef labeled "treated by irradiation" or "treated with radiation." This FDA-approved process will neither (a) make your stomach glow, nor (b) deplete the meat's nutrients. It will reduce your risk of E. coli infection, though not by 100 percent. Some microbes may survive if the initial contamination was heavy, so keep reading.

Check the temp

Is the package cold to the touch? It'd better be, given that bacteria breed in warm environments. That's also why your refrigerator should be 33° to 40°F. If there's no built-in digital thermometer, pick up the CDN Refrigerator/Freezer Professional Thermometer ($7, amazon.com). It's certified for accuracy by NSF International.

Counterattack

After you've sculpted your mound of ground beef into burgers, it's time to sanitize. Use hot, soapy water to wash your hands as well as any dishes and utensils that touched raw meat. Then wipe down the counter with an all-purpose cleaner, followed by a spritz of Clorox Anywhere sanitizing spray. (It contains diluted bleach.) Wait 2 minutes, and wipe.

Hit the digits

To be sure your meat hits an E. coli–killing 160°F, use a tip-sensor thermometer, says Shelley Feist, the director of the Partnership for Food Safety Education. Models with sensors that run the length of the probe are less accurate for thinner meats, like burgers. Try the TruTemp Cooking Thermometer ($18, amazon.com).

That's 120 million quarter-pound patties that made it as far as our grocery carts and, in some cases, our stomachs.

FOR MOST MANUFACTURERS, PROFIT is tied to production, and the industry that turns bovines into burgers is no different: The top four meat-packing companies process more than 60,000 head of cattle a day. Given this staggering amount of cow, it makes you wonder how they test all of it for contamination. They don't.

"The biggest plant I've heard of produces about 3 million pounds of trim daily," says John Munsell, manager of the Foundation for Accountability in Regulatory Enforcement. Trim, or beef destined for processing into hamburger, is then put into a "combo," a huge cardboard box that holds, literally, a ton of meat. Each of these 2,000-pound boxes is tested, says Munsell. "They just reach into the top layer and take out less than a pound of trim. They mingle it together and grind it, and that's what they sample for their microbial analysis."

And after the big processors do what is required of them under HACCP, their products are moved along to the down-line processors, and ultimately our dinner tables, with the USDA mark of inspection.

Though he's never had food poisoning, Munsell's life was still up-ended by E. coli that a major meat packer had missed. In January 2002, routine tests by the USDA's Food Safety and Inspection Service found evidence of E. coli contamination in meat he was grinding at Montana Quality Foods, the small meat-packing business his father started 56 years earlier in Miles City, Montana.

In 2007 alone, MORE THAN 30 MILLION POUNDS OF GROUND BEEF WERE RECALLED for E. coli.

According to Munsell, the meat he ground that day came in vacuum-sealed packages from two sources, one of which was the huge ConAgra Foods packing plant in Greeley, Colorado. Subsequent tests a month later found more E. coli contamination from ConAgra meat. And though a USDA inspector later testified that he had seen the meat go directly from the ConAgra packages into Munsell's sanitized grinder, there was no way to conclusively prove that the contamination hadn't origi-nated at Montana Quality Foods. USDA officials shut down Munsell's operation, despite his pleas that they send investigators so he could show them documentation verifying the tainted meat's origin.

"I was expecting a whole gang of inspectors to arrive at my plant on Monday, and no one showed up. They didn't even call."

In the summer of 2002, 5 months after the first positive test results at Munsell's facility, ConAgra voluntarily recalled 354,000 pounds of ground beef from its

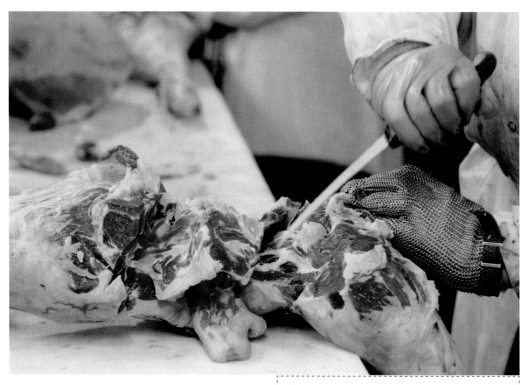
The main responsibility testing beef's safety is in the hands of the major slaughterhouses.

Greeley plant after numerous tests revealed E. coli contamination. Three weeks later, the recall was expanded to more than 18 million pounds, but it was too late to prevent 46 people across the United States from becoming ill. Of the recalled beef, only 3 million pounds were ever recovered.

Physically and emotionally spent from his one-man fight against the USDA, Munsell sold his plant in 2005. Since then, he's filed a lawsuit against the USDA, maintaining that he was retaliated against for blowing the whistle on what he sees as the agency's refusal to take on the big meat packers.

"They are too formidable a foe," says Munsell. "In the past two large-size litigations that the big packers brought against the agency, the agency lost both, so it lost interest in pressing for corrective action. What we need are people at the USDA who cannot be pressured by the large multinational companies. We need people who will simply do what is right."

To be fair, the USDA has made some strides in the wake of the latest recalls. It recently announced that it will step up the number of E. coli tests conducted each year. Those tests will focus on plants that produce the largest quantities of ground beef and trim, as well as those that trigger positive results for contaminated meat.

But critics maintain that these moves are just Band-Aids for a testing system that was broken from the beginning. "HACCP was designed to put the onus on the small processor," says Tony Corbo, a legislative representative for Food & Water Watch, a nonprofit consumer-rights group dedicated to holding the government and corporations accountable for food and water issues. "If a sample of meat comes up positive for E. coli or salmonella, the grinder is the one taking the regulatory hit, even though it may have purchased the contaminated trim or coarsely ground beef from a large supplier. The John Munsell situation is a perfect illustration of how badly the regu-

packing plants. When I go out in public, I don't order hamburger. I just don't trust it anymore."

I F THINGS CONTINUE TO GO SOUTH, the USDA has already decided who to blame: the cows.

"The amount of product we test that's positive has gone up about 33 percent this year from the past 3 years," says Richard Raymond, MD, the USDA's undersecretary for food safety. "I don't think it's that the agency has fallen asleep at the switch. I don't think it's that the industry has gotten sloppy. I think it's the cows."

The American public is hungry for beef—and for REASSURANCE THAT IT IS SAFE TO EAT.

latory system is set up."

Today, Munsell is a full-time crusader for meat-safety reform, the Ralph Nader of hamburger. He's authored the Traceback Bill, a piece of legislation he hopes will find support in Congress. The bill puts forth four commonsense measures aimed at finding the true origin of contaminated meat. However, he realizes that in the meantime there's still a public that's hungry for beef and reassurance.

"My suggestion would be for people to buy their beef from a small, local, inspected meat-slaughtering facility," Munsell says. "I no longer have any confidence in meat that comes from these big meat-

Specifically, Dr. Raymond cites high corn prices for prompting a switch to cheaper feeds for fattening cattle. "When you change their feed, their intestinal flora change."

Could an increase in the cost of corn have had such gut-wrenching consequences? Perhaps. First you have to understand that the reason corn prices have skyrocketed is because of the recent increase in domestic ethanol production, which uses corn to produce a relatively clean alternative to fossil-based fuels. Consequently, more feedlots have resorted to using distiller's grains, which is a cheap but nutritious supplemental feed left over when corn is turned into ethanol. But research shows that the monetary savings may come at a hidden cost to the consumer.

"We found that cattle consuming distiller's grains as 25 percent of their diet had about a twofold higher incidence of E. coli O157:H7," says T. G. Nagaraja, PhD, a professor of microbiology at Kansas State University and the leader of a team of researchers targeting ways to decrease levels of E. coli in cattle before they reach the slaughterhouse. "Our observation is preliminary, but we've done three studies that show a positive association between this feed and increased levels of O157."

The USDA's Dr. Raymond points to an-

Of course, this only explains why there may have been more E. coli than usual in cattle bound for slaughter, not why the bug ultimately ended up contaminating so much of the beef supply.

Michael Doyle, PhD, director of the center for food safety at the University of Georgia and one of the world's leading authorities on E. coli and other foodborne pathogens, has a theory: "There is often an increase in bacterial contamination when experienced workers on the slaughter line are replaced with less-experienced workers, such as before and after holidays," he says, "and raids . . . on illegal slaughterhouse workers by the INS led to replace-

If things continue to go south, the USDA has already decided WHO TO BLAME: THE COWS.

other possible reason for the increase in E. coli levels: flooded feedlots. When feedlots flood, that puts stress on cattle. And when they're stressed, their E. coli numbers go up.

His flooded-feedlot explanation might hold some water. "One factor associated with cattle shedding the E. coli organism is wet and muddy pen conditions," says David Smith, DVM, PhD, a professor of veterinary and biomedical science at the University of Nebraska. "I suspect the slaughterhouses may have had cattle arrive . . . with a higher probability of shedding E. coli, or the cattle had it present on their hides, which led to greater opportunities for ground-beef contamination than during droughts."

ment with less-experienced line workers."

Still, you could argue that if an adequate testing system had been in place at the slaughterhouses during this uptick in tainted meat, little to none of it would have gone out the door. And yet some experts say that it's simply unrealistic to expect that the big meat packers will ever be able to catch all the contaminated beef, no matter what new testing procedures are ultimately instituted.

"You're not going to eliminate E. coli O157:H7," says Doug Powell, PhD, an associate professor of pathobiology and scientific director of the International Food Safety Network. "Down-line processors have to be operating under the assumption that they're going to get some E. coli just like we expect consumers to operate under the assumption that they're going to have some in their product, which is why we tell them to cook it."

And really, that basic assumption could be the most important lesson we can learn from the recalls. Forget the fact that 70 percent of the cattle in America are slaughtered by just four companies, and that those companies may have managed to intimidate the USDA into inaction. Put aside theories that cattle are loaded with more E. coli because of stress or due to diet changes arising from our rush to utilize alternative fuels. What you as the consumer need to keep in mind is that beef is being contaminated in slaughterhouses and that you are your own last line of defense.

To put it another way, remember that fecal contamination will continue to occur and shit always flows downstream.

B ACK AT THE OXFORD, THE WAIT-ress brings our hamburgers just as the first bets of the night are laid on the poker table in the front room. Eric dolls up his burger with mustard and ketchup and takes a big bite.

It's impossible to tell where the meat for my burger originated, but odds are it came from one of the big packing plants. An old man walks away from his video keno machine, discouraged at having lost his money. I cut into my hamburger patty and stare at it. It looks done, but it's impossible to tell what temperature it was cooked to. A collective groan goes up from the poker table.

"What?" Eric asks, his mouth full of half-chewed meat.

I shrug my shoulders. I'm an unapologetic carnivore. I love beef, and I can't imagine giving it up. Besides, until the USDA gets data back from its new measures, until the agency begins cracking down on packing plants that consistently produce contaminated beef, and until the beef industry figures out a way to keep fecal matter from coming into contact with meat in the slaughterhouse, it's all a crapshoot anyhow.

"Pass the ketchup," I say. ■

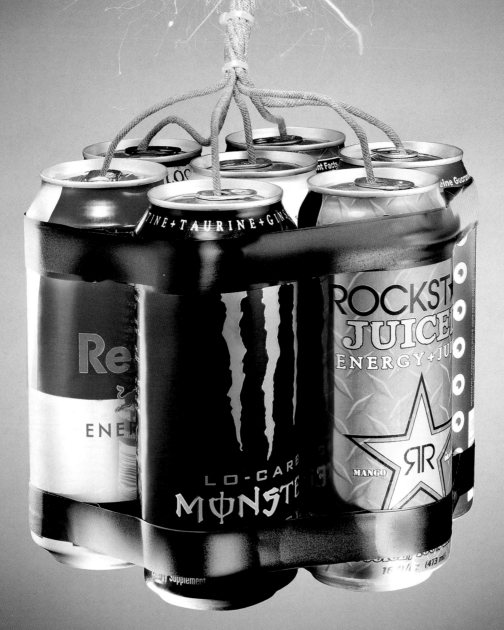

Wake Up, Already

TIRED? WHO ISN'T? ENERGY DRINKS SELL YOU ON INCREASING ALERTNESS, FIGHTING FATIGUE, AND IMPROVING REACTION TIME. BUT WHEN YOU POP THE TOP, WHAT ARE YOU REALLY POURING INTO YOUR BODY?

Apparently, it doesn't take a

NO, ACCORDING TO STARBUCKS, any guy off the street is qualified. At least that's whose opinion mattered most when the coffee giant recently created the ingredient list for its own concoction.

"There are many energy ingredients on the market, and B vitamins, guarana, and ginseng are the ones our customers are most familiar with," says Ruby Amegah, product-development manager for the team behind the Starbucks Doubleshot Energy + Coffee. Which perhaps in large part explains why the company chose them: It's smart marketing.

Trouble is, by letting consumer research influence ingredient lists, energy-drink companies are helping popularize exotic-sounding compounds that even scientists don't yet fully understand. The approach has worked: Last year, Americans spent $4.2 billion on these supposedly high-octane elixirs. And that's probably why manufacturers haven't strayed far from the best-selling recipe they used when the first energy drinks took off a dozen years ago. It's a formulation that includes a hefty dose of caffeine and sugar combined with smaller amounts of seemingly obscure substances, most notably guarana, ginseng, and taurine.

But do these beverages really energize your body and sharpen your mind? Or should you can the energy drinks for good? To help you separate the science from the sales pitch, we analyzed four key ingredients in the market's most popular potions.

CAFFEINE

WHAT IS IT? A chemical compound that stimulates your central nervous system. Most energy drinks contain between 140 and 170 milligrams of caffeine in a 15- or 16-ounce can.

DOES IT WORK? Java junkies certainly think so. As for the science, an Austrian study showed that men who swallowed 100 milligrams of caffeine had a bigger boost in brain activity after 20 minutes than those who took a placebo. Plus, a new University of Chicago study found that a 200 milligram jolt made fatigued people feel twice as alert as noncaffeinated participants.

"Caffeine indirectly affects many different neurotransmitters," says Andrew Scholey, PhD, an herb and nutrition researcher at Australia's Swinburne University of Technology.

IS IT SAFE? The most caffeine-packed energy drink contains the equivalent in caffeine of about two 8-ounce cups of coffee. If downing that much joe doesn't make you jittery, then quaffing a can shouldn't pose a problem. Of course, if you combine that with other caffeinated beverages throughout the day, then the sum total stimulation could cause headaches, sleeplessness, or nausea.

On the other hand, if you're not a regular coffee or cola drinker and you battle high blood pressure, the occasional energy drink could be trouble. Researchers in Finland reported that the caffeine in two to three cups of coffee can cause BP to spike by up to 14 points.

biochemist to formulate an energy drink.

GLUCOSE

WHAT IS IT? Sugar. Sucrose, another ingredient you'll often see on energy drink labels, is a combination of fructose (the natural sugar found in fruit) and glucose. Many energy drinks contain 50 to 60 grams of glucose or sucrose in a 16-ounce can.

Does it work? Your body runs mainly on glucose, so topping off your tank with the sweet stuff should theoretically provide an instant boost. And in fact, a recent study in the *Journal of Applied Physiology* found that men who guzzled a 6 percent glucose drink were able to bicycle 22 minutes longer than those who went sans the extra sugar.

Where glucose won't help, however, is with the fog of fatigue from too little sleep. A 2006 British study determined that sleep-deprived people who drank liquid glucose exhibited slower reaction times and more sleepiness after 90 minutes.

IS IT SAFE? Dumping empty calories down your gullet is never a great idea, and some energy drinks contain nearly as much sugar as a 20-ounce soda. Then there's the fact that a sudden infusion of glucose can cause your blood sugar and insulin levels to skyrocket, signaling your body to stop incinerating fat.

A 2006 New Zealand study revealed that caffeine combined with even the 27 grams of sugar in, say, an 8.3-ounce Red Bull might be enough to temporarily inhibit your body's ability to burn lard.

GUARANA

WHAT IS IT? A South American shrub. One seed has a caffeine content of 4 to 5 percent, while a coffee bean has 1 to 2 percent. The amount of guarana in a 16-ounce energy drink ranges from a minuscule 1.4 milligrams to as much as 300 milligrams.

DOES IT WORK? Yes, if you don't set the bar too high. A study in the journal *Appetite* reports that people who took 222 milligrams of guarana felt slightly less fatigued and were up to 30 milliseconds faster on a reaction-time test than those

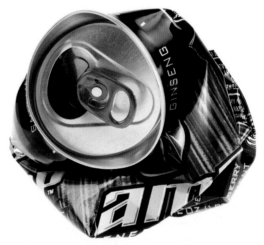

The amount of sugar in an energy drink is enough to INHIBIT YOUR BODY'S ABILITY TO BURN FAT.

who popped a placebo. Some scientists attribute guarana's effect solely to its caffeine content, but Scholey isn't so sure. His team found energizing effects with doses just under 40 milligrams, which contain very little caffeine. That means there's probably something else in guarana that produces a stimulating effect on its own or that bolsters the effect of the caffeine, he says.

IS IT SAFE? Scientists at Florida's Nova Southeastern University recently conducted tests and concluded that the amounts of guarana found in most energy drinks aren't large enough to cause any adverse effects. That said, there's still a question mark regarding the safety of higher levels, which could conceivably be consumed by downing a few energy drinks in a brief time span.

GINSENG

WHAT IS IT? An extract made from the root of the ginseng plant. Panax ginseng is the species most commonly used. The ginseng content in energy drinks typically ranges between 8 milligrams and 400 milligrams in 16 ounces.

DOES IT WORK? Not if you're hoping for energy to burn. A recent review in *American Family Physician* determined that ginseng doesn't enhance physical performance.

But there is an upside: It might boost your brainpower. Dr. Scholey and his colleagues found that people who swallowed 200 mg of the extract an hour before taking a cognitive test scored significantly better than when they skipped the supplement. They also felt less mental fatigue. Ginseng

Alternative Energy Sources

If you're looking for a quick pick-me-up, plenty of beverages provide ample quantities of caffeine or sugar—and in most cases, both. We compared amounts of these two key components in several popular drinks.

DUNKIN' DONUTS
Black coffee, 14-ounce medium

CAFFEINE	164 milligrams
SUGAR	0 grams
CALORIES	20

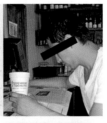

COCA-COLA
Classic 20-ounce bottle

CAFFEINE	58 milligrams
SUGAR	68 grams
CALORIES	240

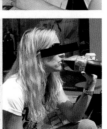

AMP ENERGY
16-ounce can

CAFFEINE	143 milligrams
SUGAR	58 grams
CALORIES	220

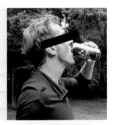

STARBUCKS
Caffé Mocha 16-ounce grande

CAFFEINE	175 milligrams
SUGAR	33 grams
CALORIES	330

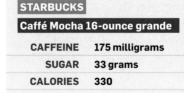
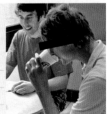

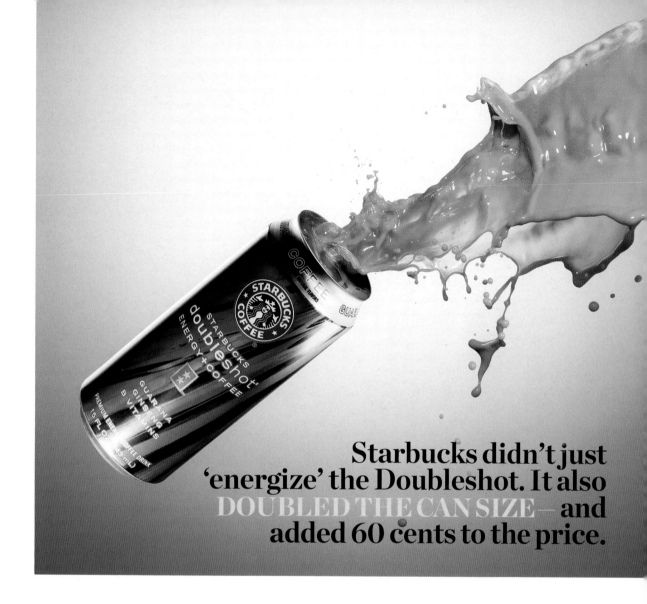

Starbucks didn't just 'energize' the Doubleshot. It also DOUBLED THE CAN SIZE— and added 60 cents to the price.

might work by increasing the uptake of blood glucose by cells in the brain and elsewhere, says Dr. Scholey.

However, the right amount is essential. Only two of the eight major energy drinks we examined contained that optimal dose of at least 200 milligrams.

IS IT SAFE? Since the amount of ginseng in an energy drink is minimal, harmful effects are unlikely. And while there have been some reports of negative side effects from ginseng—diarrhea, for example—Dr. Scholey points out that those occurred in people taking 3 grams a day.

One caution: If you're on any medications, check with your doctor before knocking back an energy drink. Ginseng has been shown to interact with blood-thinning drugs like warfarin, potentially altering their effectiveness. ∎

Get an Edge

STILL LOOKING FOR A BOOST? CONSIDER THE CAFFEINE ADVANTAGE. HERE'S EVERYTHING YOU NEED TO KNOW TO THINK FASTER, EXERCISE HARDER, AND LIVE LONGER

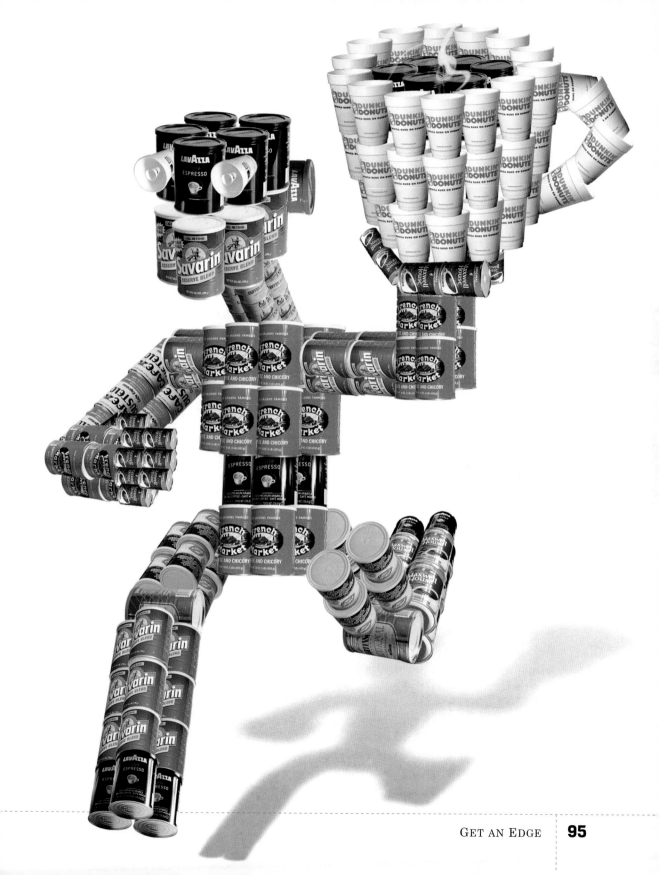

By now you'd think scientists could close the book on caffeine

and move on to other mysteries, like why anyone would ever order a chai latte. After all, coffee and related beverages have been revving people up since, oh, the 15th century. And in the past 60 years, researchers have conducted more than 21,000 studies on our favorite stimulant. That's an average of one new study a day through all of those decades. (Those nutrition scientists might have gotten into their own stash.)

If we don't know caffeine by now, you may well ask, when will we know it? And do I have time for a fix while I'm waiting?

Make it a venti, and sit down. We'll explain a few things. First off, caffeine is a complex compound. And it's made even more so by America's preferred delivery method, coffee. For instance, caffeine raises blood pressure, but habitual coffee drinkers are half as likely to die of heart failure as those who don't fill their mug daily. And while caffeine spikes blood sugar, a java habit might help you dodge diabetes.

Confused? Then use this primer to learn how to consume caffeine to your advantage—at work, in the gym, and for overall health.

THE BIOLOGY

The science: To understand how a double espresso can take you from dead tired to completely wired, you first need an introduction to the compound adenosine. Right now, adenosine is coursing through your veins, and its job is to put the brakes on your central nervous system. You might call it nature's chill pill. That's because as your day progresses, adenosine builds up naturally in your bloodstream, causing you to slow down and become sleepier—a convenient way to let you know it's time to turn off Conan and recharge your batteries.

Adenosine accomplishes this total-body shutdown by plugging into adenosine receptors—like electrical cords into outlets.

"These connections inhibit the release of neurotransmitters, which are chemical messengers that control both brain and muscle function," says William Lovallo, PhD, a professor of psychiatry and behavioral sciences at the University of Oklahoma. "As a result, both your mind and your body slow down."

But as it turns out, caffeine is an excellent adenosine impersonator. In fact, when the two rivals jockey for the same parking space, caffeine wins.

"If caffeine is plugged into the adenosine receptors, adenosine can't do its job," says Dr. Lovallo. "And this causes your central nervous system to run at a faster rate." Thus you experience the classic and often sought-after caffeine jolt. Here's how to make it work for just about every part of your body.

YOUR BRAIN

The science: Soon after your first sip, caffeine begins to work its magic by causing the release of dopamine. Dopamine is a brain chemical that stimulates the area of your gray matter responsible for alertness, problem solving, and pleasure.

"You have that feeling of being activated, sharper, and on the ball," says Lovallo. "And you can also experience a mild mood-elevating effect." All of which goes a long way in explaining why so many of us are such caffeine fiends.

Be smarter instantly. Down a cup of joe just before your next meeting. It'll boost your mind power for about 45 minutes, according to a recent Austrian study that directly measured the impact of 100 milligrams of caffeine on brain activity.

Be smarter for life. Refill your cup three times a day. Harvard researchers have determined that men who drink four cups of caffeinated coffee a day are half as likely to develop Parkinson's disease as those who skip the java—presumably because caffeine keeps dopamine molecules active. What's more, blocking adenosine might slow the buildup of amyloid-beta, which is a toxic brain plaque that's associated with Alzheimer's disease.

YOUR HEART

The science: Adenosine helps blood vessels relax. But once caffeine infiltrates the receptors that line vessel walls, your arteries constrict, causing your blood pressure to rise. In fact, research has shown that blood pressure may increase by as much as 10 points in nonhabitual drinkers. Yet when Harvard researchers tracked the coffee intake of more than 128,000 people, they determined that drinking more than six cups of coffee a day didn't boost the chance of developing heart disease. And last year, scientists at Brooklyn College found that men who drank four cups of caffeinated coffee daily had a 53 percent lower risk of dying of heart disease than those who never took a sip.

"If you don't have hypertension to begin with, the temporary blood-pressure increase from a cup of coffee isn't a problem," says Matthew Sorrentino, MD, a cardiologist and professor of medicine at the Uni-

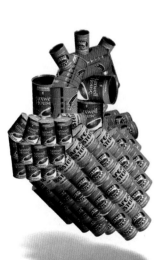

Harvard researchers found that men who drink 4 cups of coffee a day are HALF AS LIKELY TO DEVELOP PARKINSON'S.

versity of Chicago. "Plus, the impact on blood pressure tends to be smaller in habitual caffeine drinkers because their bodies become somewhat tolerant to its effects."

Take your health history into account. If caffeine makes your heart race or skip beats, you're probably genetically sensitive to the stimulant. "Although this may sound serious, symptoms such as palpitations are actually considered innocuous, unless you've had a recent heart attack," says John Kassotis, MD, a cardiac electrophysiologist at SUNY Downstate, in Brooklyn. Still, Dr. Kassotis suggests playing it safe. His rule of thumb: If you think you're caffeine-sensitive, consult your physician to determine if you should limit your intake.

Stick with antioxidant-rich java. Scientists aren't sure whether it's the caffeine or the antioxidants in coffee—or a combination of the two—that provide the aforementioned cardiovascular benefits. But unless you're caffeine-sensitive, go with the leaded variety. Research shows that antioxidant levels are decreased by about 15 percent in decaf.

YOUR MUSCLES

The science: Because caffeine revs up your central nervous system, it slightly increases your heart rate and breathing rate, both of which help prepare your body for peak performance. Caffeine may also have a direct effect on your muscles. Here's how: Calcium must be released within a muscle fiber in order for that fiber to contract, and caffeine may block the adenosine receptors attached to muscle fibers, triggering electrical activity that prompts bigger bursts of calcium.

"The result is a stronger muscle contraction," says Terry Graham, PhD, a professor of human health and nutritional sciences at the University of Guelph, in Ontario.

Jumpstart your workout. Studies show that consuming 140 to 400 milligrams of caffeine 30 to 60 minutes prior to exercise can improve both speed and endurance and make your workout seem easier. But to achieve those effects, researchers have used either caffeine pills or caffeinated soda. The reason: "Many other chemical compounds in coffee appear to counteract

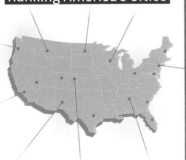

METROGRADES
Ranking America's Cities

Where Caffeine Is King

AT FIRST, we considered measuring city caffeine consumption with a seismograph. We figured the place with the worst jitters would be off the scale. But in the end, we stuck with statistics drawn from the United States Census Bureau, Simmons Research, and SimplyMap.

Starting with the number of Starbucks per capita, we crunched the data on all things coffee, from the biggest bloc of whole-bean brewers to the most java drinkers. We also compared the number of people who quaff regular and diet cola and high-octane energy drinks. Finally, because the truly overcaffeinated are short on shut-eye, we looked at hours of sleep logged per night along with rates of insomnia and other related sleep disorders. Add it all up and you can see who's wired where. The newly crowned capital of caffeine? Yonkers, New York.

MOST CAFFEINATED	
1	Yonkers, NY
2	Anaheim, CA
3	San Francisco, CA
4	Riverside, CA
5	Las Vegas, NV
6	Arlington, TX
7	Bakersfield, CA
8	Seattle, WA
9	Honolulu, HI
10	Oakland, CA

caffeine's ability to impact your exercise session," Dr. Graham says. Now you know why energy drinks were created. Looking for a boost? Try Celsius, which is sugar-free and contains about 200 milligrams of caffeine per 12-ounce can. To determine if it's enhancing your performance, be sure to monitor how it impacts your exercise session both mentally ("My workout seemed easier" or "I felt like I was dragging") and physically ("I completed more repetitions" or "I didn't improve").

Use caution. If you have heart problems or a family history of heart disease, avoid high-caffeine energy drinks for 4 hours before exercising. A 2006 study in the *Journal of the American College of Cardiology* determined that 200 milligrams of caffeine decreases bloodflow to the heart by up to 39 percent during exercise because it constricts coronary arteries.

YOUR LIVER

The science: When your central nervous system is activated, so is your body's fight-or-flight response. This causes the release of stress hormones such as cortisol and adrenaline. These in turn signal your liver to pump sugar into your bloodstream. After all, had you been in a truly stressful situation—say, face-to-face with a cranky barista—your body would need that sugar for quick energy. But in everyday life (read: sitting at your desk), extra blood sugar is the last thing you need, because it signals your body to store fat and increases your risk of diabetes.

Keep your blood sugar in check. Forgo the sugar in your coffee, and you'll actually reduce your risk of developing diabetes, according to multiple studies. For example, in 2005, Harvard University researchers determined that drinking five cups of coffee a day cuts in half the risk of developing diabetes. Scientists aren't sure why coffee may have a protective effect against diabetes, but credit its high level of disease-fighting antioxidants. While visiting Starbucks, we recommend a Caffè Americano, which is coffee at its finest: strong and flavorful, but sugar-free. ■

11 Portland, OR	31 Colorado Springs, CO	51 Little Rock, AR	71 Toledo, OH	
12 San Diego, CA	32 Orlando, FL	52 Austin, TX	72 Nashville, TN	
13 Fremont, CA	33 San Antonio, TX	53 Jacksonville, FL	73 Burlington, VT	
14 Jersey City, NJ	34 Boise, ID	54 Montgomery, AL	74 Des Moines, IA	
15 Sacramento, CA	35 Charlotte, NC	55 Spokane, WA	75 Sioux Falls, SD	
16 Fresno, CA	36 St. Petersburg, FL	56 St. Paul, MN	76 Omaha, NE	
17 Aurora, CO	37 Tampa, FL	57 Grand Rapids, MI	77 Bangor, ME	
18 Los Angeles, CA	38 Richmond, VA	58 Boston, MA	78 St. Louis, MO	
19 Miami, FL	39 Wilmington, DE	59 Baltimore, MD	79 Providence, RI	
20 Modesto, CA	40 Albuquerque, NM	60 Jackson, MS	80 Billings, MT	
21 Washington, DC	41 Columbia, SC	61 Chicago, IL	81 Lexington, KY	
22 San Jose, CA	42 Dallas, TX	62 Indianapolis, IN	82 Salt Lake City, UT	
23 Denver, CO	43 Corpus Christi, TX	63 Baton Rouge, LA	83 Cleveland, OH	
24 El Paso, TX	44 Atlanta, GA	64 Minneapolis, MN	84 Philadelphia, PA	
25 Cheyenne, WY	45 Fort Worth, TX	65 Charleston, WV	85 Kansas City, MO	
26 Tucson, AZ	46 Birmingham, AL	66 Hartford, CT	86 Wichita, KS	
27 Newark, NJ	47 Durham, NC	67 Cincinnati, OH	87 Manchester, NH	
28 New York, NY	48 Anchorage, AK	68 Pittsburgh, PA	88 Fargo, ND	
29 Raleigh, NC	49 Houston, TX	69 Oklahoma City, OK	89 Columbus, OH	
30 Phoenix, AZ	50 Norfolk, VA	70 Greensboro, NC	90 Louisville, KY	

LEAST CAFFEINATED

91	**Memphis, TN**
92	**Milwaukee, WI**
93	**Fort Wayne, IN**
94	**Tulsa, OK**
95	**Lubbock, TX**
96	**Madison, WI**
97	**Rochester, NY**
98	**Buffalo, NY**
99	**Lincoln, NE**
100	**Detroit, MI**

EXERCISE SCIENCE

GET RIPPED ON A BUDGET

Go ahead: Cut back on the amount of pricey protein powder in your postworkout shake. Half a scoop of whey protein is enough to build muscle, say Canadian researchers. In their study, men were able to stimulate the muscle-building process when they downed a drink made with just 10 grams of whey.

To shake it up like the men in the study, blend together ½ scoop of whey protein powder with a half cup of water and ice, and a cup of fresh blueberries. Drink it up to 30 minutes after your workout.

BE SORE NO MORE

Forget the mantra "No pain, no gain": A tea leaf might lead to ache-free workouts, say scientists at Rutgers University. When study participants con-

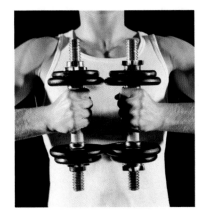

sumed about 1,800 milligrams of black tea extract a day, they experienced significantly less muscle soreness after an intense workout than those who skipped the supplement.

"Not only do antioxidants in the extract appear to reduce inflammation after a workout," says study author Shawn Arent, PhD, "but they also seem to blunt muscular strain while you're training." Look for black tea extract online at houseofnutrition.com.

BOOST STRENGTH WITH COFFEE

It's a curious example of food synergy, but consuming caffeine along with carbohydrates after you exercise refuels your muscles faster than eating carbohydrates alone, according to a study in the *Journal of Applied Physiology*. Your muscles will have 66 percent more glycogen, muscles' primary fuel source, which means better workouts and more gains, say the study authors.

In a separate study, researchers confirmed that eating a high-carb diet—8 to 10 grams per kilogram of body weight—1 to 3 days before exercising boosts workout performance.

DON'T WITHER AWAY

Eating more potassium could help protect your biceps for life. In a recent study, researchers at the Department of Agriculture's Human Nutrition Research Center on Aging at Tufts University found that foods rich in potassium help preserve lean muscle mass. After studying 384 volunteers for 3 years, they found that those whose diets were rich in potassium (more than 3,540 milligrams a day) preserved 3.6 more pounds of lean tissue than those with half the potassium intake.

"That almost offsets the 4.4 pounds of lean tissue that is typically lost in a decade by healthy men," says study author Bess Dawson-Hughes, MD.

One possible reason: Potassium-rich foods, such as fruits and vegetables, help neutralize the acid that can cause muscle to break down as you age, say the scientists. While more research is needed to confirm this finding, consider it another reason to eat more produce.

While bananas are the easiest on-the-go source of potassium (each contains about 420 milligrams), there are better sources of the nutrient. Here are 15 of the best:

Food	Serving	Potassium (in milligrams)
SWISS CHARD, boiled	1 cup	961
LIMA BEANS, cooked	1 cup	955
YAMS, cooked	1 cup	911
ACORN SQUASH, baked	1 cup	896
SPINACH, boiled	1 cup	839
PAPAYA	1 cup	781
PINTO BEANS, boiled	1 cup	746
CREMINI MUSHROOMS, raw	5 oz	636
COD, baked or broiled	4 oz	586
BEETS, boiled	1 cup	518
BROCCOLI, boiled	1 cup	457
BRUSSELS SPROUTS, boiled	1 cup	450
CANTALOUPE	1 cup	427
TOMATO, raw	1 cup	427
BANANA	1 whole	420

SHAKE IT UP

A cocktail of protein, carbs, and creatine can help you build brawn faster, according to Australian researchers. Men who consumed this mix during 10 weeks of weight training packed on 68 percent more muscle than those who took in only protein and carbs.

"Creatine helps you train harder and recover faster," says study author Alan Hayes, PhD. And drinking it with carbs and protein helps shuttle even more of the compound into your muscles. The magic formula is 40 grams each of carbs and protein, plus 5 grams of creatine. (Optimum Nutrition's After Max has that combo.) Divide your drinks into two equal servings for the day, and have one after your workout.

FIND A NEW USE FOR AN OLD SUPPLEMENT

A remedy for osteoporosis might be found in your preworkout

HARD TRUTH **3,114** THE AMOUNT OF POTASSIUM, IN MILLIGRAMS, THE AVERAGE GUY CONSUMES DAILY—NEARLY 1,600 MG LESS THAN IS RECOMMENDED, ACCORDING TO THE CENTERS FOR DISEASE CONTROL AND PREVENTION

shake. Canadian researchers recently discovered that creatine strengthens your skeleton. The likely reason: "Bone-building cells rely on phosphocreatine as an energy source," says the study's coauthor, Stephen Cornish, PhD. "Consuming creatine increases that energy source, so you boost your ability to lay down new bone."

Not surprisingly, of course, the study participants also gained muscle and strength. The magic formula is about 1 gram of creatine for every 22 pounds of body weight—taken immediately before a workout—3 days a week. (We like At Large Nutrition Creatine 500, $15, atlargenutrition.com.)

While the benefits of creatine might seem magical, they're not: The supplement simply helps provide your muscles with more adenosine triphosphate, or ATP, the compound your body uses for energy. "This allows you to work out harder for longer, the key to faster gains," says Jeff Volek, PhD, RD, an exercise scientist at the University of Connecticut. It all starts when

you supplement with creatine, which boosts the levels of creatine phosphate in your muscles. Read on for the details.

1 For a muscle to contract, it has to break off a phosphate molecule from ATP. (ATP has three phosphates.)

2 This creates a chemical reaction that causes muscle contraction, allowing you to lift weights at a high intensity.

3 But as a result, ATP becomes adenosine diphosphate, or ADP. (ADP has two phosphates.)

4 Your muscles can't use ADP for energy, and the amount of ATP stored in your muscles is limited.

5 The fix: ADP takes a phosphate from your muscles' stores of creatine phosphate.

6 ATP forms quickly, giving you more energy to train intensely.

EAT SPINACH, ADD SIZE?

A chemical in leafy greens might help you build muscle. In a test-tube study, Rutgers researchers dis-

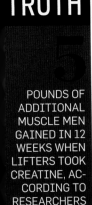

covered that treating human muscle cells with a phytoecdysteroid—a compound found in spinach—increased protein synthesis by 120 percent.

Phytoecdysteroids appear to allow muscle tissue to repair itself faster, says study author Jonathan Gorelick-Feldman, PhD. What's more, rats that consumed high amounts of the substance became stronger after just 28 days. Unfortunately, you'd have to eat Popeye-sized quantities—almost 2 pounds a day—to reap similar benefits. In future studies, the scientists hope to determine the effect of smaller quantities.

EAT MORE CHOLESTEROL?

Eggs might be the secret to more muscle—and not for the reason you think. In a study of older men in a 12-week weight-training program, researchers found that the more cholesterol the men consumed, the better their muscle gains were, regardless of their protein intake.

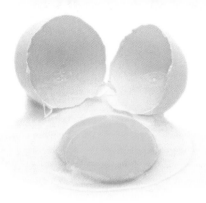

The key is combining dietary cholesterol with resistance training. The researchers hypothesize that the cholesterol might aid in muscle repair, but more research is needed to be sure.

POP SOME RAISINS

This isn't a grapevine rumor: Raisins provide the same cardio boost as energy gels do. When San Diego State scientists had cyclists down 3.5 ounces of raisins or a similarly carb-packed gel before training, they found that both enhanced performance equally.

"Raisins, however, also deliver antioxidants, fiber, and vitamins," says the study author, Mark Kern,

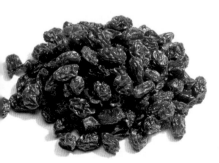

PhD. And at a fifth the cost of gels, raisins also help keep your wallet full.

Bonus: Raisins can help fight off prostate cancer, thanks to their high content of the mineral boron.

BUILD INNER FORTITUDE

Sprint to the finish line, not to the john. Finnish researchers have discovered that taking probiotics—healthy bacteria—can help protect runners from the runs. When 70 athletes consumed a daily dose of the probiotic Lactobacillus rhamnosus GG (LGG) for 3 months, their gastrointestinal episodes were significantly less severe than a placebo group's. Before a big race, down a Dannon Danimals shake, which contains about the same amount of LGG that was used in the study.

CAP YOUR C

Many athletes take vitamin C, which fuels muscle recovery. Problem is, too much vitamin C can diminish your training gains, reveals a study in the *American Journal of*

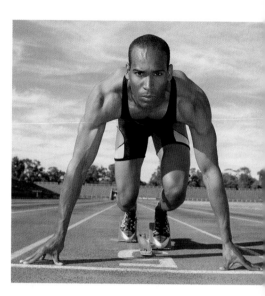

Clinical Nutrition. Men who took 1,000 milligrams of the vitamin daily while following an 8-week cardio plan increased their endurance less than those who skipped the supplement. According to the study authors, the vitamin users' muscles contained fewer mitochondria, cells that convert nutrients into energy.

Limit your vitamin C intake to 500 milligrams a day. British researchers found that this amount helped repair muscles faster than megadoses did. ■

TRAINING TIPS

Q: I just went vegetarian. Will I still be able to build muscle without eating meat?

A: Check out the bodies of NBA guard Raja Bell and six-time Ironman triathlon winner Dave Scott. Both have excelled athletically on vegetarian diets.

But that doesn't mean they achieved their physiques by eating only fruits and vegetables, which by themselves aren't complete sources of amino acids, the building blocks of muscle tissue. Milk and eggs provide all the necessary amino acids, as do combinations of beans or nuts with wheat or rice. That takes care of the quality of your protein, but you'll also need to consider quantity.

"If you're skinny and attempting to build muscle, you should eat 1 gram of protein per pound of your target body weight," says nutritionist Alan Aragon, a nutritionist in Westlake Village, California, and the *Men's Health* Weight-Loss Coach.

If you find yourself struggling to hit your target through food alone, try supplementing with a protein powder made from whey.

Q: I often give in to my cravings. Do I just lack willpower? Am I a loser?

A: "Don't be too quick to blame yourself," says Louis Aronne, MD, FACP, a clinical associate professor of medicine at Cornell University's Weill Medical College and an adjunct clinical associate professor at Columbia University's college of physicians and surgeons. "Studies show that cravings are not strongly associated with a lack of willpower. Try to identify and avoid the environmental and emotional situations that trigger your cravings."

Q: Can you suggest some snacks that won't clog people's arteries at my Super Bowl party?

A: Many guys view the Super Bowl as a dietary get-out-of-jail-free card—an opportunity to throw caution to the wind and dive into a bowl of whatever deep-fried delicacy they desire. After all, they'll be off the health wagon for only a few hours, right?

The Super Bowl is second only to Thanksgiving when it comes to the number of calories consumed by Americans in a single sitting. This, of course, isn't all that surprising when you consider the cornucopia of distractions—from touchdown jigs to halftime shows—that keep us glued to the tube and chowing mindlessly on an endless assortment of high-calorie finger foods.

Problem is, those few hours can bump you up a waist size and pack your arteries with plaque. Indeed, the average armchair quarterback consumes 1,200 calories—more than half the total number of calories he should consume in an entire day—during a typical 3-hour Super Bowl.

HERE'S HOW SOME OF YOUR FAVORITE SUPER BOWL SNACKS WEIGH IN.

Source: USDA Nutrient Database

BARBECUE-GLAZED WINGS WITH BLUE CHEESE SAUCE (3 wings and 1 ounce blue cheese)
Calories: 384
Fat (g): 34.3
Sodium (mg): 430
% of daily caloric intake: 17.5

TORTILLA CHIPS AND GUACAMOLE (3 ounces chips and guac)
Calories: 558
Fat (g): 28.3
Sodium (mg): 412.3
% of daily caloric intake: 25.4

NACHOS (6 to 8 chips)
Calories: 346
Fat (g): 19
Sodium (mg): 816
% of daily caloric intake: 15.7

PIGS IN A BLANKET (1)
Calories: 390
Fat (g): 26.6
Sodium (mg): 1,337
% of daily caloric intake: 17.7

DEVILED EGGS (2 halves)
Calories: 105
Fat (g): 8.7
Sodium (mg): 95.1
% of daily caloric intake: 4.8

BABY CARROTS AND RANCH DIP (about 6 carrots and 2 tablespoons dip)
CALORIES: 176
FAT (g): 15.5
SODIUM (mg): 310
% of daily caloric intake: 8

POTATO CHIPS (1 ounce)
Calories: 158
Fat (g): 10.9
Sodium (mg): 186
% of daily caloric intake: 7.2

BUTTERED POPCORN (100 grams)
Calories: 530
Fat (g): 30.6
Sodium (mg): 796
% of daily caloric intake: 24.1

THIN HARD PRETZELS (2 twists)
Calories: 45
Fat (g): 0.3
Sodium (mg): 163
% of daily caloric intake: 2

PIZZA (2 slices of meat lover's)
Calories: 780
Fat (g): 32
Sodium (mg): 2,260
% of daily caloric intake: 35.5

THE FOLLOWING HEART-HEALTHY snacks are low in calories, salt, and saturated fat, and they'll serve up to eight people without leaving their arteries screaming for mercy. They're also tasty enough to prevent your guests from making halftime sprints to the corner pizzeria.

BAKED SWEET-POTATO FRIES (215 calories per serving). Cut 5 large sweet potatoes into sticks and toss them in a bowl with 2 tablespoons olive oil, 2 cloves minced garlic, and ½ teaspoon cayenne pepper. Bake at 400°F for 20 minutes, or until tender, and top with freshly grated Parmesan.

CURRY SHRIMP DIP (190 calories per serving). Combine 4 ounces light cream cheese with ½ cup light sour cream and beat until smooth. Stir in chopped green onions, a handful of chopped roasted red pepper, ⅓ cup mango chutney, 1 clove minced garlic, 1 teaspoon curry powder, a pinch of salt and pepper, and 1 pound diced cooked shrimp. Stir again until ingredients are evenly blended. Serve cold and accompany with a midriff-affable dipping medium such as baked Garden of Eatin' black-bean tortilla chips or Stacy's multigrain pita chips.

THAI PEANUT CHICKEN (240 calories per serving). Cut 4 boneless, skinless chicken breasts into small cubes, and cook with 1 tablespoon olive oil in a skillet over medium heat for 5 to 7 minutes. Thread onto wooden skewers and set aside. Combine 3 tablespoons peanut butter and 3 tablespoons low-sodium soy sauce with 2 tablespoons each of water, honey, and lime juice. Add minced garlic, fresh grated ginger, and a squirt of sesame oil to the mixture. Blend until smooth, drizzle over skewers, and serve.

Q: Is it unhealthy to drink four or five diet sodas a day?

A: Worried you'll end up with a brain tumor, huh? Multiple studies have failed to turn up a cancer risk from the additives and artificial sweeteners, including aspartame, used in zero-calorie colas. Instead, you should worry about what's growing in your belly. A 2005 University of Texas study revealed that people who drank at least one diet soda every day had a 23 percent greater chance of becoming overweight than those who downed one regular soda, possibly because those going

no-cal unconsciously gave themselves permission to pig out at other times.

Then there's the toll on your teeth. According to a recent report in *General Dentistry*, the phosphoric and citric acids in soda can significantly erode tooth enamel. It happens faster with regular soda. Teeth immersed in Coke for 48 hours lost 5.9 percent of their enamel, compared with 1.6 percent for those soaked in Diet Coke.

Try using a straw so the liquid bypasses your bicuspids.

Q: I've heard that some pro athletes have started swapping their regular sports drinks for Pedialyte. Should I try it?

A: The reason some pros are pounding Pedialyte has to do with the sodium content, which is twice that of standard Gatorade. When you sweat like those guys do, the extra sodium significantly improves water retention and distribution, says Michael F. Bergeron, PhD, a professor of exercise physiology at the Medical College of Georgia.

"Overall rehydration is more complete with Pedialyte compared with water or most sports drinks," he says, "because it more effectively restores all your fluid compartments, particularly the spaces between your capillaries and muscle-cell membranes."

But again, we're talking about pro athletes, and amateurs who sweat a lot participating in endurance sports or multiple bouts of intense exercise in one day. Ordinary mortals simply won't realize enough of a benefit from Pedialyte to justify the additional cost.

Q: What's the best way to get an energy boost without coffee?

A: If you want the kick without the jitters, pop some American ginseng, says Mark Moyad, MD, the Phil F. Jenkins director of preventive and alternative medicine at the University of Michigan Medical Center.

A recent study at the Mayo Clinic found that taking 1,000 to 2,000 milligrams of the herb can provide an all-day energy boost.

Five hundred milligrams of L-carnitine—an amino acid that shuttles nutrients into cells' power plants—will also do the trick.

Another idea is to try drinks with carbs and protein, such as Accelerade ($48, accelerade.com).

All of these strategies work. Try each to see which one works best for you.

Of course, the best energy boost is weight lifting. Studies show that pumping iron three times a week can increase energy levels by up to 50 percent even on days you don't lift. You can't get those results in a bottle.

Q: Is a protein shake a sensible dinner?

A: Yes, as long as you're covering your nutritional bases the rest of the day, says Dr. Aragon. Toss some frozen fruit into your shake and eat plenty of vegetables at lunch. Protein shakes tend to be less satisfying than solid food, so expect hunger pangs if you drink one early in the evening. To make a protein shake more filling, add a little fat to it. Try peanut, almond, or cashew butter.

Q: How long should I wait to drink alcohol after exercising?

A: Ideally, you want 24 hours on either side of a workout, but in a world where cocktails go hand in hand with business, an hour is often all you have, says Lisa R. Young, PhD, a registered dietitian and the author of *The Portion Teller Plan*.

Fortunately, that's enough time for your body to eliminate some of the alcohol. That's important because alcohol is a diuretic, and for each liter of water you lose, your heart rate elevates eight beats per minute, causing it to work harder while getting less done.

Alcohol also increases levels of cortisol, a hormone that breaks down muscle. Finally, remember what you learned in college: Drink on a full stomach. Complex carbs (e.g., whole-wheat bread) will help absorb alcohol and keep you hydrated.

Q: Does alcohol kill brain cells?

A: "The concentration of alcohol in the brain of even a terrifically drunk person doesn't come close to the levels required to kill living cells," says Stephen Braun, a science writer and the author of *Buzz: The Science and Lore of Alcohol and Caffeine*. People become intoxicated with only a tenth of a percent of alcohol in their blood. But alcohol is a "dirty bomb," Braun says. Rather than zeroing in on one specific region of the brain, alcohol impacts your entire noggin. The result: A few drinks can temporarily block new memory formation, dull your thinking, and reduce muscle control. ■

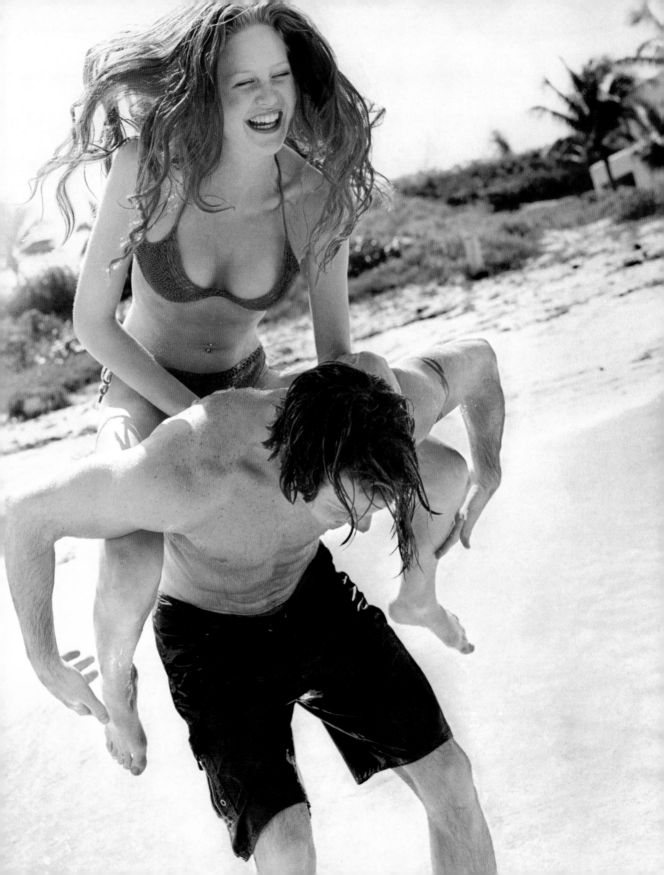

3

Muscle Up Fast

Test Your Strength

FIRST THINGS FIRST: TAKE OUR 1-MINUTE MUSCLE TEST. THEN BUILD GREATER STRENGTH AND BALANCE BY SHORING UP WEAK SPOTS YOU NEVER KNEW YOU HAD

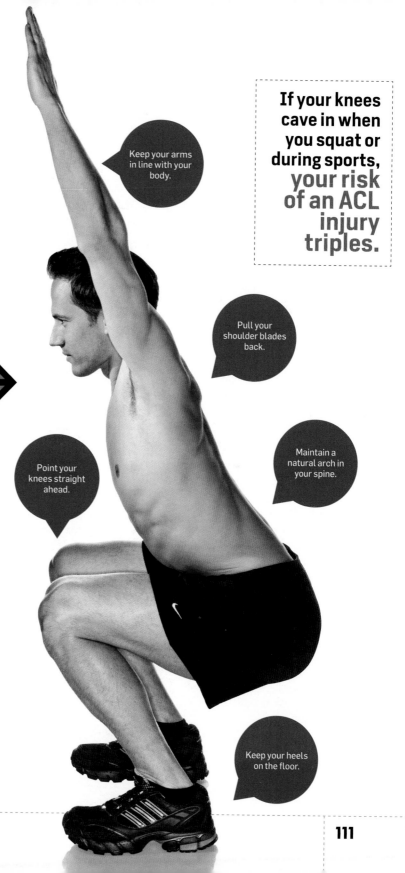

Keep your arms in line with your body.

Pull your shoulder blades back.

Maintain a natural arch in your spine.

Point your knees straight ahead.

Keep your heels on the floor.

THE OVERHEAD SQUAT TEST

When your body is in perfect balance, it stays aligned when you squat. But your workout, job, and poor posture can all cause you to develop weak or tight spots that restrict movement. To identify those areas and fix them quickly, take this test every 4 weeks.

HOW TO DO IT

Stand facing a full-length mirror with your feet shoulder-width apart and pointed straight ahead, and your arms raised overhead. Squat three times. Don't overthink this: Simply bend at the hips and knees to lower your body straight down. Hold the pose at the lowest point in your third squat and take note of your body position at the checkpoints highlighted on the next page. Repeat the test with your profile to the mirror.

111

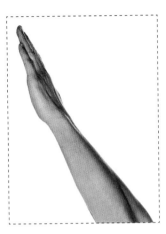 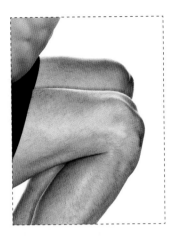 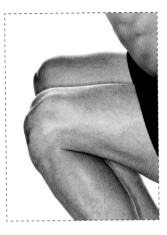

IF YOUR `ARMS` MOVE FORWARD

. . . then your chest and latissimus dorsi muscles are tight, which often leads to ailments of the neck and shoulders.

Fix yourself: Lie on the floor with a foam roll under your lats. Glide your body up and down, pausing at tender points for 30 seconds. Repeat for your chest. Stretch your lats and chest, and add the cable squat to row to your workout.

Cable Squat to Row

Stand at a low-row cable station, holding the handles with your palms facing each other. Take a few steps back. With your arms straight, squat down. Stand up as you pull the handles to the bottom of your rib cage. Do 10 repetitions.

IF YOUR `KNEES` MOVE OUT

. . . then your hips and lower back must compensate for that imbalance, which means they'll fatigue faster and might even strain during explosive sports movements.

Fix yourself: Use a foam roll behind your hips, pausing at tender points, and stretch your hips and hamstrings. Add the cable soccer kick to your workout.

Cable Soccer Kick

Attach a foot strap to the low-pulley cable of a cable station and stand with your right hip to the weight stack and the strap wrapped around your right ankle. Keeping your leg straight, sweep it across the front of your body as far as you can while rotating your foot inward, and then return to the starting position. Do 12 reps with each leg.

IF YOUR `KNEES` CAVE IN

. . . then your outer thighs are weak and your risk of injury to an ACL (knee ligament) might triple, say researchers at the Cincinnati Sports-Medicine Research and Education Foundation.

Fix yourself: Roll your inner and outer thighs over a foam roll. Stretch your inner thighs and add the lateral tube walk to your workout.

Lateral Tube Walk

Loop resistance tubing around your ankles and slide it up your legs until it's above your knees. Stand with your knees slightly bent and your hands on your hips. Keeping your abs tight, sidestep 12 to 15 times to your right and then 12 to 15 times back to your left.

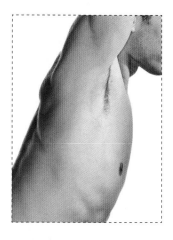

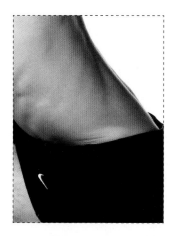

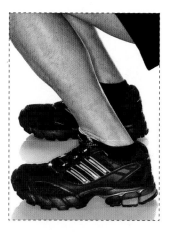

IF YOUR `UPPER BODY` LEANS FAR FORWARD

. . . then your calves are tight. Tight calves impede your ankles from bending, so your torso shifts forward in an attempt to maintain your base of support as you squat. But this throws off your center of gravity, making it harder for you to produce power during any activity.

Fix yourself: Glide your calves over a foam roll. Stretch your calves and hip flexors, and perform the Swiss-ball cobra.

Swiss-Ball Cobra

Lie facedown on a Swiss ball with your abs drawn in and your arms hanging down, holding light dumbbells. Raise your arms up and back until they're in line with your body, and pull your shoulder blades down and together. Return to the starting position and repeat for a set of 10 repetitions.

IF YOUR `LOWER BACK` ARCHES EXCESSIVELY

. . . then the fronts of your hips (your hip flexors) are tight and your abs are weak. Tight hip flexors shorten your stride, making you a slower, less efficient runner.

Fix yourself: Use a foam roll on your hip flexors and outer thighs. Stretch your hip flexors and shore up your core with the plank.

Plank

Assume a modified pushup position, with your forearms resting on the floor. Your elbows should be under your shoulders and bent 90 degrees. Keep your body straight and rigid for 10 seconds, rest for 20 to 30 seconds, and then repeat for a set of 10.

IF YOUR `FEET` TURN OUT

. . . then your outer calves are tight. This reduces your ability to produce force when you're running and jumping.

Fix yourself: Lie with the outside of your calf on a foam roll and glide up and down, pausing at any tender points for 30 seconds. Stretch your calves twice a day, and add this twist on the standard calf raise to your workout.

Calf Raise with Inversion

Hold a dumbbell in your right hand and stand on your right foot with your toes angled slightly inward. Rest the instep of your left foot across the back of your right ankle. Rise on your toes as high as you can, then descend. Do 12 reps and repeat with the other leg. ■

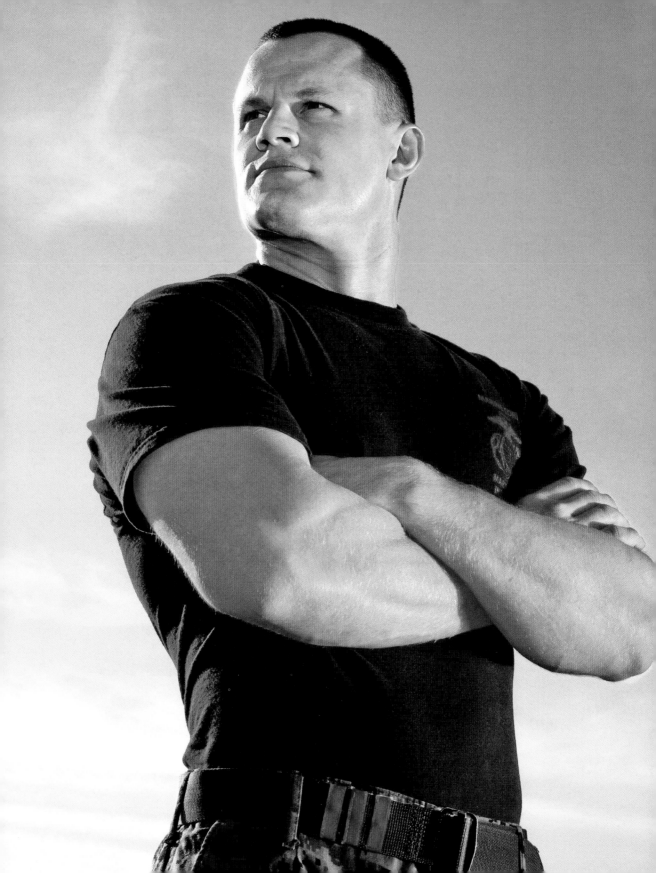

Get Semper Fit

WHAT U.S. MARINES HAVE LEARNED ABOUT COMBAT-READY FITNESS CAN HELP YOU BUILD THE STRONG, POWERFUL BODY YOU'VE ALWAYS WANTED

Raider Hall
is part gym, part museum.

The corridors in this plain brick building are lined with photos of stone-faced men from the elite U.S. Marines Raider units who were trained to sneak behind enemy lines during World War II. Medals and military insignia spill into several rooms, where today's marines are taught hand-to-hand combat.

But writer Denny Watkins wasn't in northern Virginia at Marine Corps Base Quantico for a history lesson or a guided tour. He went to experience the future of the U.S. military's physical-conditioning regimen.

The fitness standards favored by the world's most technologically advanced military force seem as old and rusty as the M1 rifle still in Okinawa beach sand on display in Raider Hall. Can you complete 3 pullups and 50 crunches, and run 3 miles in less than 28 minutes? Then as far as the U.S. Marine Corps is concerned, you can carry a gun.

But after the Corps noticed a significant number of preventable muscle strains and sprains among troops in Iraq and Afghanistan since 2003 (some 27,000 were sent home with noncombat-related injuries), it recently took a hard look at its physical-development policies and decided it was time for a change.

Specialists designed a workout that combines the latest training techniques and exercise-science research with the rigors of modern warfare.

"We're becoming stronger, more powerful, and more athletic," says Captain Justin Jordan, an experiment action officer in the Corps' Warfighting Lab, which oversees the workout.

THE FOUR TENETS OF COMBAT CONDITIONING

Armed with the workout's innovative muscle-building principles, you can put it to the test for yourself.

1. Train Like an Athlete

At Raider Hall's Martial Arts Center of Excellence, fitness experts studied elite athletes' routines and incorporated facets of those programs in the new combat workout.

For instance, marines use a common football-training technique that couples an explosive exercise with sprints.

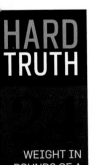

HARD TRUTH

24

WEIGHT IN POUNDS OF A FULLY LOADED M249 MACHINE GUN CARRIED BY U.S. TROOPS

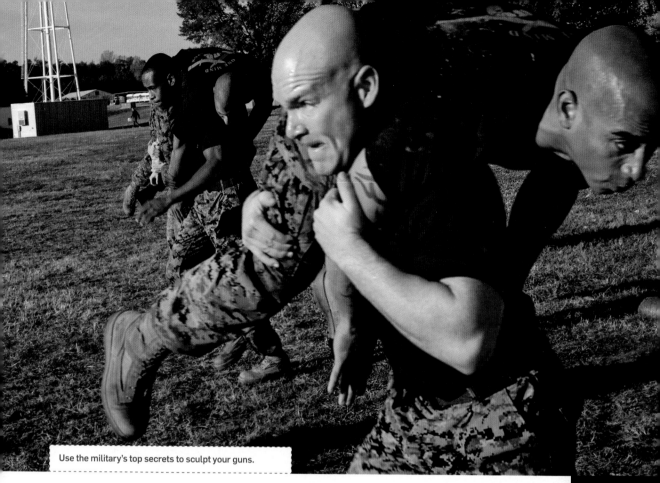

Use the military's top secrets to sculpt your guns.

"The conditioning that gives an NFL linebacker his power also helps protect him from injury," says Colonel Brian McGuire, ATC, head of the USMC's sports-medicine and injury prevention program.

Your orders: Start your workout with one of their favorite total-body power exercises, like the sandbag swing. But use a light dumbbell instead, as shown in the workout on page 120. Do 20 reps and then sprint for 40 yards. Rest 1 minute and repeat.

2. Strive for a Harder Core

After strapping on his body armor to stay alive, it's not unusual for a marine to be hauling 60 extra pounds around a blazing desert. Unless he gets used to carrying that load during training, he's likely to strain his back or sprain his knee while hopping off a low wall, McGuire says. Being overweight can put the same crush on your joints.

Your orders: Shed the spare tire and sculpt a harder core. Instead of holding weights at your sides as you lunge, try holding a barbell overhead.

"When the weight is farther from your center of mass, your core works harder to stabilize it," says Staff Sergeant Brandon Millsaps, a combat-conditioning instructor and USA Weightlifting–certified coach.

3. Take Pride in Your Exercise Technique

When your goal is a bulletproof body, the last thing you want to do is to injure yourself in the gym. That's why every marine learns the proper way to perform squats and deadlifts at the onset of training. This guarantees that the more technically challenging exercises are performed correctly and reduces the risk of injury to the back and lower-body muscles and joints.

Your orders: Stand tall with your head up and shoulders back. When pressing yourself up in a squat or deadlift, lead with your chin. This keeps your hips properly aligned and reduces injury risk, say researchers at Miami University of Ohio.

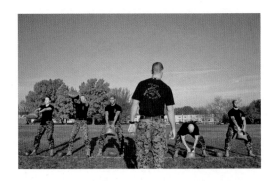

Every marine learns the proper way to perform squats and deadlifts at the onset of training.

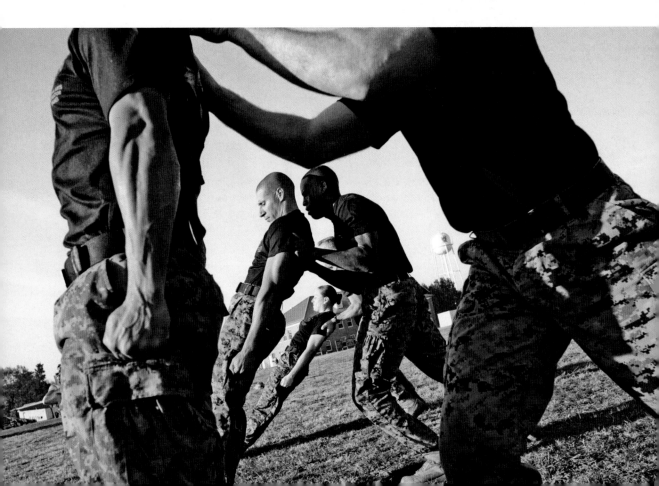

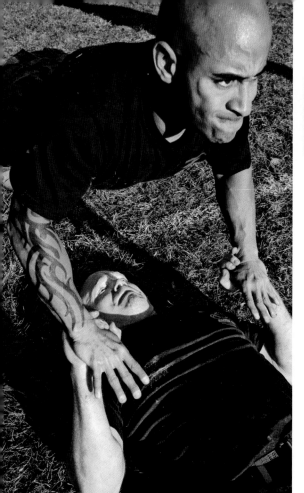

HARD TRUTH

GREATEST NUMBER OF PULLUPS EVER PERFORMED IN SUCCESSION BY A MARINE RECRUIT

4. Don't Allow for Any Weak Spots

Most marines train for the events they're tested on (pullups, crunches, long-distance runs), while ignoring other areas of their bodies, says Jordan. The solution: a complement to the physical-fitness test that measures stamina, strength, agility, and speed.

Your orders: The Marine Corps is in the process of designing its new "combat fitness test," but you can use the series of drills to measure your overall fitness. Then consult the workout on the next page for a 4-week program that can help you improve your score. ∎

PUT YOUR FITNESS TO THE ULTIMATE TEST

Use this series of athletic challenges to measure your overall strength and conditioning. Rest for 60 seconds between sprints, and give yourself ample time to rest between exercises. Complete the interval sprint test on a separate day if it's more convenient for your training schedule. Then follow the plan in the workout on the next page, and retest yourself every 4 weeks to chart your improvement.

MILITARY MEASURING STICKS

EXERCISES	WEEK 1	WEEK 4
PUSHUPS (max reps in 1 minute)		
HANGING LEG RAISES (max reps in 1 minute)		
BODY-WEIGHT SQUATS (max reps in 1 minute)		
STANDING BROAD JUMPS (average of 3 jumps)		
INTERVAL SPRINTS (total time repeating 6x50 yards)		

THE MARINE WORKOUT

The U.S. Marine Corps keeps its combat-conditioning program engaging by frequently mixing in cool new workouts and physical challenges. The routines aren't designed to wage war on a man's body, but that's exactly what they'd do if you jumped into the program headfirst. So we created a plan to gradually prepare you physically and mentally for the demands of its military training.

DURING THE FIRST WEEK, you'll master the cornerstone combat-conditioning exercises. Next, you'll improve your overall fitness by pairing power moves with sprints. For the third week, you'll take on an intense athletic drill to train your total body for strength and speed. Finally, you'll be fully prepared for a real U.S. Marine Corps fitness challenge, and you'll have the muscle to prove it.

1
Sandbag Squat

Grab a heavy dumbbell (marines use sandbags) and stand holding it vertically, by one end, against your chest. With your elbows pointing down, bend at the hips and knees to lower your body until your thighs are at least parallel to the floor. Return to the start.

2
Sandbag Deadlift

Stand holding a heavy dumbbell (or sandbag) with both hands under the top of the weight and your arms hanging down in front of you. Keep your chest up and shoulders back. Next, lower your body until the weight touches the floor. Now stand up again.

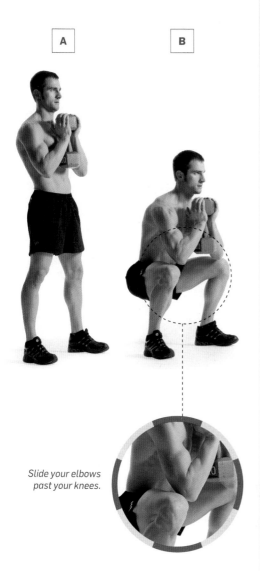

A   B

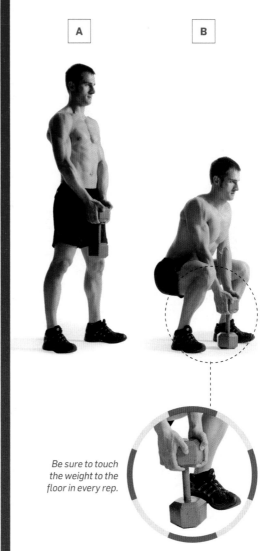

A   B

Slide your elbows past your knees.

Be sure to touch the weight to the floor in every rep.

3
Dumbbell Clean and Press

From the starting position, dip your hips and explode upward, pulling the weights up. As the weights come close to your chest, dip under and "catch" them on top of your shoulders. Stand, press the weights overhead, and then reverse the move.

4
Dumbbell Swing

Stand holding a dumbbell with both hands. Push your hips back and lower the weight between your legs until it's under your butt. Drive back up to a standing position and swing the weight up, keeping your arms straight. Return to the starting position.

A   B   C

A   B

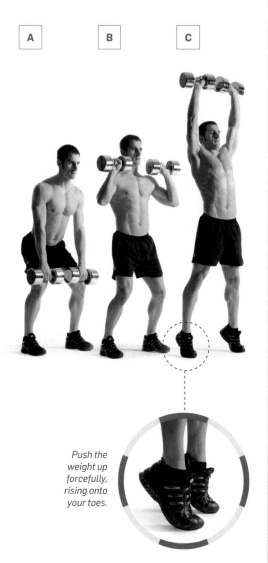

Push the weight up forcefully, rising onto your toes.

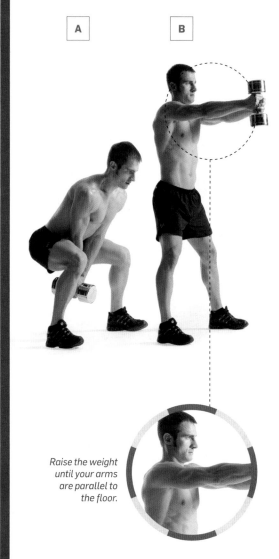

Raise the weight until your arms are parallel to the floor.

5
Pullup

Grab a chinup bar with an overhand grip (palms forward) and your hands slightly more than shoulder-width apart. Hang with your arms straight and pull your shoulder blades down. Pull yourself up, and then lower back to the starting position.

6
Front Squat to Push Press

Stand holding a barbell across the front of your shoulders and bring your elbows forward. Push your hips back and then bend your knees to lower your body. Now quickly stand back up while pushing the bar above your head until your arms are fully extended. Lower the weight. That's 1 rep.

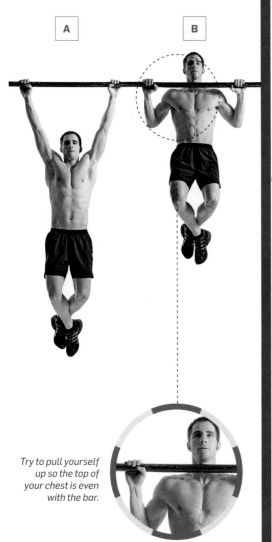

A	B

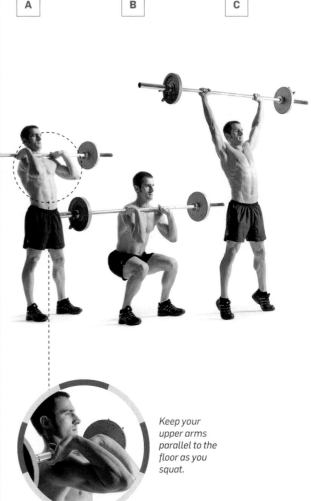

A	B	C

Try to pull yourself up so the top of your chest is even with the bar.

Keep your upper arms parallel to the floor as you squat.

7
Pushup

Assume the classic pushup position (legs straight, hands beneath your shoulders). Keeping your body rigid, bend your arms to lower yourself until your chest is just off the floor. Push back up until your arms are extended.

8
Side Bridge

Lie on your side with your forearm on the floor under your shoulder and your feet stacked. Contract your glutes and abs. Push your hips off the floor, creating a straight line from ankle to shoulder and keeping your head in line with your spine. Hold for 20 to 30 seconds and repeat on the other side.

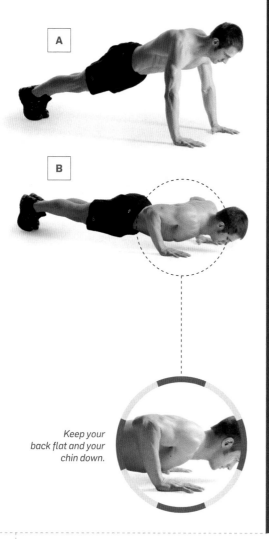

Keep your back flat and your chin down.

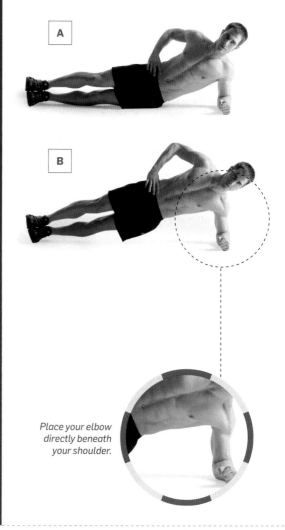

Place your elbow directly beneath your shoulder.

DIRECTIONS

Complete three workouts a week, resting at least a day between sessions. Start your routine with core moves. Marines use planks, side bridges (shown), hanging leg raises, and Supermans, among other exercises. For a complete core routine, go to **MensHealth.com/marines**.

WEEK 1

Perform each exercise in the Marine Corps arsenal in the order shown. Do 1 set of 8 to 10 repetitions for each move except the side bridge. (Hold the side bridge for 20 to 30 seconds on each side.) Rest up to 60 seconds between exercises.

WEEK 2

Using the Week 1 exercises, you'll perform A STRENGTH MOVE FOLLOWED IMMEDIATELY BY A SPRINT. THIS IS CALLED A DOUBLE.
For each set of sprints, run as fast as you can for 8 to 15 seconds. Then walk back to the starting line and begin your next set of exercises.

Day 1: Do 2 doubles of pushups and sprints. Rest 60 seconds; do 2 doubles of squats and sprints. Perform 12 reps of each exercise.

Day 2: Perform 2 doubles of pullups and sprints. Rest 60 seconds; do 2 doubles of swings and sprints. Aim for 8 pullups and 20 swings.

Day 3: Do 2 doubles of pushups and sprints. Rest 60 seconds; do 2 doubles of squats and sprints. Perform 12 pushups and 20 squats.

WEEK 3

A TRIPLE IS AN UPPER-BODY EXERCISE FOLLOWED IMMEDIATELY BY A LOWER-BODY EXERCISE AND THEN CHASED WITH A SPRINT.
For sprints, charge hard for 8 to 15 seconds and then return to the start. Do a total of 6 triples in each workout, resting 60 seconds between triples.

Day 1: Perform 20 squats followed by 12 pushups, and then sprint.

Day 2: Do 25 dumbbell swings followed by 12 clean and presses, and a sprint.

Day 3: Perform 25 reps of the front squat to push press, and a sprint. Then drop down for 20 pushups.

WEEK 4

HERE ARE TWO OF THE MARINE FITNESS CHALLENGES. Rest at least a day between them. Begin each session with the side bridge and plank (pushup position, but on your elbows). Hold each move for 1 minute, rest for 30 seconds, and repeat. Then, at the end of the week or the beginning of the next week, take the "Military Measuring Sticks" fitness test on page 119.

Marine challenge 1
Go for a quarter-mile run. This will be your sprint distance for your doubles. For your first double, do 15 reps of the clean and press, and then run. Next, do another double of 20 deadlifts followed by a run. Finish with a double of 25 squats, and then run. Try it again in a month, with the goal of beating your total time by at least 1 minute.

Marine challenge 2
Perform 20 dumbbell swings immediately followed by 20 pushups. That's a superset. Do as many supersets as you can in 20 minutes. Repeat the challenge after 4 weeks, and try to complete an additional superset.

Sculpt a Gold Medal Physique

ROMANIA'S OLYMPIC WEIGHT-LIFTING WIZARD NOW COACHES ATHLETES IN THE LAND OF OZ. HIS WORKOUTS GUARANTEE A SIX-PACK. WRITER GRANT STODDARD LEARNS ALL YOU HAVE TO DO IS SURVIVE

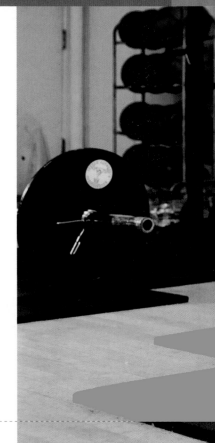

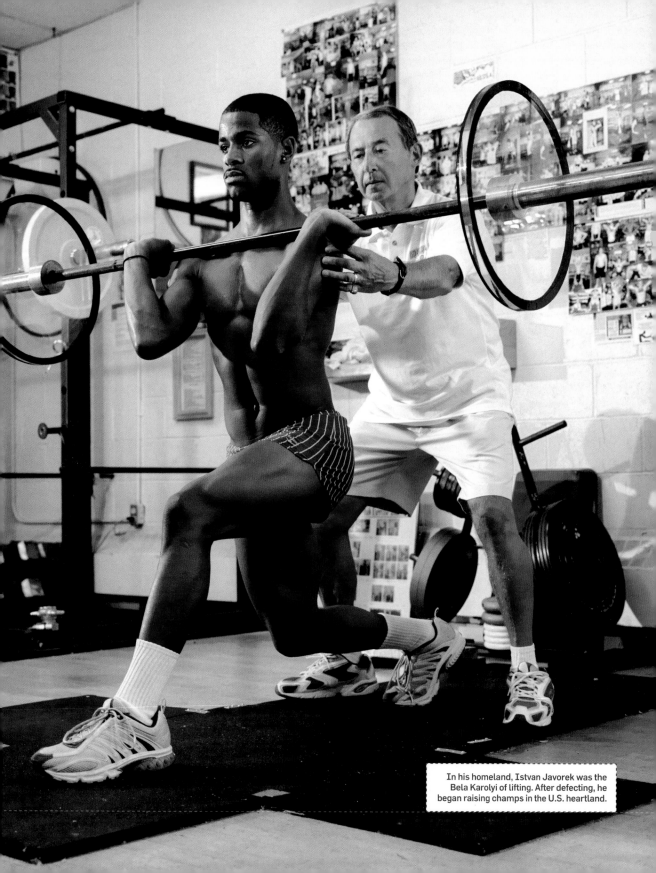

In his homeland, Istvan Javorek was the Bela Karolyi of lifting. After defecting, he began raising champs in the U.S. heartland.

"How do you say?"

asks Istvan Javorek, grinning at the freshmen he's gleefully working to the point of nausea and delirium.

"Yes, I love it!" they shout with the last of the air their Transylvanian tormentor has allowed to remain in their lungs.

This college gym class began normally enough 35 minutes ago, with Javorek dishing out pushups as reparations for a number of minor infractions, including but not limited to hat wearing, nose picking, fingernail chewing, and using nonwords like huh, mmm, and hey, the last of which he insists is "for the horse." Javorek provides musical accompaniment for the running-in-place drills that follow. He sings excerpts from Tchaikovsky's *Swan Lake* and mimics the gallop from Jacques Offenbach's *Orpheus in the Underworld*, the jolly tune usually associated with the can-can.

"Higher, higher, brrrum, dum, dum, dum, dum, dum, dum," he sings, conducting an invisible orchestra with his forefingers.

Once Javorek has them panting, he assigns the class a punishing lunge walk that incorporates short sets of dumbbell exercises. It suddenly becomes apparent why some of his students have taken to referring to their coach as Dr. Javorkian.

As these young, rosy-cheeked men and women strain to complete the drill, former pro basketball player Wayne Simien—all 6'9" of him—strides into the gym.

"Yo, old man!" he yells, grinning widely.

Javorek's eyes twinkle with pride and excitement as he turns to me. "My son! Ha-ha-ha. He is like my son!" The 65-year-old coach leaps onto a foot-high box that still fails to make up for the height discrepancy between him and his massive protégé. Then he throws an arm around the shoulders he helped widen with 15 years of training.

"You've seen *Rocky*, right?" the power forward stoops to ask me. "Well, this old dude right here? Man, he's my Mick."

As the class struggles through something called "Javorek's Special Abdominal Program No. 1"—a gauntlet of 26 gut-busting exercises—Simien cycles through a series of dumbbell exercises that look

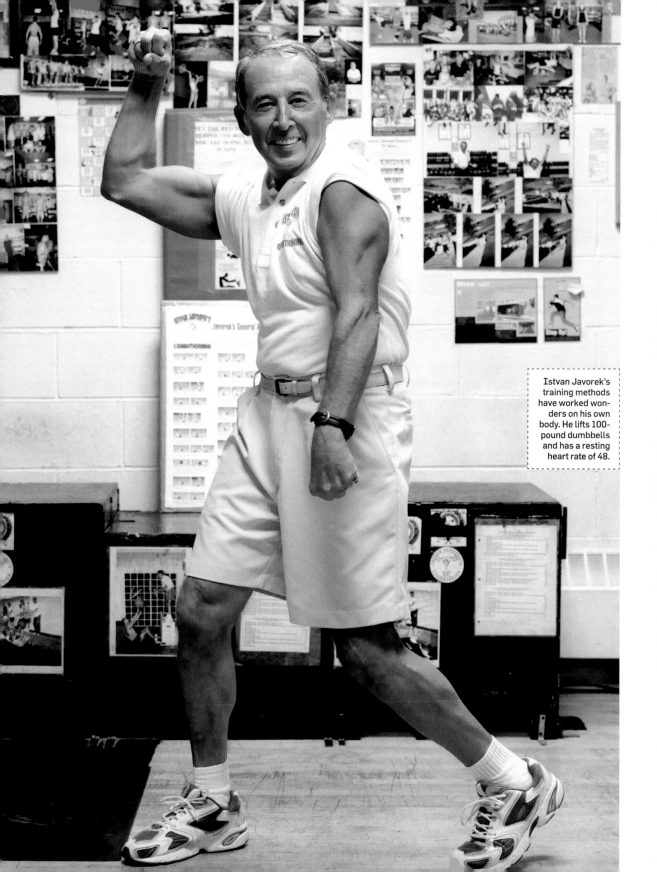

Istvan Javorek's training methods have worked wonders on his own body. He lifts 100-pound dumbbells and has a resting heart rate of 48.

more suited to a lap pool than a gym. Indeed, the coach's celebrated and often-copied dumbbell complexes are what I am here, in Overland Park, Kansas, to experience for myself.

Compressing a high volume of intense work by shrinking or even eliminating rest periods, the complexes were originally devised to combat monotony and save time while improving endurance, muscle tone, coordination, and aesthetics. As it turns out, the complexes might also be the best way possible to sculpt your abs. Your core never stops working during each full-body move, and your metabolism pegs in the red zone.

But I soon surmise that Javorek's complexes are only part of what makes the professor of fitness and all-sports conditioning coach at Johnson County Community College able to churn out world champions the way India produces software wizards.

Exhausted, the class huddles around the teacher, who disappears from my view.

"Now," I hear him say from the center,

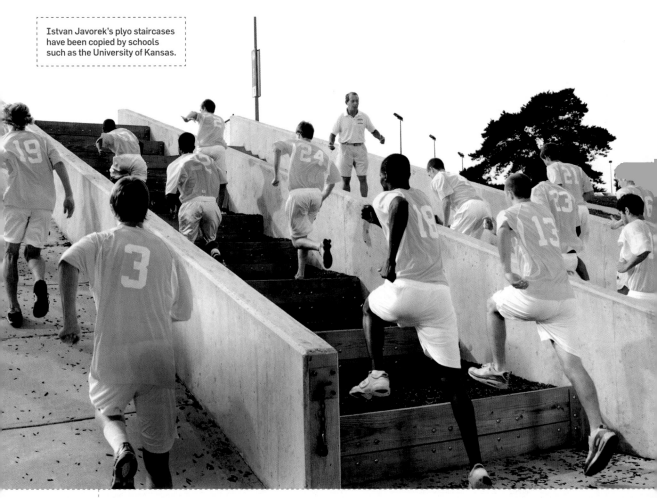

Istvan Javorek's plyo staircases have been copied by schools such as the University of Kansas.

"put your tiny, wimpy little hands on my huge, impressive biceps, and on one, two, three . . . "

"Yes, I love it!" they shout.

COACH COMRADE

Understanding how weight lifting's answer to Bela Karolyi came to be teaching at a Kansas community college begins with a geography lesson. A hasty bit of map redrawing at the end of World War II resulted in Javorek, an ethnic Hungarian, being raised in Romania. The new border was imposed just beyond his childhood backyard, dividing his family from their friends and relatives.

But cartography wasn't his only handicap. At the age of 14, Javorek, who was busy propelling himself toward a future as a violinist, weighed 99 pounds and suffered from flat feet, high blood pressure, and a congenital spinal-cord defect known as spina bifida. On the walk home from music practice one day, his sister's friends mockingly challenged him to press his violin bow over his head, an insult that sent him off to the gym. A few years later, he was accepted into the physical education department at the Pedagogical Institute at Cluj, Romania, where he developed into a serious weight lifter and track-and-field athlete.

After graduation, the gym became his laboratory, his body the subject of a self-administered, ongoing experiment. After several years, the former weakling could clean and jerk more than 340 pounds and possessed the physique of a superhero. In 1964, Javorek became the weight-lifting and conditioning head coach at Clujana Athletic Club in Romania. It was there

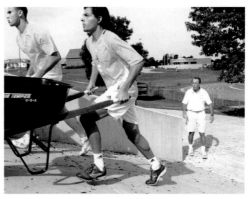

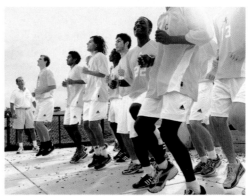

It suddenly becomes apparent why some of his students have taken to REFERRING TO THEIR COACH AS DR. JAVORKIAN.

that Coach Comrade, as he was called, met Dragomir Cioroslan, an 81-pound boy with rickets and rheumatic heart disease.

Javorek gently dismissed Cioroslan at first but relented after the boy's friends insisted that the coach allow him to join the gym.

"In the end, I say okay," Javorek recalls. "But I told him he would have to work 10 times harder than the other kids, like I did myself. The first time I saw him perform a clean and jerk, I could hardly watch." This was the less-than-promising beginning of a weight-lifting career that would culminate in a bronze medal for Cioroslan at the 1984 Olympics in Los Angeles.

As important as the medal resting against the weight lifter's heart was the transformation of the heart itself. Working for up to 5 hours a day, Cioroslan transformed himself from a sickly kid to an athlete whose heart beat only 38 times a minute.

"When the doctors examine him, they think something is wrong," says Javorek. "They don't hear *dom-dom*, but *boom* [waits two Mississippis] *boom*."

What the coach knew from measuring heart rates in his elite lifters, science has borne out. A new study published in the journal *Clinical Science* found that over 12 weeks, people achieved the same cardiovascular benefits from three weekly sessions of strength training as they did from the same amount of moderate aerobic training.

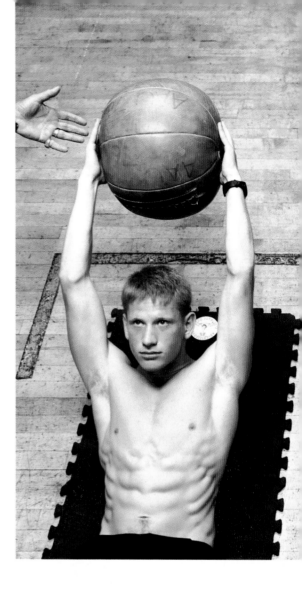

COMING TO AMERICA

Cioroslan isn't Javorek's only success story. Another Club Cluj lifter, Stefan Tasnadi, won a silver medal for Romania in 1984.

Even though Javorek had been named a coach emeritus in Romania, the political regime was strangling him. His office phone was bugged. His athletes were either under surveillance or being "flipped" by the Securitate—the Romanian secret service. The only way he could obtain a visa to visit the West was by grudgingly

At Texas A&M, Javorek unleashed the methods he'd smuggled from Romania. THE RESULT: MORE CHAMPS.

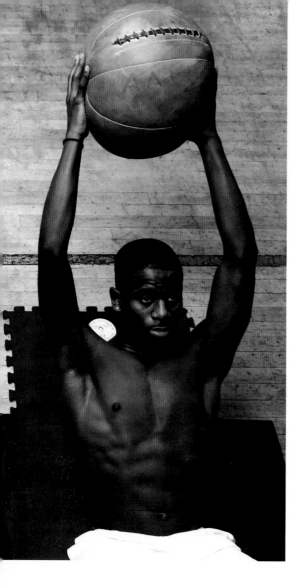

like home. His growing reputation for morphing duds into studs made him a shoo-in for a position at several better-known schools, but Javorek wanted to implement his own training system from the ground up. So in 1987, he began his current position at a wonderfully equipped but little-known community college 20 miles outside Kansas City. That he began offering conditioning training for every sport in the athletic department is remarkable.

"We have a game similar to baseball in Romania," he says, "but football was new to me."

Fortunately, weight lifting and track had given Javorek an encyclopedic training knowledge that applied equally well to sports he barely knew existed before he arrived stateside. Which leads to the next revelation from my stay: In an age of sports-specific training, athletes still need an underlying level of basic conditioning.

"General physical prep prepares all athletes for more intense training later on," says Alexander J. Koch, PhD, an associate professor of health and exercise sciences at Truman State University, in Kirksville, Missouri. "Those who train for broad-based development tend to have longer careers and suffer fewer injuries than those who train only for their sport."

THE COMPLEX MADE SIMPLE

After I witness another group of pimpletons going through dumbbell hell, Javorek invites me into his cluttered office, where he shares his lunch with me—stuffed

becoming a Communist Party member.

Sure enough, with visa in hand, he defected. After a yearlong struggle, during which he committed to learning 150 new English words a day, Javorek became conditioning coach at Texas A&M University. There, he unleashed the training methods he'd smuggled from Romania. The result: more world champions.

The relentless Texas heat eventually sent Javorek in search of a climate more

cabbage. "My wife made too much today," he says. "Please, eat."

Another of Javorek's nicknames is "the Dumbbell King," and it's also well earned. Along with more than 300 barbell movements, his workouts include 780 different dumbbell exercises. He lives to devise new programs, giving them ironic titles like "Big Fun."

"It's not actually fun," says Javorek, as if initiating me into a conspiracy. "Not until you find how strong you become."

As I eat, he excitedly shows me snapshots of his recent vacation in India as the printer spits out workout program after workout program. Some have been compiled into a book, *Javorek Complex Conditioning*, which he signs and gives to me, along with T-shirts, pens, a laser pointer, and an alarm clock, all emblazoned with his logo: an Alfred E. Newman–looking pencil neck straining under a bent barbell.

One of Javorek's stranger quirks is his fondness for crudely superimposing his face on other pictures. One of my favorite examples, from his Web site, shows Michelangelo's 16th-century masterpiece *The Creation of Adam*, but with a different smiling face pasted over God's. Now, Javorek's forefinger meets Adam's. "Give credit to the creator," demands the caption. It makes Javorek happy that people around the world use his conditioning knowledge. He becomes slightly prickly, though, when people use his innovations without crediting him.

"Okay!" he says, clapping his hands. "Now I show you what you have come to learn. Tomorrow you will say, 'Coach Javorek, I am very sore,' and I will say, 'Grant, I am very sore-y.'" He howls at his own joke for what seems like several minutes.

SWEATING THE DETAILS

Dumbbell and Barbell Complexes Nos. 1 and 2 were developed in Cluj, but Javorek has since devised a great many more, tailoring them to particular sports as well as specific goals, such as strength and endurance.

We begin where it all started, with his first dumbbell complex, consisting of five high-intensity movements that flow from one to the other and loop around. The exercises are familiar to me, but with Javorek micromanaging my form and commanding me up on my toes at the zenith of every movement, I'm sweating and sucking air. When I miscount reps, he counts for me, looking and sounding just like the Count from *Sesame Street*.

I manage to complete the work without puking, but we segue immediately into Complex No. 2. I misunderstand Javorek's thick accent, and after uttering "Huh?" my apology is pushups. Ninety perfect reps lie between a moment's rest and me.

"It's okay," he says with a laugh. "You're not supposed to like it. But you will like being strong!"

Somehow I manage to finish. My usual entire gym routine doesn't compare with the cardiovascular exertion prompted by one round of a Javorek complex. It's all I can do to stay on my feet.

"So life is . . . ?"

"Huh?" I ask.

Ten grueling pushups later, Javorek repeats the question: "So, again, life is . . . "

"Complex?" I ask, vaguely recalling one of his earlier call-and-answer routines.

"Ha-ha!" he says, clapping his hands. "You are learning about life! I am a great

Athletes call Javorek "THE DUMBBELL KING" because his workouts include 780 different dumbbell exercises.

teacher! Now we move on to Barbell Complex Number 1!"

Javorek takes me through another 15 exercises, gauging the maximum amount of weight I can use while I complete 5 reps of each. This data will allow his computer program to spit out my own customized 12-week workout program.

"Now, we will go to my house," he says.

I enter to find the home teeming with art and curiosities collected by Javorek and his wife during their world travels. He's providing context for one piece when he stops midsentence.

"By the way, did I tell you that the Romanian deadlift was named after me?" he asks. "If the guys at Texas A&M could pronounce my name, it would be the Javorek deadlift."

Over an espresso on his deck, I ask him if his workouts have ever killed anyone. Overtraining was studied in Cluj, right?

"Overtraining comes from bad technique, bad diet, not enough sleep," he says. "But if you eliminate these things, it's difficult for overtraining to be the real issue."

Javorek's overtraining-is-underrecovering mantra also holds up to scientific scrutiny. After all, Olympic athletes can train every day for hours because they sleep and eat the rest of the time. His full-body approach is mirrored in today's functional-training movement. Dr. Koch agrees that training while sore offers recuperative benefits, as long as the workout is 10 to 20 percent less intense than the one that made you sore.

The next day, as promised, Javorek hands me my program. The first session features 10 dumbbell and plyometric exercises, plus an ab routine. It takes me 25 minutes to complete a circuit, after which I feel like I've been at the mercy of the Securitate myself.

"My 103-year-old grandmother can do better!" He chuckles and points to a framed picture. It shows a muscle-bound Javorek curling a 50-pound dumbbell, wearing a white wig, a string of pearls, and spectacles.

"As you progress with my program," says Javorek, "you should be able to complete each circuit in 13 minutes."

"Come and see my greatest invention," says the coach excitedly as he leads me out of the gym. Javorek's "conditioning hill" has three sections, each designed for plyometric exercises, which train the fast-twitch muscle fibers that normal gym workouts overlook. Research shows that fast-twitch fibers decrease 43 percent as you age and slow-twitch fibers decrease less than 33 percent. An older man struggling up from a chair can blame the wasting away of fast-twitch fibers.

The All-in-One Abs Workout

Istvan Javorek's dumbbell complexes build the entire body while pegging metabolism in the red zone. He designed them to help create Olympic champions in Romania, but you'll enjoy the effects: more muscle, less fat, and a six-pack core.

THE DRILL

Three times a week, do either complex. For Complex No. 1, do 6 reps of each exercise and move to the next without stopping. For No. 2, do 3 reps of each exercise and move to the next without stopping, building to 3 total circuits. As you advance, increase the number of circuits.

THE PROGRAM

1. Upright Row	2. High Pull Snatch	3. Squat Push Press	4. Bent-over Row	5. High Pull Snatch

THE TECHNIQUE

Upright row

Stand with your knees slightly bent and hold a pair of dumbbells at arms' length in front of your thighs, thumbs facing each other and palms facing your thighs. This stance turns your elbows slightly outward and your shoulders slightly inward. Look ahead with your chest up, back straight, and abs tight. Bring the weights up to neck level, keeping the pair aligned. Your elbows should be flared out to ear level. At the top, rise up on your toes. Return to the starting position.

High pull snatch

Stand with dumbbells as if you're about to perform an upright row, but lean forward to lower the weights to knee level, keeping your head and neck aligned. This is the starting position. Now raise the weights as you did with the upright row, but don't pause at the top; instead, flip your wrists back to bring the weights overhead, extending your arms fully while rising up on your toes. Return to the starting position. Keep the weights as close to your body as possible throughout the lift.

Squat push press

Stand upright and hold dumbbells at your shoulders, palms facing forward. Maintaining this position and looking straight ahead, bend your hips and knees to lower into a full squat, thighs at least parallel to the floor. As you rise from the squat, begin pressing the weights overhead, rising up on your toes at the top, at which point your arms should be fully extended overhead. Return to the starting position.

Bent-over row

Stand holding dumbbells at arm's length in front of you, palms facing back. Bend your knees slightly, and bend at the waist so that your back is flat and angled 45 degrees to the floor. Once your body weight is centered on your heels, you're in the starting position. Without altering this position—no swinging your trunk—bend your elbows to bring the weights quickly and explosively into your armpits. Return to the starting position at a slower pace.

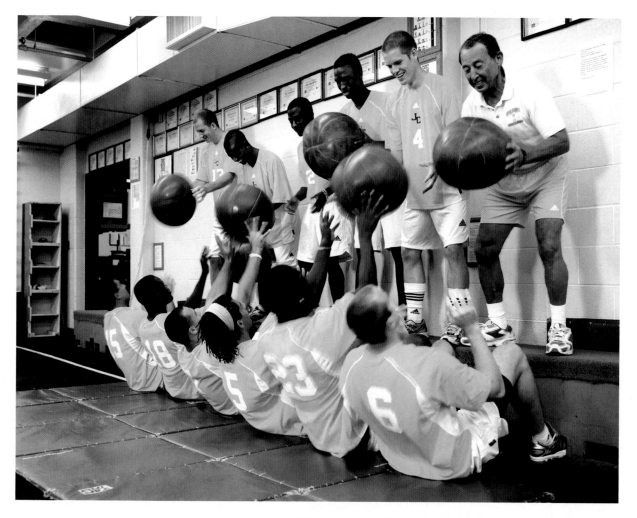

Coach Javorek CAN STILL OUTMANEUVER AND OUTLAST many of his college athletes.

Javorek can still outmaneuver and outlast many of his college athletes. Joined by Simien on the hill, he runs us through a few sets of double-leg bounding on the steps, sprinting up the ramp, and leaping up through the tiers of rubber-filled boxes.

"Look at this campus," says the coach after the workout ends. "I like it here," he says with a shrug. For the faculty members, students, and burgeoning athletes I've met during my stay, the feeling is mutual. ∎

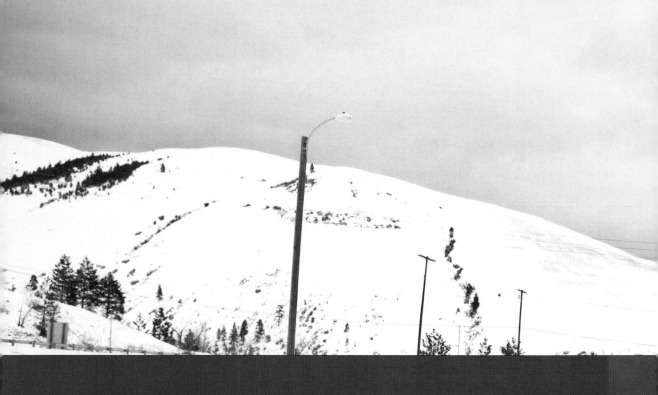

Build the Body You Want

HERE ARE SECRETS FROM AMERICA'S BEST GYMS: 30 NEW WAYS TO GET STRONGER, FASTER, BETTER

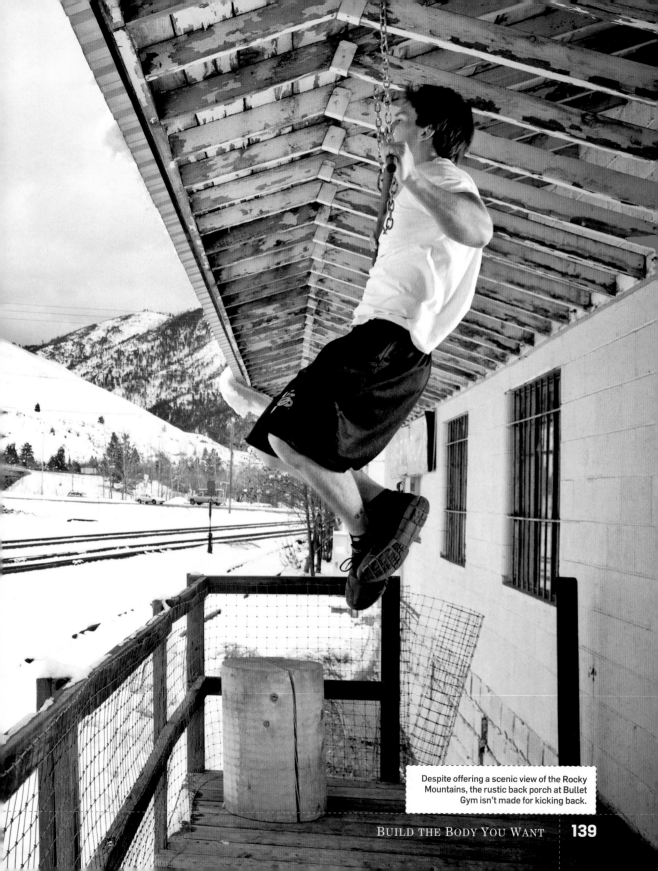

Despite offering a scenic view of the Rocky Mountains, the rustic back porch at Bullet Gym isn't made for kicking back.

Our list of the country's 30 best gyms—as selected by our panel of fitness advisors—is defined by the only criteria that truly matter: results. Make that big results. The kind that can help you get fit now and live longer and better later. But because these gyms might lie outside your ZIP code, we've gathered elite advice from their top fitness experts and offer it to you here, for free—no membership fee required. After all, doesn't your body deserve the best?

MASTER THE PULLUP

● Of the four pullup bars at **Bullet Gym in Missoula, Montana**, the one shown in the photo on page 139 on the back side of its building is the most challenging. A chain suspension forces your core to work harder to leverage your body. But it's not just the equipment that sets this old-school gym apart from most places; it's the way the men who train here use it.

"Ask people where they feel fatigued most during pullups or lat pulldowns, and they usually mention shoulders and arms," says the owner, Mike Casey. But if you can keep those areas from giving out too soon, the pullup becomes the ultimate move for building wider lats.

The key to limiting fatigue is relaxing your hands and pulling your shoulder blades back and down. Focus on hooking your fingers over the bar rather than squeezing it, and apply pressure with your middle finger, ring finger, and pinkie. Then squeeze your shoulder blades down and think about pushing your elbows down into your lats instead of pulling up with your arms.

Once you've completed a pullup, move to another exercise in your routine. Return for another pullup after each exercise. By workout's end, you'll have completed twice as many repetitions as if you were doing them all at once.

PUMP OUT MORE REPS

● "When bench-pressing, keep your wrists as straight as possible," says Joe DeFranco, the owner of **DeFranco's Training Systems in Wyckoff, New Jersey**. "When your wrists bend back too much, your triceps fatigue faster because the bar is farther from your center of gravity."

LEARN TO SKY

● "To jump higher, concentrate on pushing the ground away from you," says Jamie Hale, CSCS, the owner of **Total Body Fitness in Winchester, Kentucky**.

For even better results, combine this strategy with an exercise called the depth jump: Stand at the edge of a 12-inch box and then simply step off it so that you land on the balls of both feet simultaneously. (Don't allow your heels to touch the floor.) When you make contact with the floor, jump as high as you can. That's 1 rep. Step back onto the box and repeat. Do 4 to 5 sets of 3 to 5 reps, resting for 60 to 90 seconds between sets.

LUNGE FOR SPEED

● Instead of holding dumbbells at your sides when you lunge, try holding one dumbbell out in front of your chest with your arms extended.

This should stop you from leaning forward as you fatigue, says David Donatucci, MEd, CSCS, a performance specialist at **International Performance Institute in Bradenton, Florida**. As a result, you'll train your glutes harder with each repetition, a key for generating more power when you sprint.

REV UP YOUR ENGINE

● Try this simple 2-minute warmup: Do high knees, jumping jacks, skips, and side-to-side hops for 15 seconds each. Then drop to the floor for 15 seconds each of pushups, crunches, mountain climbers, and squat thrusts.

"You've just activated your entire backside, core, and shoulders, and added a little running," says David Jack, life and sport

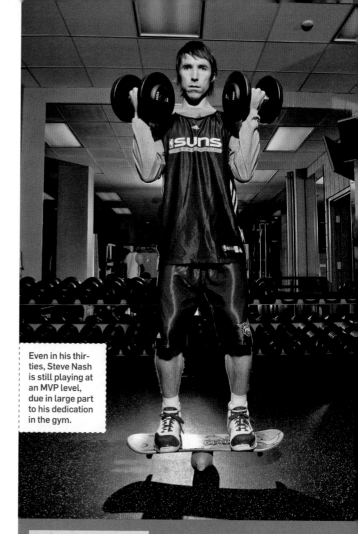

Even in his thirties, Steve Nash is still playing at an MVP level, due in large part to his dedication in the gym.

Achieve Balance

■ Steve Nash knows his way around a weight room. "I've spent half my life in gyms," says the two-time NBA MVP and the owner of a sports club in Vancouver. But he's not showing off in the **Suns Strength Room** (above).

No, Nash is demonstrating his ability to perform nearly his entire strength routine on a Vew-Do balance board, which is like a skateboard without wheels. This feat requires core strength, ankle stability, and lots of practice. It's one reason the Suns consistently rank among the most injury-free franchises in the NBA.

"Striking a balance between stability and strength is the basis of basketball training, as well as most other sports," says Erik Phillips, MS, ATC, the Suns' head strength and conditioning coach. He says that simply performing some of your exercises with a split stance—one foot forward, the other back—will add balance to your training and help shore up your core. Try it with squats, overhead presses, and rows. Just stagger your stance and then do the exercise. Switch leg positions each set.

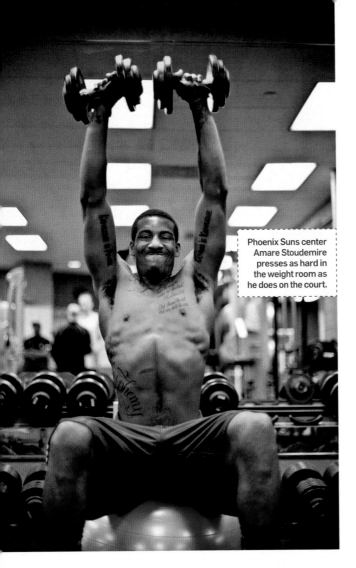

Phoenix Suns center Amare Stoudemire presses as hard in the weight room as he does on the court.

In this case, frustration is a good thing. "An awkward bag requires you to use more muscles and expend greater energy to lift it." Pick up inexpensive sandbags from your local home-improvement store and use them for presses, curls, squats, deadlifts, and power cleans.

END SHOULDER PAIN

● "The cause of your pain is not always where it hurts," says Michael Boyle, ATC, the owner of **Mike Boyle Strength & Conditioning in Winchester, Massachusetts**. "If your shoulder hurts in front, then massage, ice, and stretch the back of your shoulder."

Try this stretch: Lie on your right side with your right upper arm on the floor perpendicular to your body and your forearm pointing straight up. Keeping your shoulder blades pulled together and your el-bow in place, rotate your palm toward the floor as far as you can, then return. Do 10 repetitions.

PULL FOR POWER

● "When you lower your body during a dip, try to pull yourself down very slowly," says Robb Wolf, the owner of **NorCal Strength & Conditioning in Chico, California**. "This forces both your biceps and triceps to fire si-multaneously and may cause an over-spill of the chemicals needed for muscle contraction."

The end result: You'll be able to press yourself back up with less effort.

LOSE THE SHOES

● Running or jumping rope barefoot on grass or sand strengthens your arches and Achilles tendons, helping to restore proper mechanics to flat-footed runners. Barefoot

director at **Teamworks Centers in Acton, Massachusetts**.

The payoff: Researchers at the United States Military Academy at West Point found that this type of warmup helped men sprint faster, jump higher, and throw harder.

START SANDBAGGING

● "There's no equipment that frustrates guys as much as a sandbag," says Mike Morris, CSCS, head strength and conditioning coach for the **Tampa Bay Buccaneers Physical Development Center**.

BREAK THROUGH STRENGTH BARRIERS

■ Kettlebell training is ideal for improving the explosive power you need to run faster, jump higher, and perform better.

What appears to be a log cabin in the photo on page 148 is actually a room for mixed martial arts training on the second floor of a warehouse called **Total Performance Sports in Everett, Massachusetts**.

This room is also used for explosive exercises like the kettlebell snatch. Mastering the snatch (imagine that you're throwing a weight from the floor toward the ceiling but without letting go of it) will require your neurological system to recruit more muscle fibers, says the owner, C.J. Murphy. So it's the perfect exercise for breaking out of a strength slump.

Most men who fail to derive the full benefit from the snatch haven't mastered the technique, or they select a weight that's too light. Your brain will allow only the maximal number of muscle fibers to fire in power movements when you use very heavy weight, Murphy says. So what's heavy enough? Find a pair of dumbbells that allows you to complete no more than 5 shrugs and challenges your grip by the last rep. Then go 10 pounds lighter. This is the ideal weight for the snatch. Do sets of no more than 5 reps.

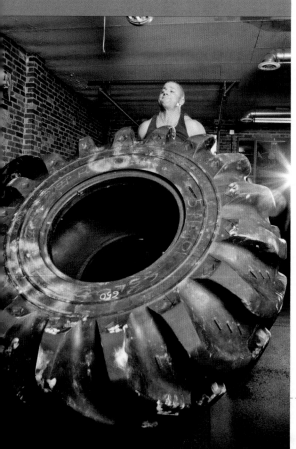

training will also make you faster by developing the smaller muscles in your feet, says Kurt Hester, CSCS, the director of training for **D1 Sports Training in Nashville, Tennessee**.

ADD 10 POUNDS TO YOUR BENCH

● "To boost your bench press, raise your head and upper back off the bench as you lower the barbell to your chest, almost like you're doing a situp," says Mark Bell, CSCS, the owner of **Super Training Gym in Sacramento, California**. "As soon as the bar touches your T-shirt, drive your head and torso into the bench and press the bar up as forcefully as you can."

The result: Your body uncoils like a loaded spring, helping you push more weight. (Always use a spotter.)

FINISH LIKE A CHAMP

● "After the last full rep of your final set, do 4 to 8 more reps through the last quarter of the range of motion. Then hold the weight in the final position for 5 to 10 seconds, flexing hard," says Brian Dobson, the owner of **Metroflex Gym in Arlington, Texas**, the training home of eight-time Mr. Olympia Ronnie Coleman.

RAISE THE DEAD

● "Before you perform a deadlift, warm up by first doing the movement while standing on a 4-inch box or step," says Mark Philippi, CSCS, a seven-time World's Strongest Man competitor and the owner of **Philippi Sports Institute in Las Vegas, Nevada**. "When you start your regular sets, the exercise will seem easier because you won't have to move the weight as far."

(continued on page 146)

Prepare Your Muscles for Any Challenge

■ Before Rayne Gray was a firefighter for the Phoenix Fire Department, he was a triathlete.

"I don't have a set date to race now, but I need to be ready to perform my best at any moment," he says.

To determine ways to stay fit at all times despite a volatile work schedule, exercise scientist Matthew Rhea, PhD, studied Gray and his colleagues. He discovered that the best workout for the day depends on a lot of variables—sleep patterns the night before, nutrition for several days prior, stress levels, and motivation, to name a few.

"A savvy exerciser will pay attention to all of these factors and ad-just his or her training accordingly," says Dr. Rhea, who is the director of human movement at **A.T. Still University in Mesa, Arizona**. Or you can take them into account ahead of time and use a method called "daily undulating periodization." With this technique, you vary your sets and reps with each workout—3 sets of 10 reps on Monday, 4 sets of 5 reps on Wednesday, and 2 sets of 15 on Friday. By using a different training scheme each session, you'll automatically vary the volume and intensity of your workout, allowing for faster recovery and less chance of overtaxing your body.

In fact, Dr. Rhea found that this approach increased strength in men twofold compared with the traditional method of gradually increasing sets and reps. While the firefighters often train with unconventional equipment, the principle of varying your workout applies equally as well to training with free weights.

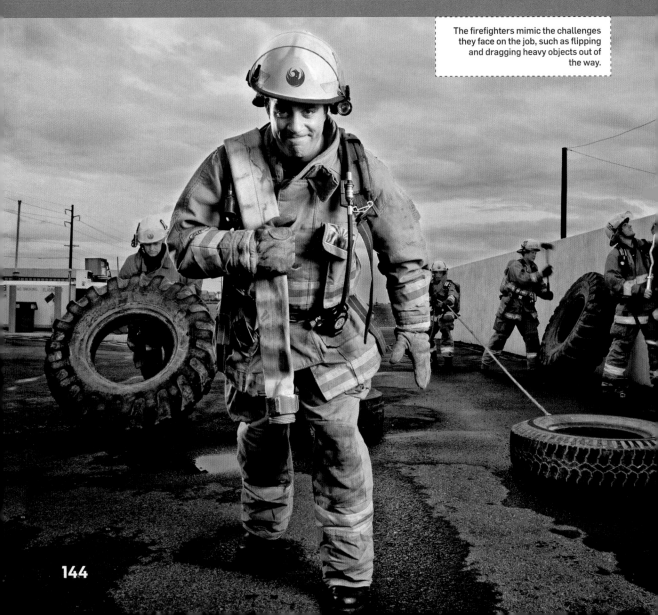

The firefighters mimic the challenges they face on the job, such as flipping and dragging heavy objects out of the way.

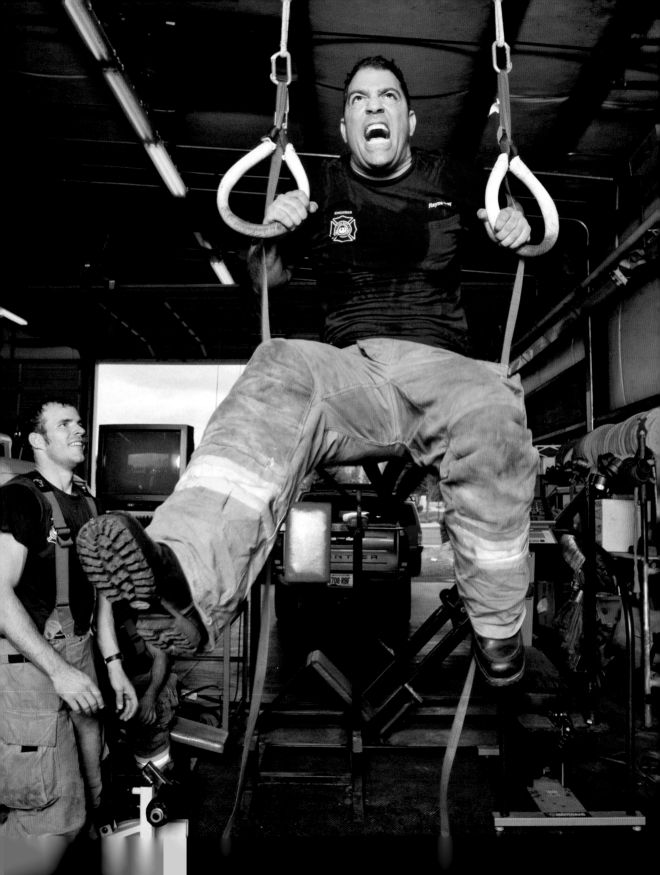

For your elevated warmup, do 3 sets of 3 reps, using a weight that's 50, 75, and 90 percent, respectively, of the weight you plan to work out with.

CARVE YOUR ABS

● For total ab development, employ an improved version of the classic cable woodchop, an exercise that mimics the swinging of an ax.

"Instead of pulling the cable from your shoulder to the opposite knee, try chopping in every line of action," says Jim Liston, founder of **CATZ Competitive Athlete Training Zone in Pasadena, California**. Your start and end points are your eyes, shoulders, waist, knees, and ankles. Choose one point and pull the handle to another. Do 12 reps in one line, switch sides, and repeat. Then choose a new line for each of 2 more sets.

JUMPSTART YOUR WORKOUT

● Can't get up for your training session? "Make an ankle-deep ice-water bath—as cold as you can bear—and stand in it for 20 seconds," says Mark Verstegen, CSCS, the owner of **Athletes' Performance in Tempe, Arizona**. Then dry off and hit the gym.

"The cold water will shock your nervous system, giving you an immediate rush of energy," he says.

PERFECT YOUR FORM

● "Once you're in the starting position of the squat, push your hips back as far as you can before you allow your knees to bend," says Brian Schwab, CSCS, the owner of **Orlando Barbell in Oviedo, Florida**. "This recruits the often-neglected muscles of your hamstrings and glutes while reducing the strain on your knees."

LOOK UP FOR LATS

● "When you're doing pullups, fix your eyes on the ceiling," says Logan Hood, the owner of **Epoch Training in Los Angeles, California**. "This causes you to pull your chest instead of your chin toward the bar, which better engages your lats."

CHEAT FOR 4 WEEKS

● Start your presses, rows, or curls with your elbows bent about 6 inches, and return to that point with each rep. "The tension on your muscles is greatly reduced near the end range of motion," says Juan Carlos Santana, MEd, CSCS, owner of the **Institute of Human Performance in Boca Raton, Florida**. "So this strategy keeps tension on your muscles to spur faster growth."

Do 3 to 4 sets of 10 to 15 reps, and try this technique for a month. Then return to standard full range-of-motion training to boost strength and flexibility.

BURN MORE FAT

● "If you want to become lean, finish off your weight workout with a 'leg matrix,'" says Alwyn Cosgrove, CSCS, the owner of **Results Fitness in Santa Clarita, California**. "It's a body-weight circuit that's highly effective for both fat loss and cardiovascular conditioning."

Without resting between exercises, perform each movement for 15 seconds. Then repeat the circuit once or twice. As you progress, gradually increase the duration of each set to 30 seconds.

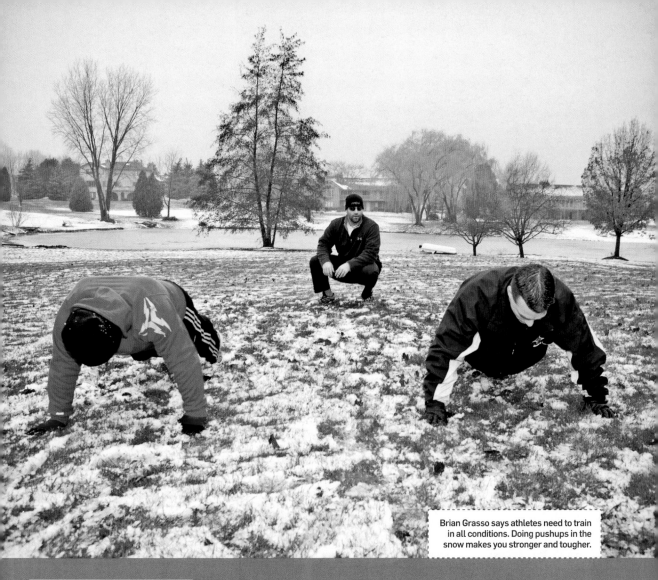

Brian Grasso says athletes need to train in all conditions. Doing pushups in the snow makes you stronger and tougher.

Simplify Your Workout

■ The CEO of the International Youth Conditioning Association trains all his clients, from Little Leaguers to professional baseball players, with $50 worth of equipment in his backyard.

"I've owned several nice facilities," says Brian Grasso (squatting in the photo above), "but I've learned that anyone can produce great results with virtually no equipment." That's the idea behind his current training facility, **Brian Grasso's backyard in Hawthorn Woods, Illinois**. There, Grasso takes a gladiator's approach to making muscle.

"We take heavy objects—a wheelbarrow, sandbags, or cement bags, for instance—and pick them up, walk with them, and lift them overhead. And we use a sturdy tree limb or swing set for pullups," he says. But don't just lift up and down or forward and backward. Muscle grows best when you train in "nonlinear" patterns, says Grasso.

For example, try clockwork pushups. Keep your feet planted and move around an imaginary clock with your hands, completing 5 pushups in each position. Another option: Create stations with markers so you can run, jump, and skip rope in a variety of patterns. For instance, you might stagger 10 hurdles (boxes, cones, milk cartons) and jump over them 10 times. Then place sticks in an octagonal pattern, stand in the middle of it, and sprint to each corner. Next, zigzag all over your yard while jumping rope. You'll slash fat and improve athleticism, all within shouting distance of your family.

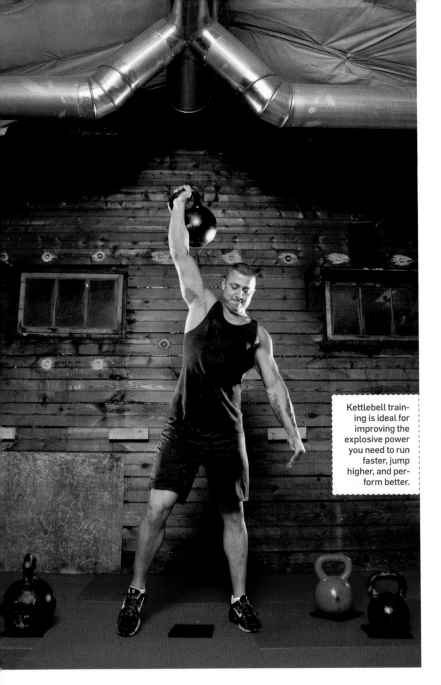

Kettlebell training is ideal for improving the explosive power you need to run faster, jump higher, and perform better.

for 1 second in the down position.

4. **Squat hold:** Lower yourself into a squat, and hold for the duration of the set.

FIRE UP YOUR MUSCLES

● Try this tweak with just about any exercise. "Hold the weight in the starting position for 3 to 5 seconds before performing your first rep and again when you've finished your last rep," says Marc Bartley, CSCS, the owner of **South Carolina Barbell in Columbia, South Carolina**. "This stimulates your central nervous system to activate more muscle fibers, which allows you to generate more force."

STAY FOCUSED

● Don't stare at yourself in the mirror when you squat," says Matt Wenning, the director of athlete training and testing at **Westside Barbell in Columbus, Ohio**. "It'll cause you to lean farther forward, which increases the strain on your lower back and reduces overall strength."

His advice: Before you descend, find a mark that's stable and just above eye level, and stay focused on it throughout the movement. Just as important, have your training partner watch for flaws in your form.

THE LEG MATRIX

1. **Jump squat:** Squat, leap as high as you can, and repeat.
2. **Speed squat:** Do each rep as fast as possible.
3. **Pause squat:** For each rep, pause

BLAST YOUR BICEPS

● "Imagine you're holding a grapefruit between your shoulder blades as you do arm curls," says Michael A. Clark, DPT, the CEO of the **National Academy of Sports Medicine in Calabasas, California**.

Standing tall with your shoulder blades squeezed back and down allows your rotator cuff to properly control the head of your humerus, or upper-arm bone. As a result, you'll be able to produce a greater amount of force with your biceps, says Clark. This will allow you to complete more reps with more weight for greater strength and size.

KEEP LIFTING

● "Take advantage of your 30s and 40s," says Bob Bonham, the owner of **Strong & Shapely Gym in East Rutherford, New Jersey**. "Because your metabolism starts to slow, it actually becomes easier for skinny men to pack on muscle compared with when they were in their 20s." Bottom line: You can build muscle at any age.

CREATE AN OBSTACLE

● Try this Polish abs exercise called the hanging hurdle. "It works your entire core," says Mark McLaughlin, the owner of **Performance Training Center in Beaverton, Oregon**.

Here's how to do it: Place a bench under and parallel with a chinup bar. Now hang from the bar with your feet together, knees slightly bent, and legs to one side of the bench. Without changing the bend in your knees, simply lift your legs over the bench to the opposite side. Repeat back and forth for 10 to 15 seconds. Your goal: 2 sets of 60 seconds, with 30 to 90 seconds' rest between sets.

FIX YOUR WEAK SPOT

● "Nine out of 10 guys don't specifically train their lower back," says Jim Hoskinson, the owner of **IronWorks Gym in Callahan, Florida**. "And that's unfortunate because it's the key to total-body strength."

Hoskinson's remedy: Perform the seated good morning at least once a week, after you train your lower body. Holding a barbell across your upper back, sit down on a flat bench with your torso upright. Keeping your lower back naturally arched, bend forward at the waist as far as you can. Then lift your torso back to the start. That's 1 repetition. Do 5 sets of 10 repetitions, resting 60 to 90 seconds between sets.

GET MORE ON THE FLOOR

● "When you do a pushup, make your body as stiff as a board by bracing your abs, and flexing your glutes and quads," says Lance Mosley, owner of **HardCore Fitness in Boca Raton, Florida**. "Then lower yourself until your chin, chest, and thighs simultaneously touch the floor." This is what Mosley calls a "true pushup."

TRY A BAND-AID

● "I have an 8,200-square-foot gym filled with high-dollar exercise equipment," says Jean-Paul Francoeur, the owner of **JP Fitness in Little Rock, Arkansas**. "But my favorite training tool is a giant rubber band that costs about 20 bucks."

Francoeur explains that large bands—like those at resistancebandtraining.com—are as effective for building muscle as free weights, and they also allow you to take your gym anywhere. ∎

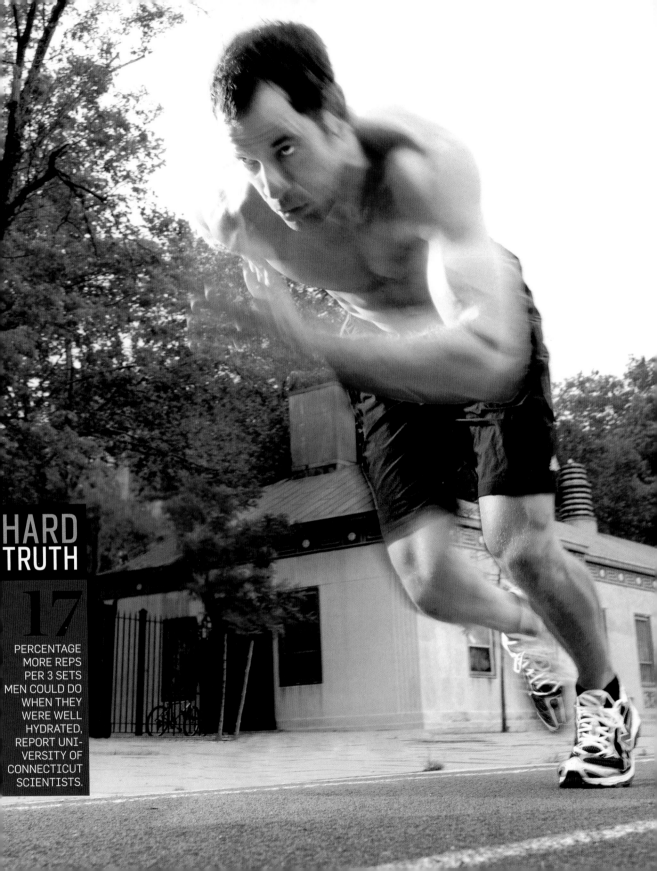

HARD
TRUTH

17

PERCENTAGE
MORE REPS
PER 3 SETS
MEN COULD DO
WHEN THEY
WERE WELL
HYDRATED,
REPORT UNI-
VERSITY OF
CONNECTICUT
SCIENTISTS.

Get Huge in a Hurry

THESE FIVE NEW MUSCLE RULES WILL MAKE YOU BIGGER, LEANER, AND STRONGER—IN LESS TIME THAN EVER BEFORE

Ask the average guy in the average gym how to build bigger muscles, and chances are he'll tell you to do exactly what he's doing: lots of sets and reps of lots of redundant exercises. Except . . . well, you notice it's not working particularly well for him.

Worse, you realize you're already doing workouts similar to his, and it's not happening for you, either.

The old playbook doesn't work for most people who use it. It's the fitness equivalent of "3 yards and a cloud of dust." There's a better, faster, more streamlined way to get bigger, leaner, and stronger. Think of these five principles of size—borrowed from the book *Men's Health Huge in a Hurry*—as the spread offense for gym rats.

Principle 1:
LIFT BIG TO GROW BIG

The longer you've been lifting weights, the heavier the weights need to be in order for you to see results. On one hand, it's a stupidly obvious point—of course you use bigger weights as you become stronger. But that's not exactly what we're talking about.

When you were a beginner, you could gain size and strength as long as the weight you used on any given exercise was at least 60 percent of the amount you could lift for a single max-effort repetition. It's a weight you could lift 15 to 20 times

in a single set. By any definition, that's pretty light.

That percentage, though, increases with experience. Most gym regulars need to use at least 80 percent of their 1-rep max to grow bigger and stronger. Now, we're talking about a weight you could probably lift about 8 times in an all-out set before there's nothing left in your tank.

Be honest: Do you really use weights heavy enough to fall into that range? If you typically perform multiple sets of 8 to 10 repetitions for each exercise, you don't. To use 80 percent of your max for 3 or 4 sets, each set would probably consist of 5 or 6 repetitions.

It becomes even harder from there. If you're beyond the intermediate stage—if you're a serious gym rat and have been lifting consistently for much of your adult life—you might need 85 to 90 percent of your 1-rep max to see genuine progress. In a normal workout with multiple sets of each exercise, we're talking about 2, 3, or 4 repetitions per set.

You can see the problem: Nobody can lift near-max weights on every exercise of

HARD TRUTH

78 PERCENTAGE MORE LIKELY MEN WHO PERFORM POORLY IN A PUSHUP TEST ARE TO GAIN 20 POUNDS OF FLAB OVER THE NEXT TWO DECADES, ACCORDING TO A CANADIAN STUDY.

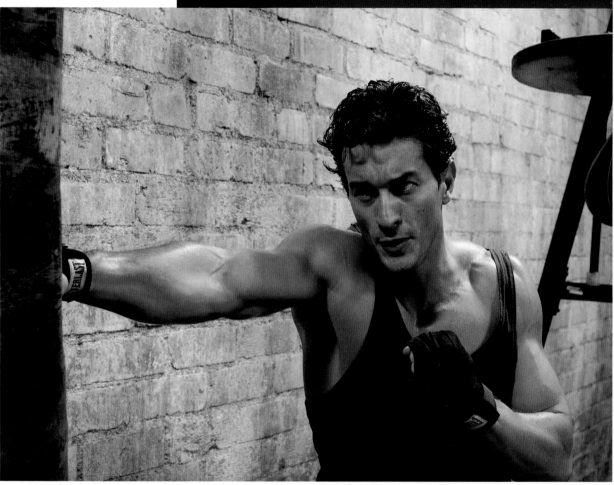

every workout. You'd either burn out or hurt yourself, and it wouldn't take long.

Fortunately, there is one loophole.

Principle 2:
LIFT FAST TO GET BIG

You know you're supposed to lift weights slowly and deliberately and under control. We have no problem with the "under control" part; good form requires it. But we

ANYTHING WORTH LIFTING IS WORTH LIFTING FAST, as long as you can control the weight.

want to take serious issue with "slowly and deliberately."

The faster you lift, the better the results. If you're trying to increase size, fast lifts activate more of the muscle fibers that have the most potential to grow. If you're trying to become leaner, fast lifts do more to crank up your heart rate—and by extension your metabolism—than anything else. And if you're trying to grow stronger . . . well, how many feats of strength can you list that are performed slowly and deliberately? Even if something looks slow from the outside, you can bet that the guy performing the feat is trying like hell to get it done as fast as possible.

cle fibers poop out really fast—usually in 15 seconds or less. Once they've quit on you, you're left to struggle with the weight using fibers that aren't up to the task.

Your body has two ways of tipping you off:

1. The speed of your repetitions slows.

2. Your form changes, and you either shorten your range of motion or have to cheat to accomplish the full range.

At that point, it makes more sense to end the set than to keep going with compromised speed or bad form. We say that knowing it's one of the most unnatural things we could ask you to do in the weight room. After all, if the goal is to do sets of 8 reps and your speed slows down on the

Focus on total reps per exercise, and let the sets take care of themselves. THE REWARD IS A BETTER WORKOUT.

Anything worth lifting is worth lifting fast, as long as you control the weight and don't let it control you. That means you'll lower the weight a bit more slowly than you lifted it. You don't have to lower it at any particular tempo; just make sure you return it to the starting position without dropping it or shifting your body out of proper alignment.

Principle 3:
QUIT WHEN YOU'RE AHEAD

A fast lift with a heavy weight uses more muscle fibers than a slower lift with a lighter weight. But those big, strong mus-

sixth, it takes discipline to end the set before grinding and shaking through those seventh and eighth reps. And it works only if you're also willing to follow Principle 4.

Principle 4:
DON'T SWEAT THE SMALL SETS

Every page of the old muscle-building playbook includes some prescription for sets and reps: a fixed number of sets of each exercise and a fixed number of reps in each set.

But if you follow Principle 3 and quit each set when your speed slows down or your form changes, you can't complete a fixed number of repetitions.

MONDAY
BENCH PRESS

CHINUP

DEADLIFT

Do 25 total reps of each exercise, using a weight you can lift 4 to 6 times before your speed slows down or your form changes. Rest about 60 seconds between sets.

TUESDAY REST

WEDNESDAY
DUMBBELL SINGLE-ARM SHOULDER PRESS

DUMBBELL SINGLE-ARM ROW

DUMBBELL LUNGE OR STEP-UP

Do 40 total reps of each exercise with each arm or each leg, using a weight you can lift 10 to 12 times before your speed slows down or your form changes. Do all the reps of each exercise before resting. Rest 45 seconds between sets.

THURSDAY REST

FRIDAY
BARBELL BENT-OVER ROW

DIP

SQUAT

Do 15 total reps of each exercise, using a weight you can lift 2 to 3 times before your speed slows down or your form changes. Rest about 90 seconds between sets.

The new playbook says this: Focus on total reps for each exercise, and let the sets take care of themselves. Say you're doing a workout that specifies 5 sets of 5 reps. That's 25 reps total. Now let's say you use our method of doing all your reps perfectly: It might take you 6 sets instead of 5 to hit your 25-rep goal. The reward is a better workout, because you're doing more work with your biggest, strongest muscle fibers.

Principle 5:
THINK BIG TO GROW BIG

Our final revision of the weight-lifting playbook makes it dramatically shorter and lighter: We've eliminated almost all the exercises that work only small muscles or single muscle groups in isolation. Instead, our workouts begin and end with the exercises that work your biggest muscles, with the goal of working as many of them as possible every time you lift.

Each workout is built around one lower-body exercise—squats, deadlifts, lunges, or step-ups—and two upper-body exercises, one for pushing and one for pulling. Gone are the leg extensions and biceps curls.

If you're wondering how you're supposed to build big arms without curls, we have a simple assignment for you: Grab a chinup bar and try to pull yourself up without using your biceps. Impossible, right? So if you work your biceps with chinups or lat pulldowns, using an underhand grip, or any type of rowing exercise, why would you need to do curls? What benefit does a curl offer that you can't achieve with a chinup or row? As a bonus, you burn a lot more calories when you train your biggest muscles.

The greatest surprise isn't that these new-school workouts give you more benefits in less time. It's that the old-style playbook survived as long as it did. ■

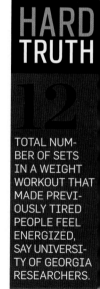

HARD TRUTH

12

TOTAL NUMBER OF SETS IN A WEIGHT WORKOUT THAT MADE PREVIOUSLY TIRED PEOPLE FEEL ENERGIZED, SAY UNIVERSITY OF GEORGIA RESEARCHERS.

Build Bigger Biceps

CAN RUBBER BUILD MUSCLE AS WELL AS IRON DOES? SUPERTRAINER J.C. SANTANA CHALLENGES YOU TO STRETCH THE LIMITS OF CONDITIONING

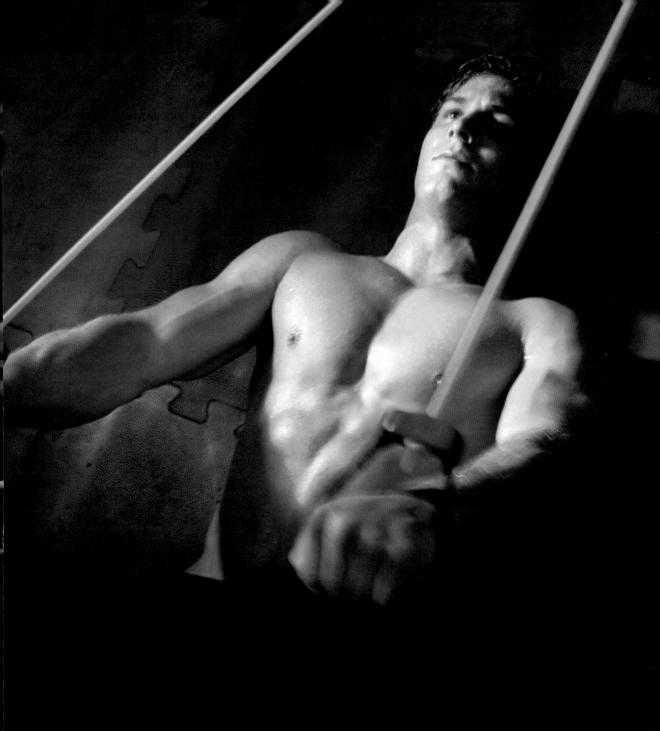

When it comes to growing strong and building muscle, real men need clanking iron and leather kidney belts. We need to stare down an imposing piece of steel, spit on our hands, and then conquer it.

Or do we?

JUAN CARLOS SANTANA, MEd, CSCS, stands in his gym—the Institute of Human Performance in Boca Raton, Florida—and laughs. Unlike most other 49-year-olds, Santana doesn't jiggle when he giggles. At 5'10" and 212 pounds, he's as solid and looming as that hunk of limestone in Gibraltar.

"I ain't no long-distance-running, yoga-posing, Pilates-training, VO_2-pumping, aquatics-floating, 150-pound sissy boy," he snarls. "I train like a beast and have competed in Olympic weight lifting, wrestling, judo, and kickboxing all my life. Bring me the biggest guy you can get your hands on. I will put him in a fetal position, with him sucking his thumb, in less than 30 minutes—with nothing but these elastic bands."

In Santana's meat packer hands, he holds out a tangle of what looks like giant rubber bands and tubes, of various widths and colors. Over the years, he's learned to manipulate these bands as masterfully as another man named Santana twangs guitar strings. And the result, you could argue, is the same in both cases: a perfectly tuned body of work.

Skeptical? So were we. We sent writer Joe Kita to see for himself. Here's his story:

I came to Boca Raton as a 170-pound, aerobic-training "sissy boy." With achy knees and flagging enthusiasm for my life sports of running and bicycling, I was looking for a new way to stay fit and become stronger. Plus, I travel a lot, so I was hoping this workout would be portable enough to help me maintain fitness on the road. Here are the benefits Santana promised if I hopped on his bandwagon.

1. You will become strong.

2. You will pack on muscle.

3. You will improve your aerobic conditioning without running.

4. You will improve your sports performance (golf, basketball, baseball) while reducing your risk of injury.

5. You will work out for only 30 to 40 minutes every other day.

6. You will be able to train anywhere, anytime, with a piece of equipment that fits in your pocket.

It was sounding better all the time.

(LOSING) BREAKFAST WITH J.C.

The weird thing about band training is that done correctly, it makes you feel simultaneously strong and sick, as I quickly learn when I show up for a morning workout with Santana, or J.C., as just about everyone calls him.

"This isn't going to be easy," he warns. "The band doesn't stretch itself. You have to work, and you have to work hard. Once you commit to doing that, you'll see remarkable results. I'll prove it. One of my favorite exercises is the 30-second pump. You're about to see what curling 60 reps in 30 seconds can do for you. Ready?"

I step on his 3-foot-long, half-inch-wide SuperBand ($13, ihpfit.com) with both feet, grasp the upper part of the band with both hands (palms up), and then, on J.C.'s signal, commence a pace of two biceps curls a second for 30 seconds. The resistance feels manageable at first, but by the 20th second

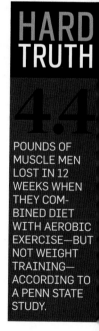

HARD TRUTH

4.4

POUNDS OF MUSCLE MEN LOST IN 12 WEEKS WHEN THEY COMBINED DIET WITH AEROBIC EXERCISE—BUT NOT WEIGHT TRAINING—ACCORDING TO A PENN STATE STUDY.

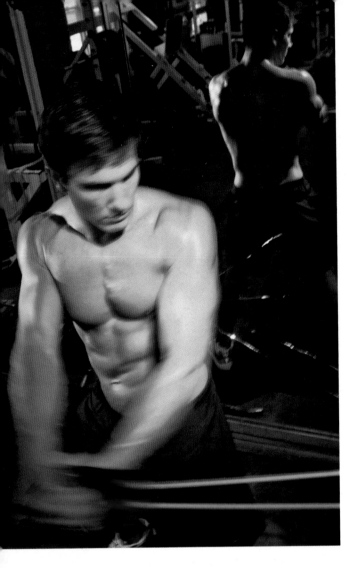

a door or hooking it around a doorknob or other stationary object, you can do standing crunches until you're crying for absolution from not exercising enough. Indeed, just about any exercise done with conventional weights can be done with bands.

Besides building strength, band training boosts cardiovascular endurance and calorie combustion. To prove this, Santana had me wear a heart-rate monitor. The highest I can usually peg my ticker is the mid- to upper 140s, when I'm cranking uphill on a mountain bike. But just 15 minutes into J.C.'s workout, my heart rate hit 144 beats per minute and, even after I stopped exercising, continued climbing to 154. This phenomenon is called EPOC, or "excess postexercise oxygen consumption." It's a great benefit of resistance training; your body can burn calories up to 48 hours after a workout. The fact that bands can produce the same effect as traditional weights is a testament to their value.

Another advantage I immediately noticed was that bands are infinitely variable in direction as well as resistance. Unlike Nautilus machines and traditional cables, these elastic bands can be used in any plane of movement to mimic tennis, golf, and baseball swings, or even swimming and poling strokes. If you're creative enough, any key sports movement can be replicated with bands.

LEARNING A PAINFUL LESSON

Enlightened, inspired, and armed with a specific training program, I headed home for 8 weeks of workouts. The plan was to

I'm curling in painful slow motion. He then commands me to immediately do 30 seconds of "speed extensions," which are triceps presses done at the same pace with a suspended band. When I'm finished, my arms feel blasted—but also big.

Cruelly, this feeling can be replicated for every muscle group. For instance, by standing on the same band and wrapping it over your shoulders or stretching it overhead, you can do full-body squats until your legs are in knots. By wedging the band in

"At first, the weight felt manageable. But when I was done, MY ARMS WERE BLASTED."

spend the first 4 weeks building a foundation and then the next 4 (the so-called metabolic stage) focusing on explosiveness. I cut back dramatically on my running and biking. Instead, I took my bands into the basement every other day. At first I had trouble climbing back up those stairs after the workouts. My legs were quivering like Nana's Jell-O, but eventually I began to feel a kind of strength I had never felt before. It seemed more inherently core, like I was becoming powerful.

My family was intrigued by my somewhat unorthodox experiment. My 23-year-old son, who was home from college, ridiculed me at first. Then he joined me for a few sets and became addicted. My wife and 19-year-old daughter were also curious, largely because it looked like a more accessible, less testosterone-charged form of strength training. They, too, gave it a try.

But then something horrible happened. In fact, I'm fortunate to be here today with my manhood still intact. I was doing bent-over rows with the "JC Travel Bands" ($20, ihpfit.com), a beefier model with two rubber grips attached to a pair of thick tubes. I thought I had adequately wedged one end into a door frame, but just as I stretched the band to its fullest it broke free and snapped into my thighs, inches from my groin. I doubled over, screaming. There was no blood, but over the next few days my thighs changed color from red to purple to yellow, and I was seriously hobbled. Neither my daughter nor my wife ever picked up a band again. But I learned a valuable lesson: These things can be lethal. You need to secure them properly, as I had foolishly failed to do.

Nonetheless, after a brief respite, I resumed training. After the prescribed 2 months, I had added 5 pounds of muscle and noticeable definition. I was feeling stronger while running, biking, driving golf balls, and jumping for rebounds. What's more, when I got a last-minute story assignment and had to hop a plane, all I needed to throw in my suitcase were a few pieces of elastic. Suddenly, even a cheap motor lodge had a pretty nice gym.

Although Santana admits that band training isn't the best way to add lots of bulk (classic free-weight training is still tops for that), I've found it to be a solid option for maintaining and building muscle and endurance when I don't have access to my normal equipment, or simply want to change pace or train a specific sports movement. In fact, bands are a great addition to any workout, even if you already pump iron the old-fashioned way.

"Exercise fads come and go," says Santana. "One year it's stability balls, the next it's cardio-kickboxing, the year after that it's medicine balls. . . . It's always the next big thing, and guys often end up going from one fad to the next and not making any progress. It's better to think of all these exercise alternatives as different tools in your toolbox. Don't use a hammer for everything. Instead, use the right tool for the right job." ∎

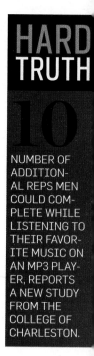

HARD TRUTH

10

NUMBER OF ADDITIONAL REPS MEN COULD COMPLETE WHILE LISTENING TO THEIR FAVORITE MUSIC ON AN MP3 PLAYER, REPORTS A NEW STUDY FROM THE COLLEGE OF CHARLESTON.

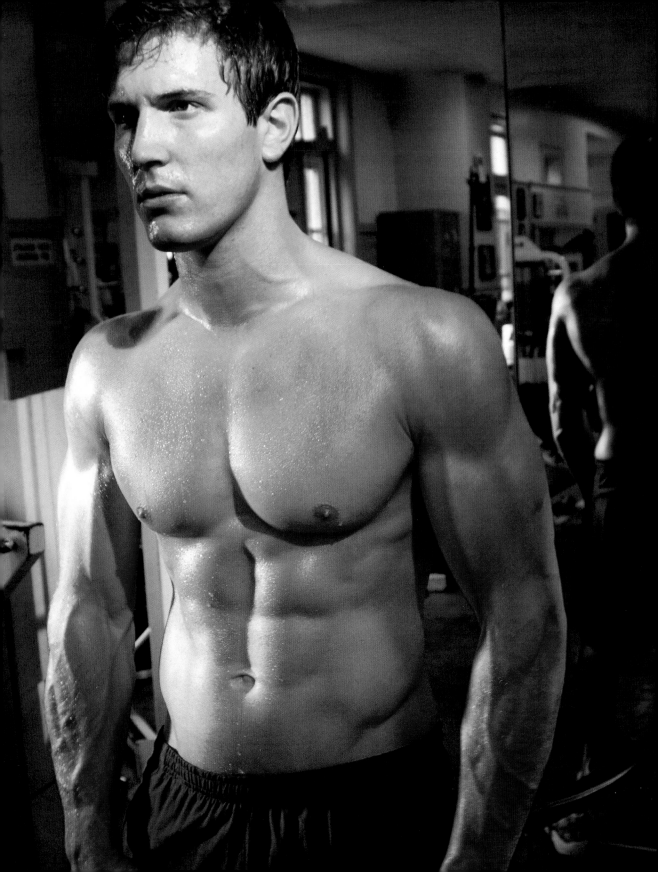

SEIZE YOUR SIX-PACK

Exercising to lose your gut is simple: It's all about your muscles. Let us explain: Contracting your muscles requires fuel, like an engine does. So the more muscle you work, the more calories you burn. This is one reason why the best way to lose your gut is with total-body weight training. But that's just the start.

Because pumping iron also builds muscle, you're simultaneously increasing the size of your engine, which helps you burn even more calories in each workout. Plus, lifting weights boosts your metabolism for hours after you train. Our point: Don't dismiss this workout because it has only six exercises. They're all you need to burn fat, build muscle, and look better than ever.

Your 4-Week Fat-Loss Plan

This fast-paced workout will help you shed fat, build muscle, and boost your fitness levels to an all-time high—in just 90 minutes a week.

DIRECTIONS

Complete the workout 3 days a week, resting at least a day between sessions. So you might train on Monday, Wednesday, and Friday.

Do the exercises in the order shown.
Perform the workout as a circuit, doing 1 set of each exercise before resting for 2 minutes. Once you've done 1 set of each

movement, repeat the entire circuit 1 or 2 times. That way you'll do a total of 2 or 3 sets of each exercise. When you've completed the weight workout, finish with 5 minutes of high-

intensity cardio. Choose any cardio machine you like—treadmill, rower, stationary bike, VersaClimber—or simply hit the streets.

YOUR CHARGE

Exercise for 60 seconds at the highest effort you can maintain for the entire duration. Then slow

to an easy pace—say, about 30 percent of your top intensity—for another 60 seconds. Alternate

back and forth for the entire 5 minutes.

THE EXERCISES

1
Inverted Row

Secure a bar 3 to 4 feet above the floor. Lie under the bar and grab it with a shoulder-width, overhand grip. Hang at arm's length from the bar with your body in a straight line from your ankles to your shoulders. Keeping your body rigid at all times, pull your chest to the bar by bending your arms and squeezing your shoulder blades together. Pause, and then lower yourself back to the starting position. That's 1 repetition. Do a total of 10 to 12 reps.

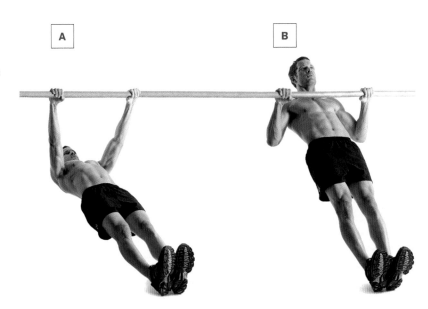

A

B

2
Mountain Climber

Kneel on all fours, your hands in line with but slightly wider than your shoulders. Straighten your left leg completely and lift your right knee toward your chest. You should be on the balls of your feet, positioned like a sprinter in the starting blocks. Now quickly switch leg positions as many times as you can for 30 to 45 seconds. That's 1 set.

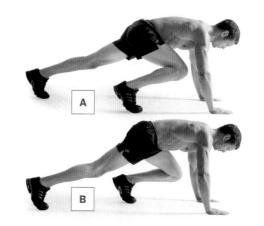

3
Split Squat to Push Press

Hold a barbell at chest level with an overhand grip that's just beyond shoulder width. Stand in a staggered stance, your left foot in front of your right. Keeping your torso upright, lower your body until your front knee is bent 90 degrees, and then simultaneously push yourself back to the start as you press the bar over your head. Lower the bar to the start. That's 1 rep. Do a total of 8 to 10 reps, and then switch leg positions and repeat. (If desired, you can use dumbbells instead of the barbell.)

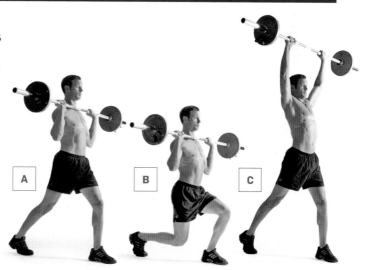

4
Dumbbell Woodchop

Hold a light dumbbell with a hand-over-hand grip, your arms extended above your right shoulder. Keeping your arms nearly straight, bend at your knees and forcefully rotate your torso to the left as you draw your arms down and across your body. (You should move as if you're chopping wood.) When your hands reach the outside of your left ankle, quickly reverse the movement with the same intensity. That's 1 repetition. Do 10 to 12 repetitions, then switch sides and repeat.

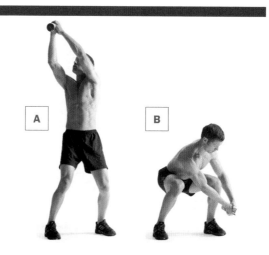

5
Squat Thrust-Chinup Combo

Squat on the floor beneath a chinup bar and lean forward so that your hands are on the floor and you're on the balls of your feet. To begin, quickly kick both legs back behind you into a pushup position. Immediately reverse the move and go back to the squat position. From there, jump up and grab the chinup bar with an underhand grip. Pull your chest to the bar. Drop back down and repeat. That's 1 rep. Do a total of 8 to 10 reps.

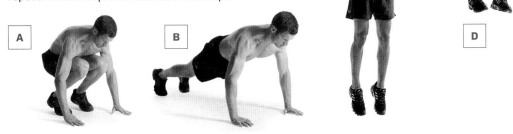

6
Pushup-Traveling Lunge Combo

Assume a pushup position, but instead of placing your hands on the floor, brace them on a pair of dumbbells. Now do as many pushups as you can. Then stand up with the dumbbells and perform a traveling lunge: Keeping your torso upright, take a step forward with your right leg and lower your body until your front knee is bent 90 degrees. Push from your front foot and step forward into a standing position. Next, repeat, lunging forward with your left leg. That's 1 rep. Do a total of 6 to 8 reps, and then turn around and do the combo in the other direction.

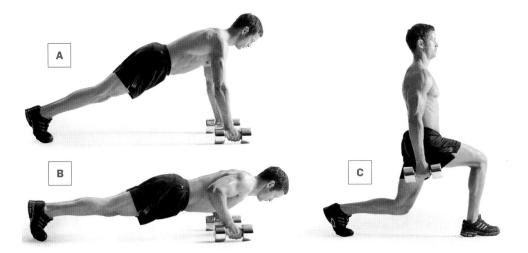

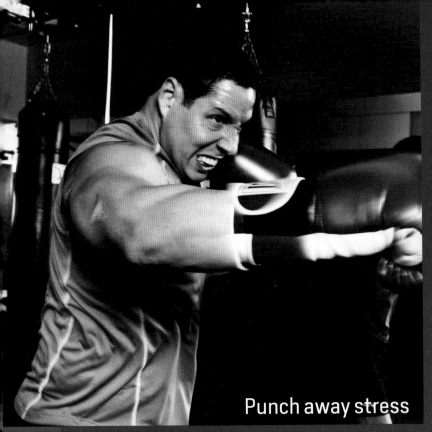

Punch away stress

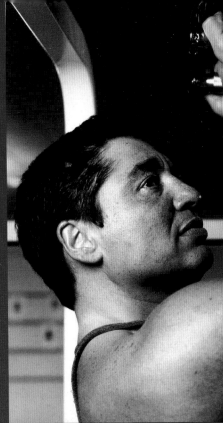

Get into the Best Shape of Your Life

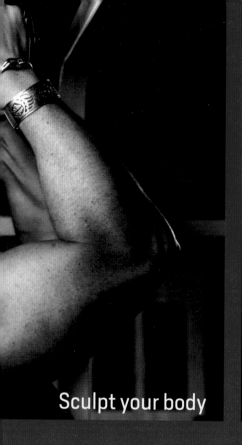

Sculpt your body

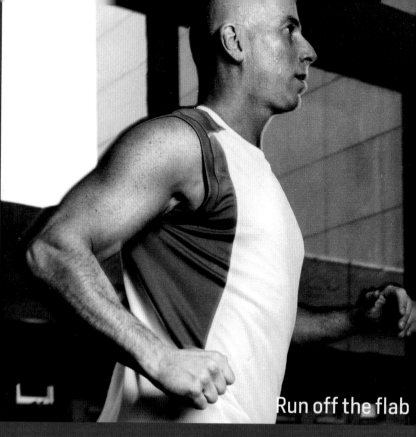

Run off the flab

HERE'S HOW THREE BUSY MEN PUT IT ALL TOGETHER IN THREE FITNESS AND NUTRITION PLANS. **THEIR STRATEGIES CHANGED THEIR LIVES—AND JUST MIGHT CHANGE YOURS**

With each rung he climbed on the corporate ladder,

commodities and equity trader Alex Gordon also loosened his belt a notch.

Gordon served as an officer in an Israeli Defense Force paratrooper unit in his early 20s, where the strict regimen trimmed his weight to 185 pounds and his waist to 32 inches.

"They train you until there is no fat left on your body," he says. "It was like wringing water from a wet towel."

Then he stayed lean on a diet of triathlons and marathons. The Manhattanite clocked his personal best of 3:26 in the New York Marathon at 28 years old and 190 pounds. But with success at the trading desk came added responsibilities.

"Business lunches, ideas dinners . . . every opportunity I had, I took clients out," says the 40-year-old. "It was steakhouses back to back to back: Smith and Wollensky's, Del Frisco, Peter Luger."

Gordon's visits to the gym went from medium rare to rare, and his weight slowly crept up until it reached 231 pounds and his waist measured 38 inches. "I still went to the gym, but I didn't have a training plan, so I had no consistency, no focus."

"I still went to the gym, but I didn't have a TRAINING PLAN."

Bill Stanton hit his 40s midstride, but he, too, was tripped up by success. The former New York City policeman had transitioned from street cop to bodyguard to private detective, earning a position as a security and safety expert for a major TV network and the moniker Wild Bill.

"The more successful you are, the more your ambition grows in other ways: You want to go on nicer holidays and eat in fancier restaurants," he says. "I was lulled into a false sense of security. I was doing the same old workouts, no problem, but it's the law of diminishing returns."

Once a ripped 175-pounder who competed in amateur bodybuilding contests, Stanton had ballooned to 222 pounds. "I could still bench 350," he says, "but my face was puffy, my heart raced when I climbed stairs, and my clothes were too tight. One day I looked in the mirror, and it hit me: I was fat. I wasn't comfortable with my body. It didn't fit me."

Mario Polit's battle with fat started in his 30s. That's when he switched career tracks, leaving his managerial job at a department store to become a New York City firefighter. Polit, who weighed 195 pounds in college, embraced the firehouse's all-you-can-eat culture and packed on the pounds.

"We scarfed down huge plates of rich food: Philly cheesesteaks, chops with gravy

The Power Circuit

MARIO POLIT **40, 6'1", Firefighter**

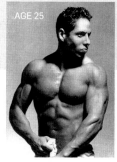
AGE 25

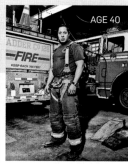
AGE 40

THE PLAN

THE POWER-CIRCUIT WORKOUT: Full-body cardio strength training with boxing (or another cardio activity such as running, basketball, cycling, or basketball)

WHO IT'S BEST FOR: Guys who are looking for an easy-to-learn weight circuit that uses common gym equipment and who also thrive doing solo cardiovascular training

THE GOAL: Reduce body fat to 15 percent, strengthen the core, add muscle tone, and improve cardiovascular fitness

DAILY ENERGY EXPENDITURE:
3,500 calories (basal metabolic rate, or BMR, factoring in exercise)

DAILY CALORIE BUDGET:
2,500

TRAINING PLAN

To help Mario Polit reclaim the 195-pound body he had in college, trainer Jean Jourdain, who is certified by the National Academy of Sports Medicine, designed a timed full-body strength circuit with an additional boxing component, because that's Polit's favorite kind of cardio.

"I wanted Mario to keep his heart rate up while exerting specific muscle groups," says Jourdain. "The combination of a timed circuit and boxing drills achieved that."

Boxing is an ideal core-strengthening and weight-loss exercise because the training demands a range of fast, intense movements. Plus, it's fun.

"Mario would power through the circuit, knowing he could then lace up the gloves. With other athletes, I'd swap boxing for running

or hoops or whatever it was they felt passionate about."

The program also suited Polit's desire to blend traditional free weights with modern fitness devices. "Guys in the firehouse laughed when I said I was doing pushups on a stability ball," says Polit. "But the truth is that I could bang out 30 pushups easily on the ground, and I struggled to do 10 on the ball. Now I can do 30 on the ball, and a lot of my colleagues can't even do five." Polit says the pace of the circuit surprised him—there's no time for watching TV or chatting—while the repetitive action of the boxing drills proved meditative and honed his coordination.

THE RESULTS

	BEFORE	AFTER
WEIGHT	240 LB	220 LB
BODY FAT	29%	19%
CHOLESTEROL		
TOTAL	170	150
HDL	60	50
LDL	94	86
TRIGLYCERIDES	73	69
WAIST SIZE	38 INCHES	35 INCHES

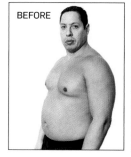
BEFORE

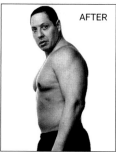
AFTER

NUTRITION PLAN

"I'd often sit down for dinner and eat two baskets of bread, soaking each piece in olive oil," says Polit. "When I start *(continued)* eating, I go full bore."

At the firehouse, he's often surrounded by pasta, doughnuts, and soda. Skolnik, who regularly works with lineman-size appetites, advised Polit to eat smaller portions up to six times a day and replace soda with water.

"I've found that it helps big guys to know they can eat again in a few hours," she says. "With Mario, it was a matter of explaining the portion sizes and emphasizing more vegetables and protein, and then finding snacks that would tide him over between meals."

Polit's lipid profile was good at the start of the program, and it improved, thanks to the exercise and diet changes. But his doctor would still like to see Polit's body-fat percentage drop by a point or two. (Polit was ill for 2 weeks near the start of the diet and lost early momentum, but he has since edged under 18 percent.)

"It was tough," says Polit. "I used to eat until I was full. Now, I eat the right portion size and I savor every bite. I sometimes chew 30 times before swallowing. If I'm still hungry, I don't sweat it, because I know I can snack again soon."

The Power Circuit

WARMUP (5 to 10 minutes): Jump rope, spin on a bike, or cruise on the elliptical trainer at a gentle pace. You should be able to hold a conversation.

CARDIO STRENGTH CIRCUIT: Do each exercise for 1 minute (use a weight that you can lift for that amount of time, usually 60 percent to 70 percent of your 1-repetition max) with no rest between exercises. Aim to keep your heart rate elevated for the entire circuit. Once you complete one cycle of exercises, rest for 90 seconds. After 4 weeks, reduce the rest to 60 seconds, and after another 4 weeks, reduce to 45 seconds. Complete each cycle three times. Aim for one rest day between Days 1 and 2, and 2 days after Day 3.

DAY 1

Part 1: Total body with emphasis on chest, back, legs, core, and arms

STABILITY-BALL DUMBBELL CHEST PRESS: After 1 minute, reduce the weight by half or a third (depending on your fatigue level) and do an-other minute.

LOW ROW USING DUMBBELL: After a minute, reduce the weight by half and do another minute.

BODY-WEIGHT SQUAT: After 4 weeks, add dumbbells. After 8 weeks, try one-legged squats.

HIP BRIDGE: Aim for 30 seconds on each leg. If you are strong enough, you can progress to 45 seconds or 1 minute on each leg.

STABILITY-BALL PUSHUP

Part 2: Boxing (or another full-body cardio workout)

HEAVY BAG (15 minutes): Punching a heavy bag incorporates core movement and explosiveness and helps loosen the body after weight training, says trainer Jean Jourdain. A typical workout involves four 3-minute rounds, with 1 minute of rest, and the boxer performs drills for throwing different combinations of speed and power punches.

MITT WORK (10 minutes): During mitt training, the boxer fires punches at the trainer, who also counterpunches. "It's a total-body workout," says Jourdain. "Plus, it tests reactions, coordination, and speed."

Note: Boxing can be replaced by another full-body cardio workout, such as interval training on a rowing machine, spin bike, treadmill, or elliptical trainer, or activities such as basketball, soccer, or a martial art.

DAY 2

Part 1: Total body with emphasis on core

ABS CRUNCH ON STABILITY BALL

OBLIQUE TWIST RIGHT ON STABILITY BALL

OBLIQUE TWIST LEFT ON STABILITY BALL

HANGING LEG RAISE

SUPERMAN

Part 2: Boxing (or another full-body cardio workout)

DAY 3

Part 1: Total body with emphasis on shoulders, biceps, triceps, and core

STABILITY-BALL DUMBBELL SHOULDER PRESS

DUMBBELL ALTERNATING LATERAL RAISE

LYING TRICEPS EXTENSION (a.k.a. skull crusher)

DUMBBELL BICEPS CURL

PLANK ON A BOSU BALL

After 4 weeks, start to tilt the ball from side to side, as this will fire different muscles in your abs.

Part 2: Choose from cardio menu.

and mash, penne with chicken parm," says the 40-year-old. "Chased by Entenmann's cakes and chocolate-chip cookies, of course!"

While some of the younger firefighters stayed trim, Polit's weight increased rapidly and topped out at 240. "Some of my family members are on the heavier side," says Polit. "I realized that I could let myself go very easily. My wife had been nagging me to lose the flab, and turning 40 gave me the impetus. The alarm bell was ringing: It was now or never."

Like many guys in their 40s, these three men found themselves perched precariously on a slippery slope. Science tells us that the 40s are the critical decade to arrest the spread of fat and build muscle. By 40, the body's metabolism has slowed 4 percent since age 20, which means it doesn't burn as many calories. Sarcopenia, the inexorable deterioration of muscle mass that starts at 25 and advances at about a pound a year, is also kicking in, stealing the results of hours spent at the gym. Body-fat percentage is creeping up and with it our size. Muscle is about 20 percent denser than fat, so 1 pound of muscle is roughly the size of a base-ball, while 1 pound of fat equals a softball. Combined, these factors cause a snowball effect, which softens the physiques of many men and deposits their bloated selves into the La-Z-Boy of middle age.

We presented Alex, Bill, and Mario with a challenge: Try to wind the age clock back 20 years in 12 weeks. We teamed up with trainers at the Sports Club L.A. and Reebok Sports Club, both in New York City, to create three customized workouts; enlisted certified dietitian Heidi Skolnik, a fellow of the American College of Sports Medi-

Muscle is about 20 PERCENT DENSER THAN FAT. One pound of muscle is around the size of a baseball.

cine and team nutritionist to the New York Giants, to consult on each man's diet; and tapped Stephen Lamm, MD, a clinical professor of medicine at New York University and the author of *The Hardness Factor*, to provide medical guidance.

The goal wasn't for these men to drop as much weight as possible, but to reshape their bodies in a healthy way by replacing fat with muscle and lowering their body-fat percentages.

"Fat cells are like toxic dumps in your body. They increase inflammation and the risk of heart disease and cancer," says Dr. Lamm. "Reducing your body-fat percentage is the best way to reduce the most dangerous kind of fat, visceral fat, which marshmallows around your organs."

That 1-pound baseball of muscle also burns 50 calories more per day than the softball of fat. So by lowering your body-fat percentage, you rev up your metabolism, which reverses that snowball effect.

Each of the workouts in this chapter blends elements of cardio and resistance training—the combination that experts say is essential to full-body health, but each achieves it in its own way. Turns out they all work. Pick the one that suits your goals and reclaim your body today. ■

The Pump and Burn

ALEX GORDON **40, 6', Stock Trader**

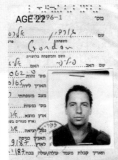

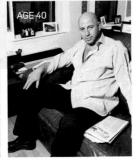

AGE 22

AGE 40

THE PLAN

THE POWER-CIRCUIT WORKOUT: High-intensity free weights and interval training with resistance

WHO IT'S BEST FOR: Guys who want to upgrade their weight-training workouts and progress beyond standard gym machines and who have a strong cardio background

THE GOAL: Reduce body fat to 15 percent and build a lean, powerful body with a rock-solid core

DAILY ENERGY EXPENDITURE:
3,400 calories (basal metabolic rate, or BMR, factoring in exercise)
DAILY CALORIE BUDGET: 2,600

TRAINING PLAN

Alex Gordon, a former tri-athlete, expected trainer Greg Gurenlian to stick him on a treadmill and have him slog away for hours. Instead, Gurenlian treated him like a sprinter and created a workout that's heavy on free weights and intense intervals.

"Alex told me he wanted to lose weight, but didn't want to look emaciated," says Gurenlian. "That requires resistance training, so I had to teach him how to lift."

Gurenlian, who previously worked as a strength trainer at Penn State University, says his mantra is effort and efficiency.

"Everything Alex did was done at a very high pace, using the most amount of muscle possible for short bursts. First he pumped iron, then he burned through intervals." The workout is based on undulating perio-dization, which, simply put, trains the two main kinds of muscle fiber on a set schedule. It involves varying the number of repetitions (from 3 to 5 to 8 to 10) over time, not every set, as in most workouts.

"I have never felt this strong," says Gordon. "My energy has sky-rocketed, and I feel supercreative." He also noticed another benefit: better sleep. "Now, when my head touches the pillow, I'm gone."

NUTRITION PLAN

Dietitian Heidi Skolnik realized Gordon had three major bad habits: big nights at the steakhouse, binge snacking, and beer guzzling. She taught him a smarter approach to eating out: Start with soup to curb his appetite and order lean cuts, such as filet mignon. She also helped

THE RESULTS

	BEFORE	AFTER
WEIGHT	231 LB	196 LB
BODY FAT	26%	16%
CHOLESTEROL		
TOTAL	182	162
HDL	63	76
LDL	75	64
TRIGLYCERIDES	222	64
WAIST SIZE	38 INCHES	33 INCHES

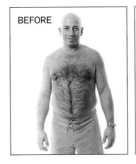

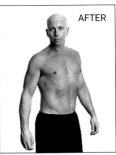

BEFORE

AFTER

him implement a snack strategy—stash yogurt in the fridge, trail mix in his briefcase, and instant oatmeal in his desk drawer—so that if he missed a meal, he wouldn't be scavenging for Snickers bars.

"Cravings tend to last 20 minutes," says Skolnik. "Knowing that can help you wait it out. Another trick is to drink water, because it can help you feel full." Gordon also replaced the three or four beers he drank every night with two glasses of wine.

After 12 weeks, Gordon had trimmed 5 inches off his waist and halved his triglyceride levels, factors which reduce his risk of developing a metabolic disorder. At the end of the program, Gordon didn't celebrate with a feast.

"I had a glass of cabernet and a 7-ounce filet," says Gordon. "It's all about discipline."

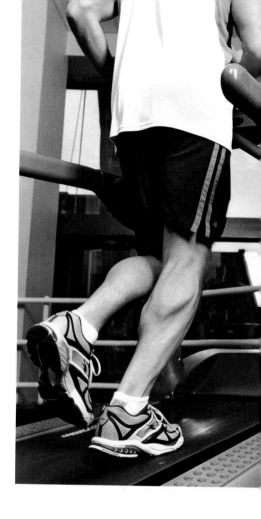

The Pump and Burn Regimen

Trainer Greg Gurenlian divided each session into three or four exercises followed by 15 or 20 minutes of interval training with a resistance element. The odd-numbered weeks are heavy: Do 7 sets of 2 to 5 repetitions of a weight that is 85 to 95 percent of your 1-repetition max. On even-numbered weeks, flip the sets and reps: Do 3 sets of 8 to 10 repetitions of a weight that is 70 to 80 percent of your 1-rep max.

In between sets, Gurenlian had Alex Gordon choose from the following core-training menu: 10 crunches, 10 incline crunches, 10 bicycle crunches, 10 hanging leg raises, or a 1-minute plank.

WARM-UP Jump rope or run for 5 minutes at a gentle pace. You should be able to hold a conversation easily.

DAY 1

Part 1: BARBELL BENCH
Active rest: 10 crunches

BARBELL DEADLIFT
Active rest: 1-minute plank

PULL-UP Depending on your ability, add weights on odd-numbered weeks. Active rest: 10 hanging leg raises

Part 2: 20-MINUTE RUNNING INTERVAL Jog for 5 minutes at a conversational pace, and then increase the incline to steep and do five 1-minute intervals at 85 percent of your max heart rate (or as fast a pace as you can sustain for 1 minute). Do 2 minutes of active recovery between each 1-minute interval. After 6 weeks, cut the recovery time to 1 minute.

DAY 2

Part 1: INCLINE BENCH
Active rest: 10 bicycle crunches

BARBELL SQUAT
Active rest: 10 incline crunches

PUSH PRESS
Active rest: 10 hanging leg raises

ROMANIAN DEADLIFT
Active rest: 1-minute plank

Part 2: 20-MINUTE CYCLING INTERVAL Spin for 5 minutes at a conversational pace, and then do five 1-minute intervals at 85 percent of your max heart rate (or as fast a pace as you can sustain), with 2 minutes of active recovery between each 1-minute interval. After 6 weeks, cut the recovery time to 1 minute.

DAY 3

Part 1: DIP Depending on your ability, add weights on odd-numbered weeks. Active rest: 10 incline crunches

LEG PRESS Active rest: 1-minute plank

BARBELL BENT-OVER ROW
Active rest: 10 hanging leg raises

Part 2: 20-MINUTE ROWING INTERVAL Row for 5 minutes at a conversational pace, and then do five 1-minute intervals at 85 percent of your max heart rate (or as fast a pace as you can sustain for 1 minute). Do 2 minutes of active recovery between each 1-minute interval. After 6 weeks, cut the recovery time to 1 minute.

The New School

BILL STANTON **44, 5'8" Security expert**

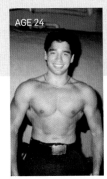

AGE 24

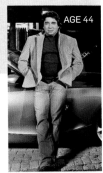

AGE 44

THE PLAN

THE NEW-SCHOOL WORKOUT: Full-body functional strength training with high-intensity cardio-sculpt classes

WHO IT'S BEST FOR: Guys who are bored with the traditional gym experience and who are not afraid of trying a completely different kind of workout

THE GOAL: Reduce body fat to 15 percent and build a lean, powerful body with a rock-solid core

DAILY ENERGY EXPENDITURE:
3,300 calories (BMR, factoring in exercise)
DAILY CALORIE BUDGET: 2,300

TRAINING PLAN

"Bill had overtrained his arms and chest muscles for 20 years, so his posture was out of whack and he was at an enormous risk for injury," says strength and conditioning coach, athletic trainer, and physical therapist Kimberly Caspare. "He was so weak that he couldn't do a single plank. He was on his knees after eight seconds."

Caspare sees many 40-year-olds who jump into new regimens and injure their rotator cuffs or herniate a disk, so she created a three-phase workout for Stanton, starting with 4 weeks of full-body drills to strengthen his stabilizer muscles.

"The pace and the movements shocked my system," says Stanton. In Phase 2, Caspare dialed up the weights and intensity to forge new muscle mass. "Phase 1 is the jackhammer, and Phase 2 is the building blocks. In Phase 3, I break

out the chisel to etch definition," she says. Throughout, Stanton also went to a cardio-sculpting class run by instructor Stephanie Levinson, creator of the Extreme Games workout. It consists of nonstop cardio and strength-training drills that incorporate dumbbells, body bars, medicine balls, and steps.

NUTRITION PLAN

"I knew my cholesterol was high," says Stanton, "but not 282!" In consultation with a doctor and a dietician, Stanton radically changed his diet and drinking habits.

Before the program, Stanton admits he sometimes ate bacon at every meal: draped on waffles, layered on cheeseburgers, and wrapped around shrimp. Plus, he gorged on fast food and guzzled soft drinks. While his wine consumption was a healthy glass or two a

day, he was prone to weekend binges.

Dietitian Heidi Skolnik recommended that he eat five or six small meals a day, replace rich foods with grilled fish or lean meat and salads, drink water instead of soda, and limit his binge drinking to once a month. After 7 weeks, Stanton was on track. "Now I think of my workout and diet like balancing a checkbook. If I put in more, then I know I have to take out more. There's no way to cheat the math." ∎

THE RESULTS

	BEFORE	AFTER
WEIGHT	222 LB	197 LB
BODY FAT	24%	16%
CHOLESTEROL		
TOTAL	282	205
HDL	41	48
LDL	172	140
TRIGLYCERIDES	346	84
WAIST SIZE	37 INCHES	33 INCHES

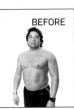

BEFORE

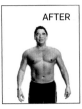

AFTER

The New-School Regimen

PHASE 1
Part 1: Weeks 1 to 4, days 1 and 3

Muscle-Balancing Drills
These exercises are low in intensity and high in repetitions. Rest for no more than 30 seconds between sets and exercises.
Warmup: Do 5 minutes on the elliptical trainer, bike, or treadmill. Then do these six exercises:

1. HIGH-KNEE WALK (20 yards)

2. WALKING BACKWARD LUNGE WITH ARMS ON HEAD (20 yards)

3. WALKING FORWARD LUNGE WITH ARMS ON HEAD (20 yards)

4. OVER/UNDER HURDLE WITH LATERAL LUNGE (20 on each leg)

5. SPIDERMAN STRETCH (10 on each leg)

6. PUSHUP (10 reps)

THE EXERCISES:
PLANK Hold the position for 30 seconds per repetition (use your knees if need be) and build up to 60 seconds. Do 3 reps.

BOSU SQUAT with cable row: Do 3 sets of 10.

INVERTED ROW with heels on a Bosu ball: Do 3 sets of 12.

STABILITY-BALL DUMBBELL CHEST PRESS: Do 3 sets of 12 at 70 percent of your 1-rep maximum.

DEADLIFT with bar: Do 3 sets of 12 at 70 percent of your 1-rep max.

STANDING EXTERNAL CABLE ROTATION: Do 3 sets of 12 per arm.

BRIDGE on a Bosu ball: Do 3 reps of 30 seconds or until your form is compromised.

Day 2 High-intensity cardio-sculpting (45 to 60 minutes) Man up and take a class at your local gym: You're looking for a description that includes the key words "strength training" and "interval workout."

PHASE 2
Weeks 5 to 8, Days 1 and 3

Building Muscle Mass and Explosive Strength
The number of repetitions is reduced, and the amount of weight is increased. Do the exercises as 3 supersets (i.e., do each exercise back to back with no rest in between). Rest for 90 seconds before repeating each superset two more times. **Warmup:** See Phase 1.

THE EXERCISES:
Superset 1
PLYOMETRIC CROCODILE BOSU PUSHUP: Aim for 15 reps per set.

BARBELL BENCH PRESS: The first set is 15 reps at 70 percent of your 1-rep max. The second set is 10 reps at 80 percent of your 1-rep max. The third set is six reps at 90 percent of your 1-rep max.

SQUAT THRUST TO PULLUP
Aim for 10 reps per set.

Superset 2
SIDE PLANK WITH DUMBBELL TORSO ROTATION: Aim for 3 sets of 10 on each side per set.

BARBELL BENT-OVER ROW: The first set is 15 reps at 70 percent of your 1-rep max. The second set is 10 reps at 80 percent of your 1-rep max. The third set is six reps at 90 percent of your 1-rep max.

SKATER'S SINGLE-LEG SQUAT
Aim for eight reps per leg per set.

Superset 3
SINGLE-LEG DUMBBELL DEADLIFT
The first set is six reps per leg at 90 percent of your 1-rep max. The second set is 10 reps per leg at 80 percent of your 1-rep max. The third set is 15 reps per leg at 70 percent of your 1-rep max.

MOUNTAIN CLIMBER
One 45-second rep.

HANG CLEAN WITH PRESS
Do 8 reps per set.

Day 2 High-intensity cardio sculpting (45 to 60 minutes). See Phase 1.

PHASE 3
Weeks 9 to 12, Days 1 and 3
Combining Toning, Endurance, and Power Exercises
The exercises are performed as 3 supersets (back to back with no rest). Rest 90 seconds before repeating each superset 3 more times.
Warmup: See Phase 1.

Superset 1
CABLE CHEST FLY in lunge position: Aim for 8 repetitions per leg per set.

STANDING CABLE CROSSOVER: Aim for 10 reps per set.

SIDE PLANK with reverse-fly pulley: Aim for 12 reps per side per set.

Superset 2
KAYAK ON A BOSU BALL with a 15-pound bar: Aim for 25 seconds per set.

BAR OVERHEAD BILATERAL LEG LOWERING: Aim for 10 reps per leg.

SQUAT on a Bosu ball with a medicine ball overhead: Aim for 12 to 15 reps per set

Superset 3
SINGLE-LEG SNATCH
with dumbbell: Aim for 7 reps per leg per set.

OBLIQUE CABLE WOOD CHOP
on Bosu ball: Aim for 15 reps per side per set.

STABILITY-BALL CRUNCH
with medicine-ball thrust: Aim for 45 seconds per set.

Day 2 High-intensity cardio sculpting (45 to 60 minutes). See Phase 1.

EXERCISE SCIENCE

DON'T BE A STATISTIC

While the number of men with gym memberships has increased 16 percent since 2003, the number who hit the weights has dropped by an alarming 15 percent. Why is that alarming? Because lifting weights 3 days a week can:

1. Cut your risk of diabetes in just 4 months, according to a Tufts University study. Weight training decreases blood-glucose levels and improves insulin sensitivity.

2. Treat depression, according to Harvard researchers who compared the benefits of weight training and cardio exercise over 10 weeks. The lifters experienced a greater mood boost.

3. Spike your testosterone levels by up to 49 percent, according to Finnish scientists. The hormone plays a key role in your overall mortality risk and, of course, your sex drive.

4. Save your brain from a stroke, according to a University of Michigan study. Lifting weights decreases blood pressure, reducing the risk of a stroke by 40 percent.

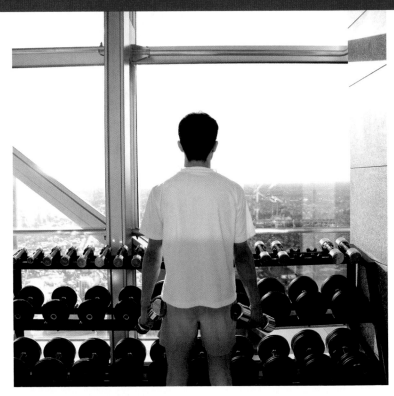

GET FIT TO LIVE LONG

The jiggle around your waist might not be the death sentence it has been made out to be. A study in the *Journal of the American Medical Association* found that overweight and obese people who are physically fit, as determined by an exercise test, are 50 percent less likely to die prematurely than their thin but out-of-shape peers.

ARM YOURSELF

Doing biceps curls can increase your life span. Men who have the highest muscle mass in their upper arms are 36 percent less likely to die from any cause of death than those with smaller arm muscles, according to a new study in the *American Journal of Clinical Nutrition*.

THINK LIKE THIS

Thinking about the benefits of exercise isn't as motivational as thinking about specific actions that would make exercise more doable, says a new study in the *Journal of Applied Biobehavioral Research*.

"Imagining being active triggers positive and realistic steps," says lead researcher Laura Ten Eyck, PhD.

THOUGHTS THAT MAKE EXERCISE MORE LIKELY:

1. I'll listen to music or a book, or watch TV, while working out.
2. I'll set a goal.
3. I'll make exercise interesting (such as choosing a treadmill with a good view).
4. I'll exercise in a comfortable environment (such as an air-conditioned, uncrowded gym).
5. I'll make a schedule.

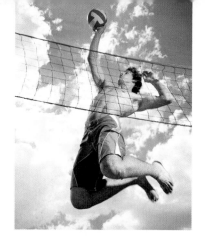

THOUGHTS THAT WON'T MOTIVATE YOU TO EXERCISE

1. I won't feel tense or like a failure.
2. I'll have more energy.
3. I won't be grumpy with other people.
4. I'll set a good example for my kids or friends.
5. I'll be in a better mood.

WORK OUT WITH WATER

Just because you're not an endurance athlete doesn't mean you're off the hydration hook. Water is a powerful lifting aid. University of Connecticut researchers discovered that men who hydrated with water before lifting completed 17 percent more reps per set during a lower-body workout than thirsty exercisers. Turns out, your central nervous system slows your muscle activation when you're not adequately hydrated. So drink 16 ounces of water just before training, and then 8 ounces for every 20 minutes of hard work.

BUILD A HARD BODY WITH HARD ROCK

Music can make you stronger, report researchers at Dalhousie University, in Canada. In a recent study, they discovered that people who listened to tunes as they lifted weights experienced significantly greater strength gains in 4 weeks than lifters who wore noise-blocking earplugs.

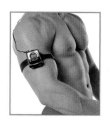

"The music may have reduced people's perception of effort during training, allowing them to work harder," says the study author, Jo M. Welch, PhD. The secret to song selection: Simply download the music you think is most motivational.

TRAIN YOUR ABS—FAST

Want a six-pack sooner? Do your core exercises explosively. Spanish scientists found that performing ab exercises at a fast tempo activates more muscle than doing them slowly. The reason: To speed your movement, your muscles have to generate higher amounts of

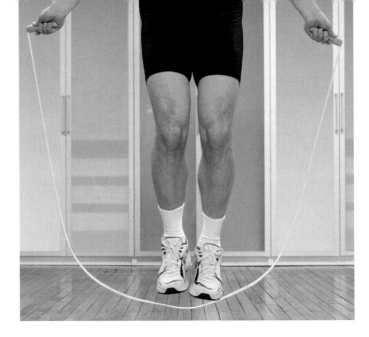

force, say the researchers.

Try it with the medicine ball slam: Grab a ball with both hands, and in one move, raise it over and behind your head, tighten your core (and keep it braced), step forward, and slam the ball to the floor. Do as many reps as you can in 20 seconds.

ELEVATE YOUR GAINS

Fast lifting can lead to fast strength. In a 2-month study, researchers at the College of New Jersey had men do explosive chest exercises, such as plyometric pushups, prior to a heavy bench-press workout 1 or 2 days a week. The result: The men benched 5 percent more weight than those who

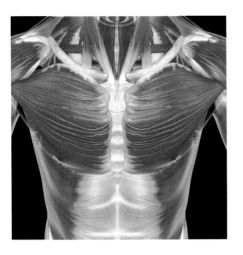

skipped the power exercises.

"Explosive training helps you press through weak spots by teaching your muscles to contract faster," says study author Nicholas Ratamess, PhD. Try the pushup: Simply push up as forcefully as you can so that your hands leave the floor each rep.

For explosive exercises, do 5 sets of 3 to 6 repetitions, resting 3 minutes between sets.

GAIN MORE MUSCLE...FASTER

Circuit training (doing short continuous sets of anaerobic exercise) spurs greater gains in explosive power than combining circuit training with endurance workouts, according

to a study in the *Journal of Strength and Conditioning Research*. Volunteers who did a circuit routine of lunges, drop jumps, hurdle jumps, single-leg hops, and arm, back, and hip extensions for 12 weeks saw greater strength improvements than did peers who combined the circuit routine with five high-intensity intervals.

EASE YOUR PAIN

Tired of having sore muscles? Combine your cardio and weight workouts, say researchers at the University of California at Santa Cruz. By performing a 30- to 45-second cardio burst prior to each resistance exercise, men reduced soreness instantly. And after 4 weeks, they were sore no more.

"This method accelerates muscle repair," says W. Jackson Davis, PhD, the lead study author. Start by increasing the intensity of your warmup until you reach a vigorous pace. Then continue with your weight routine, but before each set, jump rope or do sprints for 30 seconds.

Your cardio should be intense enough to keep your maximum heart rate between 76 percent and 93 percent throughout your training.

DON'T WORRY, BE STRONG

Here's another reason to forget about your problems: Stress can make you weak.

In a recent study, University of Texas researchers found that lifters who were stress-free showed greater strength gains in the bench press and squat than those who were stressed out.

One theory: People who are highly stressed tend to follow unhealthy diets and sleep less, both of which may affect their workout performance, says John Bartholomew, PhD, the study's coauthor. What's more, elevated stress-

hormone levels can hamper muscle recovery. So if you've quit making gains in the gym, assess your lifestyle: Maybe it needs more attention than your exercise plan does.

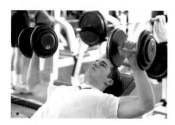

DON'T CAVE IN TO PAIN

Don't let soreness derail your fitness program. Stick with a new workout plan for 8 weeks, and the aches will probably subside. Japanese scientists found that out-of-practice martial artists who resumed training and kept at it suffered less post-workout muscle damage and inflammation after 2 months. It takes time for muscle tissue to strengthen to the point where you can endure an intense exercise regimen without experiencing muscle pain, say the study authors.

When starting a fitness program, mark the 2-month point on a calendar. Soreness should be tolerable by then.

UNBUCKLE THIS BELT

Even if you don't think weight belts look ridiculous (they do), you should know that there is no benefit to wearing lumbar support.

After reviewing 15 trials involving some 15,000 people, Dutch researchers discovered no convincing evidence that weight belts help prevent or treat back injuries. If anything, wearing one of these guy girdles might give you a false sense of security about your ability to lift heavier loads.

Drop the weight belt: The best way to shore up your back is by strengthening your core muscles. Learn proper weight-lifting techniques at MensHealth-Trainer.com. ■

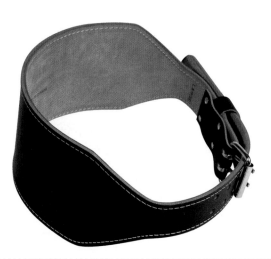

TRAINING TIPS Q&A

Q: What's a good warmup before I lift weights?

A: Doing two types of warmup is probably your best bet, and neither of the two steps below involve much cardio, says Mike Mejia, MS, CSCS, author of *The Men's Health Gym Bible.*

Step 1

First, complete a total-body circuit of five exercises (jumping jacks, squats, lunges, rows, and pushups, for example), but do only a few reps of each.

Why: You'll increase bloodflow, improve your range of motion, and activate muscle fibers, so you can exert more force in your workout.

Step 2

Now move to your first exercise and use a lighter-than-usual weight. Try 6 to 8 repetitions with 50 percent of your 1-rep max, followed by 3 or 4 reps at 65 percent to 70 percent. You need to warm up each muscle group only once.

Why: Lighter-weight sets let your muscles know what you're about to ask them to do. That way you're prepared for peak performance before you start.

Q: How often should I push my muscles to complete failure?

A: Training to failure means you can't perform one more repetition. Such extreme exertion can sabotage your muscle gains by making it difficult for you to recover between workouts—almost like running a car until it's out of gas, says Meija. Also, exhaustion can lead to poor form, which increases the likelihood of injury.

But used sparingly, training until your tank is empty can help promote growth. Try going to complete failure once every 4 to 6 weeks, but not on every set, or you'll run those risks of overexertion. Instead, find a spotter, complete 2 or 3 warmup sets, and then do 1 set to failure, staying within the range of 6 to 8 repetitions. Just make sure that you maintain perfect form from start to finish.

Q: Do isometric exercises work?

A: Sure. An isometric routine is a great addition to your workout if you're looking for a simple technique to build muscle. The concept is incorporate pausing or holding a weight so that the length of your muscle doesn't change—holding a biceps curl in a contracted position, for example. Keeping your muscle in a fixed position increases the time it's under tension, which can promote muscle growth.

Try it: After your last set, grab a lighter weight and hold it at the halfway point of a biceps curl (your forearm should be perpendicular to your upper arm) for 40 to 60 seconds. If you can't hold it for 40, the weight's too heavy; if you can hold it longer than 60, it's too light.

Q: Are the new vibration plates I saw at the gym a gimmick?

A: No, but don't believe everything you see in advertisers' "before" and "after" photos, says Neil Wolkodoff, PhD, developer of the PhysicalGolf training program.

Vibration plates aren't actually all that new. The Russians began using them back in the '60s to keep their cosmonauts strong during space travel. The benefit of using these plates was confirmed more recently by NASA, which showed that using vibration platforms during squats makes muscles work harder and thus grow faster. This is mostly due to the fact that, to keep your body steady, the muscles in your legs must fire each time the plate vibrates, which happens up to 60 times per second. Studies also suggest that the physical stress caused by the vibrations can increase bone density, reducing the risk of osteoporosis.

That said, some experts worry that vibration plates might facilitate a range of injuries from back pain to cartilage damage. Similarly, if you have cardiovascular issues or artificial joints, you'd be smart to remain on terra firma. The current generation of plates also won't do an ounce of good for upper-body strength (although keep an eye out for future models with vibrating handles to tone muscles above the waist).

Bottom line: If you're already in good health, using plates can help strengthen your legs, but don't think they'll shorten your workout time, as many manufacturers claim. There's no substitute for hard work in the gym.

Q: Is the *Wii Fit* a legit conditioning tool?

A: It depends how fit you already are, says H. James Phillips, PhD, an assistant professor of physical therapy and athletic training at Seton Hall University in New Jersey. *Wii Fit* uses a balance board to interact with yoga, strength, and aerobic programs and is well suited to unconditioned sorts: video-game-addicted kids, couch potatoes, people just getting into fitness, and those rehabbing from injuries. For such people, the board gives tremendous feedback regarding core stability, and the pushups, lunges, squats, and other exercises in the strength program will offer a mild to moderate workout.

If you're interested in building muscle and increasing aerobic endurance, however,

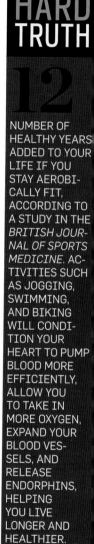

HARD TRUTH

12

NUMBER OF HEALTHY YEARS ADDED TO YOUR LIFE IF YOU STAY AEROBICALLY FIT, ACCORDING TO A STUDY IN THE *BRITISH JOURNAL OF SPORTS MEDICINE.* ACTIVITIES SUCH AS JOGGING, SWIMMING, AND BIKING WILL CONDITION YOUR HEART TO PUMP BLOOD MORE EFFICIENTLY, ALLOW YOU TO TAKE IN MORE OXYGEN, EXPAND YOUR BLOOD VESSELS, AND RELEASE ENDORPHINS, HELPING YOU LIVE LONGER AND HEALTHIER.

don't waste your time. In fact, the aerobic program is the Wii Fit's weakest link. Fancy graphics will never make up for the fact that you're running in place. If you insist on sweating to a video game, pop in the boxing program that comes with the Wii, or gather your kids and play Dance Dance Revolution, which is making its way into school physical education programs across the country.

The bottom line, however, is that fitness video games simply can't compete with conventional weight and aerobic training if you're an active adult.

Q: If squats and lunges work the same muscles, do I really need to do both?

A: Yes. And here's why: The squat allows you to use heavier weights, since both feet remain firmly planted on the floor throughout the move, says Meija. So it's great for packing on strength and size. During a lunge, your glutes must work especially hard to decelerate your body as you sink down, which boosts performance in sports such as basketball.

But doing both the squat and lunge in the same workout can be brutal. Instead, try doing the squat for 3 or 4 weeks, and then swap it out for the lunge in the following 3 or 4 weeks of training. Do 3 sets of 6 to 8 repetitions. Then you can try including both exercises in your leg workout, but scale back your sets. Do 2 sets of 6 to 8 reps of each move. Squat first, and then lunge.

Q: What exercise at the gym receives too much hype?

A: The triceps kickback provides little benefit. This exercise--you bend over, pin your arm at your side in a right angle, and extend it straight back--places your arm in a position that makes it hard to overload your muscles, and limits resistance for all but the last quarter of the move. Instead, challenge your triceps with body-weight extensions, which keep your muscles under constant tension.

Adjust a Smith machine bar so that it's level with your lower chest. Step back and grab the bar as if you're about to perform a pushup, but keep your hands closer than shoulder width apart and in line with your head. Bend at your elbows and bring your forehead toward the bar, keeping your body straight from head to ankles. Pause at the lowest point possible, usually inches from the bar, then press back up. Perform 3 sets of 8 to 10 repetitions.

Q: Can I build a big chest with dumbbells?

A: Definitely. Try this spin on the dumbbell chest press: Lie faceup on a bench and hold the dumbbells at your chest, palms facing each other. As you raise the weights, rotate your hands so your palms face your feet. To make this effective, train your chest twice a week. Do 5 sets of 5 reps in your first workout, resting a minute or two between sets. The next time, do 3 sets of 8 to 12 reps with rest periods of 45 to 60 seconds.

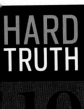

HARD TRUTH

10 YEARS YOUNGER YOUR BODY WILL FEEL IF YOU EXERCISE VIGOROUSLY FOR THREE HOURS A WEEK (WORKING UP A SWEAT) COMPARED WITH THOSE WHO EXERCISE FOR 15 MINUTES A WEEK, ACCORDING TO A STUDY IN THE *ARCHIVES OF INTERNAL MEDICINE*

Q: **Can using a fitness trail really accelerate my muscle gains?**

A: Absolutely. The beauty of fitness trails is that they encourage cross training, which combines strength training, core muscle building, and cardiovascular conditioning in a single workout. Weaving such training into your routine will reduce your risk of injury, boost athletic performance, and help balance the musculature of your body.

The key is to find a trail with upper-body exercises (pullups and pushups), middle-body exercises (planks and situps), and lower-body exercises (squats and lunges).

Q: **I'm in good shape, but I run out of energy quickly at the gym. What's going on?**

A: If you lose steam before you can even begin to impress your local gym vixen, you're probably suffering from exercise-induced hypoglycemia.

When people with the condition consume too many fast-digesting carbohydrates just before they work out, their blood sugar spikes and then free-falls as they start to exercise. The prescription?

"If you're prone to hypoglycemic symptoms, such as weakness, irritability, and fatigue, you must avoid fast-digesting carbohydrates prior to your workout," says Cassandra Forsythe, MS, an exercise science and nutrition researcher at the University of Connecticut.

She recommends fueling up instead with a meal consisting of 15 to 30 grams of protein and 40 to 50 grams of slow-digesting carbohydrates, such as a scoop of whey protein in cooked steel-cut oatmeal, or ground turkey with whole-wheat pasta and sugar-free tomato sauce. Do this approximately 1 to 2 hours before you start your gym routine.

If that doesn't do the trick and you find you're still bonking too soon, add some fat in the form of a tablespoon of natural nut butter (peanut or almond) or olive oil to the menu; it'll help put the brakes on your blood sugar.

Q: **Should I skip sleep to make time for a workout?**

A: If you're sleep deprived and not just groggy, stay in bed. University of Chicago researchers report that lack of sleep can torpedo weight loss by slowing metabolism, increasing appetite, and decreasing the number of calories burned.

Along the same lines, a 2006 study from the University of Hull, England, found that sleep-deprived participants who worked out had slower reaction times and were more susceptible to negative moods later in the day. And if you think a workout will wake you up, think again.

"Going to the gym when you're tired will only improve your alertness for a short time," says Kenneth Wright, PhD, an assistant professor of integrative physiology at the University of Colorado at Boulder. On the bright side, opting for the extra shut-eye could actually create time during the day for a workout. When you're well rested, your productivity and efficiency increase, Dr. Wright says. So use that to your advantage by leaving work earlier or taking a longer lunch break to go to the gym. ■

HARD TRUTH

7

THE LUCKY NUMBER OF HOURS OF SLEEP TO AIM FOR. A 22-YEAR STUDY OF 21,268 ADULTS PUBLISHED IN THE JOURNAL *SLEEP* FOUND THAT SLEEPING FOR FEWER THAN 7 HOURS A NIGHT IS ASSOCIATED WITH A 26 PERCENT INCREASE IN THE LIKELIHOOD OF EARLY DEATH IN MEN. SURPRISINGLY, THE STUDY ALSO FOUND THAT GETTING MORE THAN 8 HOURS IS DANGEROUS FOR MEN TOO: IT RAISES THE SAME RISK BY 24 PERCENT.

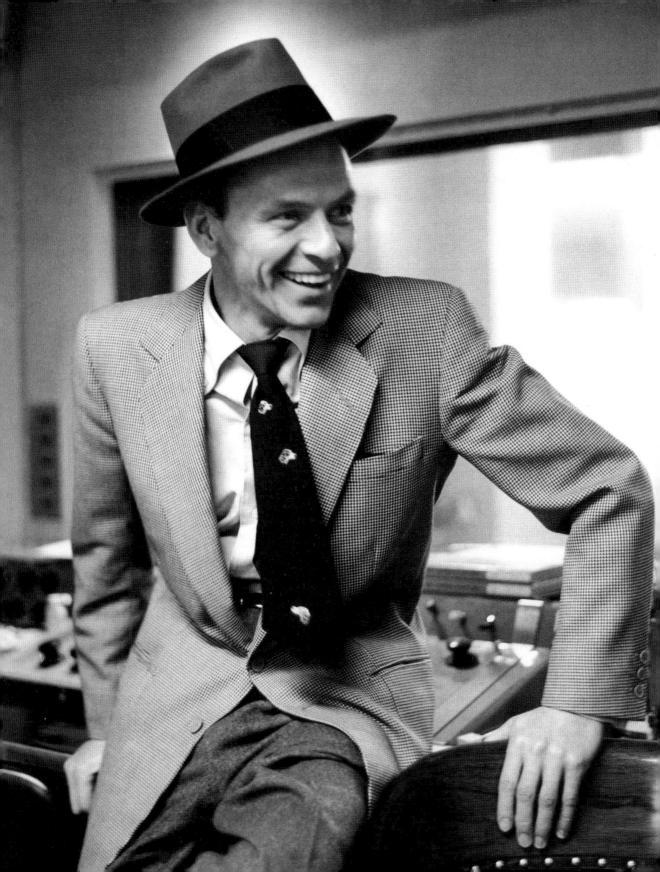

4

Look Better Instantly

Dress to Impress

THE 19 ESSENTIAL RULES OF MALE STYLE

Style principles are made to be broken. That's a bold proclamation, considering the fact that you're holding a guide chock-full of rules for dressing well. But building a wardrobe isn't like flying a passenger jet or erecting a skyscraper. In those endeavors, if you disregard the laws of gravity, people complain.

The rules on the following pages provide your style road map. But the stylish diversions you pursue should be your own.

Rule 1

BUILD ON A CLASSIC FOUNDATION

Writer Mike Zimmerman spent some time with actor Matthew McConaughey on the grounds of Frank Sinatra's Palm Springs California home. At this house—a bastion of midcentury modern architecture and a nod to the creative use of money in the desert—two big-mama palm trees stand in the backyard, near the pool. As the story goes, there was a flagpole next to those trees. When Sinatra was in town and in the mood for some company, he didn't use the phone to summon Lawford and the boys over for drinks. He ran a Jack Daniel's flag up that pole. When the flag flew, the party was on. Sinatra's friends would simply show up.

"Now that's a cool idea," says McConaughey, poolside at the estate. "Wonder what Frank's doin' tonight? Whup, flag's up! Let's go!"

McConaughey is an admirer of the old-school Rat Pack style. Today he'll make his

> ## "I like to do things right. That's what a man does."

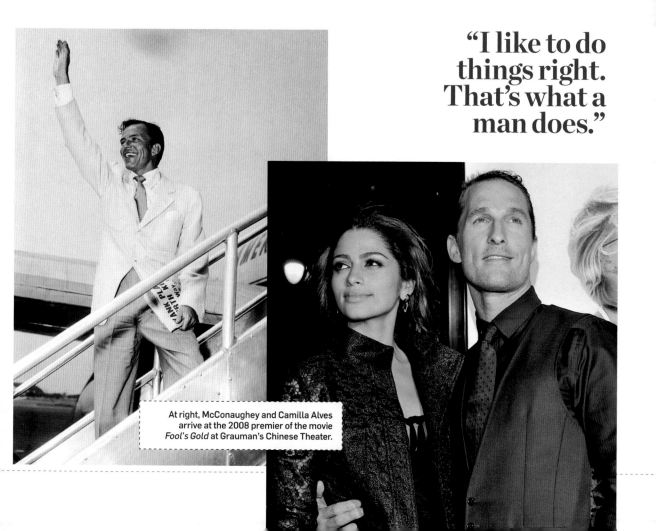

At right, McConaughey and Camilla Alves arrive at the 2008 premier of the movie *Fool's Gold* at Grauman's Chinese Theater.

way through several rooms of this single-level, 1950s-era pad, the Sinatra catalog pumping on the restored sound system. He soaks it in. It's clear the best parts of Frank's spirit are alive and well in the man.

"They were a small fraternity of the hippest, coolest cats out there, man," McConaughey says of the Pack. "They were talented, played hard, played classy, and always looked sharp. And they never wasted their time. They are what I like best about the limelight lifestyle. Those guys weren't going to the show unless they *were* the show."

McConaughey, the face of Dolce & Gabbana's new men's fragrance The One, is no stranger to looking sharp. But it's a funny thing: The paparazzi have made it look like the man's style is board shorts and flip-flops. Blame the work schedule, says McConaughey.

"In the past year and a half, I've lived three consecutive summers." First it was Malibu '06; then in the last half of that year, he headed to Australia to film the recently released *Fool's Gold* with actress and free spirit Kate Hudson. That was during the Southern Hemisphere's summer. Finally, he came back for Malibu '07 and another beach shoot, *Surfer Dude*. If it seems as if McConaughey hasn't had a shirt on in 2 years, well, basically, he hasn't. Both movies were filmed near the water, in the water, or under the water. Can you blame him?

The beach-bum label is where people start to get McConaughey wrong. He might seem like the happy-go-lucky man-child of the beach, but even his whims are shot through with logic. Example: When the shooting day ends, instead of sitting

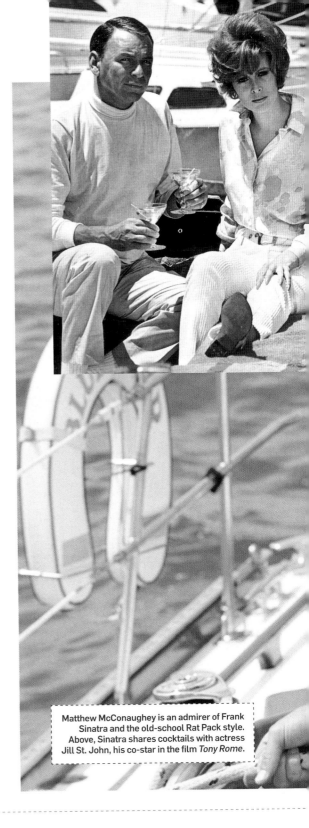

Matthew McConaughey is an admirer of Frank Sinatra and the old-school Rat Pack style. Above, Sinatra shares cocktails with actress Jill St. John, his co-star in the film *Tony Rome*.

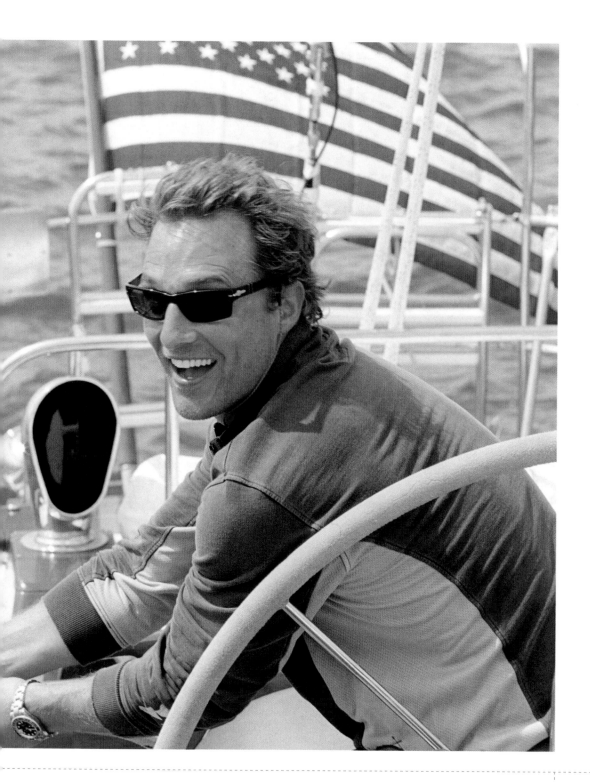

"There's a cool responsibility that comes with BEING A MAN."

down for the usual chat, McConaughey offers an unexpected suggestion. "How about we drive back to L.A.? We can talk it out on the road," he says. And just like that, a day at Frank's morphs into an impromptu desert road trip in one of McConaughey's customized conversion vans. I soon learn that one of his primary customs is to customize.

"Some of the best conversations I've ever had were while I was sitting in this seat," McConaughey says as he swings the van west toward L.A. He's done the long haul between southern California and his native Texas many times, and he fills the driving hours with good talk. If he's alone, he'll talk into a microphone hanging down from the van's ceiling. That's right: A recorder embedded in the upholstery above his head gets it all—ideas, plans, fixes. And I see now that he really does prefer to talk behind the wheel, that this was no random invitation. It's the best way he knows how to shoot some serious shit.

You'd think a guy who takes so much snark from celeb blogs about his lifestyle, his film work, and his shirt allergies would have more to gripe about. But we cover just about every subject—style, fitness, business, friendship, fraternity, and more—and it's clear he's not wasting brain space on the bad stuff.

"Cynicism can be funny. But it's the easy way. You'll forget to enjoy anything," he says. "I try to make the evolving choice, the forward-moving, life-giving choice."

McConaughey has the same approach to belongings: Keep the best, toss the rest. "A year ago, I got my life down to one big backpack," he says. "I just did a big spring cleaning and said, 'What do you really need, McConaughey?' I attacked the little things that don't matter."

The flip side? He's surrounded only by things he can depend on. Like the van we're riding in, Cosmo. He treats Cosmo as a cowboy treats a horse. A beaded curtain bops me in the head the whole way to L.A. as I kick back in the captain's chair.

One of the qualities McConaughey admires most about Sinatra, he explains, is that the guy wasn't afraid to be a man. Men today are scrutinized for the kind of stuff that ought to come naturally: wooing beautiful women, partying, surfing, even kicking around with your friends.

"Males, whether we like it or not, are one big gender fraternity," he says. "Bottom line, men need male friends, whether it's card night, going to the game, going for a run. I have great male friends and I need their friendship. When I get together with my guy friends, we end up talking about how we can be the best men possible. 'Man, I tried this and it didn't work right,' or 'This is something I'm working on, what do you think about it?' It's crucial for men to fraternize like that, because maybe you have insight or experience with something they don't. So you share: dreams, accomplishments, strategies. Lance [Armstrong] and I are good friends, because we have positive and deliberate approaches to life and we're both working

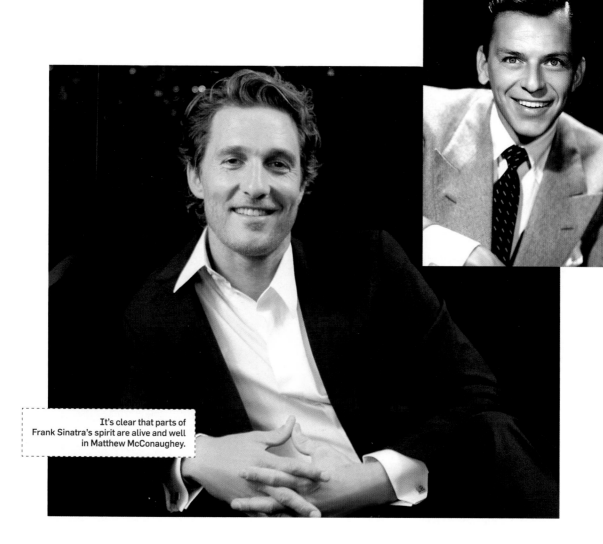

It's clear that parts of Frank Sinatra's spirit are alive and well in Matthew McConaughey.

to be the best men we can be. That's what we're talking about." Then he grins. "As well as which chicks are hot."

Which reminds him: "You can have a fraternal bond with a lady, too. Yeah, let's make love, but let's also remember to high-five sometimes. If I can't get psyched with my girl about something she accomplished and high-five and go, 'F--k YEAH!' then that relationship's not going to work. I need that."

To McConaughey, style is the combined result of how a man carries himself, what he values, and what he projects. On our journey, he throws around words that are to cynics what sunlight is to vampires: individuality, sincerity, responsibility, goals, achievement. He sees these things as the trappings of a man who respects himself, as classy as an earth-toned Italian suit with a bright tie (one of his favorite combinations). That's what matters, not the opinions of the folks who seem to get masturbatory pleasure from rolling their eyes.

"There's a cool responsibility that comes with being a man," he says. "Society needs good men who've been through a lot of victories and a lot of shit."

Rule 2
FASHION SHOULD BE FUNCTIONAL

When shopping for shades, choose the right fit.

Ultraviolet rays don't always come in the front door. "The frame makes a major difference," says Rene Soltis, an optician and the director of training for the Vision Council of America. "Wider frames block light even at oblique angles and protect sensitive skin around the eyes from sun damage."

Aviator frames are among the most protective of styles. But go with a plastic frame to help you stay ahead of the fashion-saturation curve; metallic frames are so 2007.

Find the right fit. A gap of just 6 millimeters between the lens and your forehead can allow up to 45 percent of ultraviolet light to reach your eyes, according to a University of Massachusetts study. Look for a shape that rides high on the bridge of your nose and stays put through Iron Maiden-caliber head banging.

Consider your surroundings. Radiation comes at you from all angles.

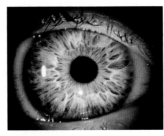

Aviator frames are ONE OF THE MOST protective. Choose a plastic frame.

Snow bounces back 85 percent of the UV rays that hit its crust, for example, and water re-flects them all. Sand and concrete kick back about 25 percent.

If you're in the wild, UV-blocking, polarized lenses and a hat may be in order, says Paul T. Finger, MD, a professor of ophthalmology at New York University School of Medicine. The lenses dampen surface glare, while a 4-inch brim can reduce the UV radiation that reaches your face by an extra 70 percent.

Take a tint. The tint, or "transmittance," of a lens doesn't affect its UV defenses. Cover up too much, though, and you'll risk a much quicker death. A transmittance of less than 10 percent is considered too dark for driving, for example. A study published in the *Journal of the American Optometric Association* found that a 23 percent tint provides the best visibility. Read the label or ask a salesperson for more info.

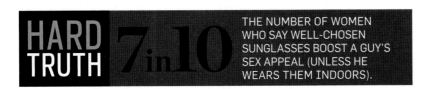

HARD TRUTH 7 in 10 THE NUMBER OF WOMEN WHO SAY WELL-CHOSEN SUNGLASSES BOOST A GUY'S SEX APPEAL (UNLESS HE WEARS THEM INDOORS).

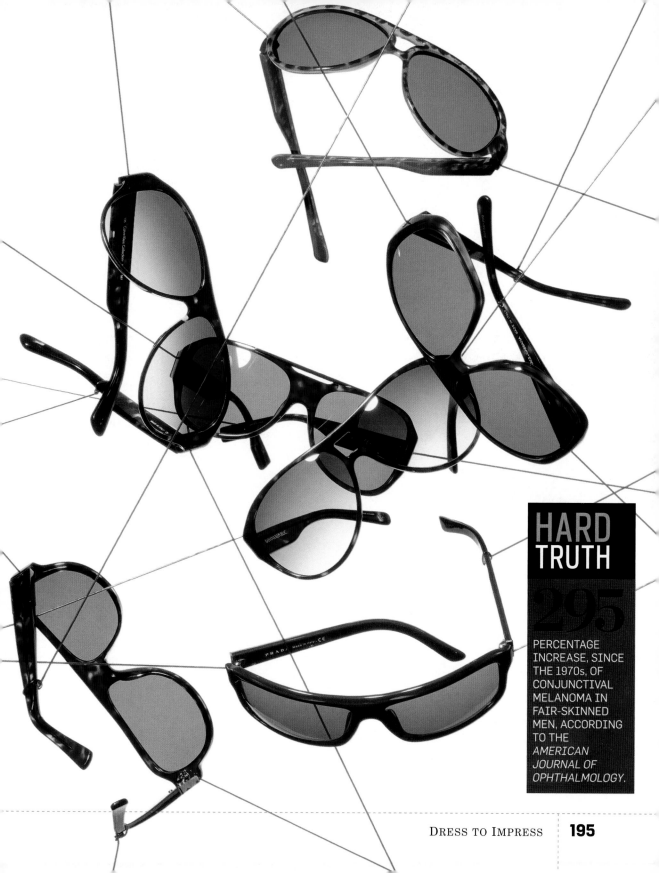

HARD TRUTH

295

PERCENTAGE INCREASE, SINCE THE 1970s, OF CONJUNCTIVAL MELANOMA IN FAIR-SKINNED MEN, ACCORDING TO THE *AMERICAN JOURNAL OF OPHTHALMOLOGY*.

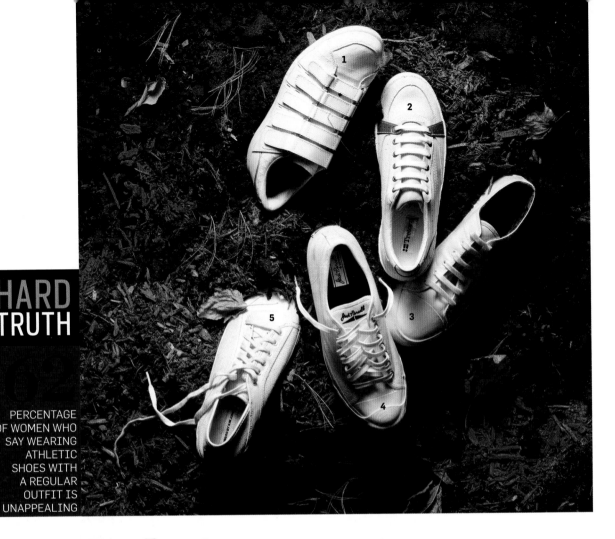

Rule 3
BE CASUAL, NOT CARELESS

Ignore what's on your feet and you risk tripping yourself up with the ladies.

"Mixing the sports wardrobe with the everyday wardrobe has become quite stylish, but when you get it wrong, it looks so inappropriate," says Sarah Whittaker, a Georgia-based image consultant.

That doesn't mean you should strike sneakers entirely from your to-wear list. These kicks will keep you comfortable and looking smart.

1. Velcro straps hug your foot—and create a style statement.
2. The brown leather accent says serious enough for the office.
3. This classic, clean shoe keeps it simple.
4. The side mesh allows your toes to breathe on the go.
5. Shiny leather uppers elevate this sneaker to a Saturday-night option.

Rule 4
USE SCENT TO SNARE HER SUBLIMINALLY

Scent is the ultimate romantic lure.

"Fragrances are linked to our emotions," says Rachel Herz, PhD, a visiting professor at Brown University medical school and the author of *The Scent of Desire*. "That's because the brain's smell center, the limbic system, also underlies learning and emotion." Here, find our favorite new scents, plus tips for deploying them.

Go easy on her nose. One whiff of a man's fragrance causes a significant rise in genital bloodflow in a woman, according to researchers at the University of Indiana. But don't bathe in the stuff.

"We have more receptors for smell than we have for any other sense except vision," says Dr. Herz. If your scent is discernible to anyone farther than 2 feet from you, dial back the amount you use.

Spin your scent. A man's smell is the single most important physical factor influencing a woman's sexual attraction, according to Dr. Herz's research. But "women don't differentiate much between real body odor and a fragrance," she says. If a woman thinks a man smells great, she will find him attractive whether it comes from his body or a bottle. The key is to allow your own musk to mix with your spritzed-on accents. One spray to your chest before you dress will allow the fragrance to mix with your natural scent and keep the smell subtle.

Stifle old olfactory flames. If a woman is already passionate about a scent, think twice about adopting it for yourself. "Once an association to an odor has been formed, it's difficult to reassociate that odor with something different," says Dr. Herz.

Translation: She might connect a fragrance to a slew of intensely sexual or deeply emotional experiences with an ex. The human nose can tease apart 10,000 different odors. Our advice: Turn her on to something new.

Pair smells with occasions. An aroma is inherently meaningless until it's paired with an experience, says Dr. Herz, so plan

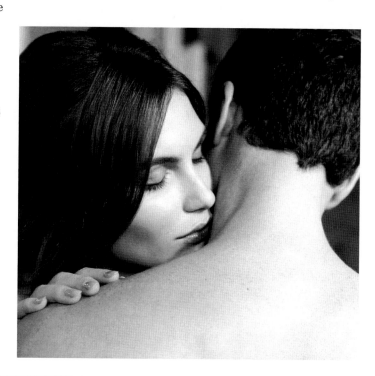

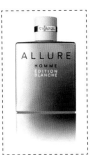

***Chanel* Allure Homme Édition Blanche**
$75, chanel.com

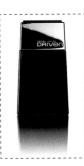

Derek Jeter Driven Black
$26, avon.com

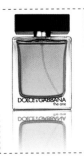

***Dolce & Gabbana* The One for Men**
$70, Dolce & Gabbana boutiques

something novel or significant when you break out a new cologne. Another context-dependent trick: Swap scents to match the occasions, using one cologne for date nights, another for outdoor activities, and another over lazy, romantic weekends. She'll begin to associate those great times with each fragrance—like an on-demand scrapbook of pleasant memories.

Leave a parting gift. In a 2006 University of Pittsburgh study, 72 percent of women said they had cuddled up at night with a partner's clothing. The most common reason given? "To remember him."

The habit is an opportunity, says Dr. Herz. Leave a well-worn T-shirt at her place after a night spent watching movies, or let her keep the sweatshirt she nabbed from you the night before to stay warm.

"It's most effective if you use a cotton shirt that you've worn for a day or so—better overnight than out at a bar," says Dr. Herz. "That gives your natural scent time to soak into the cotton."

Rule 5
ACCENT YOUR ANKLES

Socks can reveal your true colors.

"They have become the new tie," says Simon Mendez, president of the British Apparel Collection, a distributor of Pantherella socks. "They are one of the few ways you can make a style statement." Mendez and Frank Lucia, executive director of the sock brand Royal Bermuda, show you how to stand out.

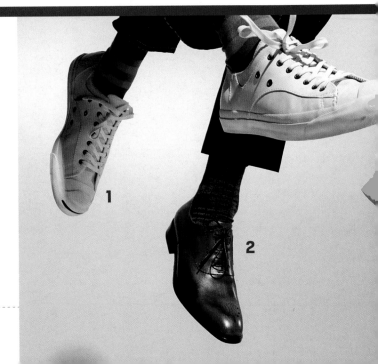

Rule 6

FOCUS ON THE FINER POINTS

A mangled tie or a misjudged trouser hem can sabotage even the finest sartorial intentions. Here's how to nail three simple but essential details.

TIE DIMPLE

Italo Zucchelli, of Calvin Klein Collection for men, on how to get it right: Hold an index finger on the tie shaft just inside the knot and then push in and squeeze the edges as you tighten.

SHIRT CUFF

The shirt cuff should extend a quarter inch to a half inch past your suit sleeve. Ask your tailor to measure both arms and adjust for your watch, says Simon Keen of Brooks Brothers.

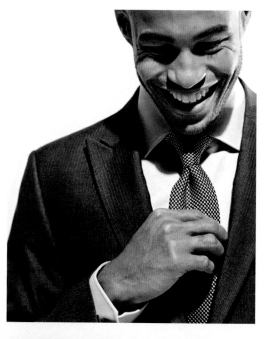

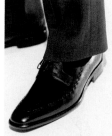

TROUSER BREAK: Your pant leg should stop just at the top of the heel of a dress shoe, naturally breaking over the front. Wear dress shoes to the tailor and walk around to ensure that the legs "flow" properly, says Zucchelli. "You shouldn't see too much of the ankle during your stride," he says.

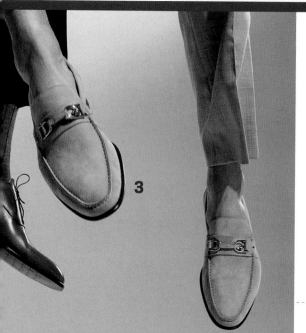

3

1. THE EXTREMIST

Go big with unexpected combinations—argyle socks with pinstriped pants, for example. Like tie-and-shirt combinations, the colors and patterns must play well together.

2. THE TRADITIONALIST

Match the weight of the sock to your shoe: Thin goes with dress shoes, medium with more casual shoes. Pair thick athletic socks with sneakers.

3. THE EXHIBITIONIST

Italian-cut suit trousers (read: high-rise) or slim-cut jeans allow you to show some ankle. The sock-free look requires forethought, though: You'll need foot powder to sop up the moisture and broken-in shoes to lessen the likelihood of blistering.

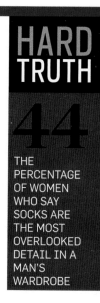

HARD TRUTH

44

THE PERCENTAGE OF WOMEN WHO SAY SOCKS ARE THE MOST OVERLOOKED DETAIL IN A MAN'S WARDROBE

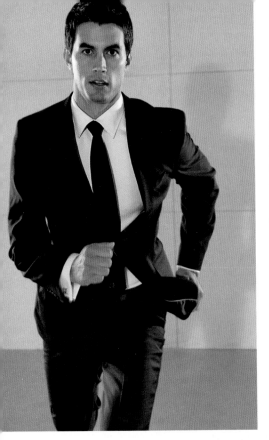

Rule 7
BE FORMAL BUT FLEXIBLE

Strict dress codes at black-tie events have gone the way of pleated trousers. Most celebratory soirees today allow for "festive" dress, or attire that you can more flexibly recruit from your existing wardrobe. Here's how.

THE SUIT: A solid suit in black or midnight blue is a small step below the staid tux, and a workhorse like this should already be in heavy rotation in your wardrobe. A peak lapel creates a more formal look.

THE SHIRT: Colorful or patterned shirts are too casual. Go with a standard-issue white dress shirt with a spread collar for a more formal turn.

THE TIE: Bow ties are for tuxedos only. A solid black necktie, sans pattern, works well.

THE SHOES: A polished, classy dress shoe (think wing-tip or cap toe) is a suitable surrogate for patent-leather kicks, and often far more comfortable.

THE TIMEPIECE: A high-end watch can elevate your ensemble and your attitude. The complicated models favored by the wealthy can be gaudy; choose a classic gold watch with a leather strap. Your look will be refined and elegant.

CUFF LINKS: French cuffs are a must-have detail at formal events. Look for gold or semiprecious stones.

Rule 8
COMFORT EQUALS CONFIDENCE

Our intrepid reporter grabbed a lab notebook and poured himself into 35 different pairs of underwear to find out which are worth stocking—and a few you'll want to avoid.

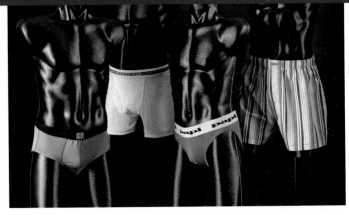

THONG: Wear these and you'll burn through your self-esteem like a Hummer through low-octane gas.

ATHLETIC BRIEF: Gym visits call for something smooth to stop bunching yet strong enough to keep the marbles in the bag.

BOXER BRIEFS: They're probation for your convicts, offering a mix of supervision and freedom. Bonus: no saggy diaper-butt feeling.

LOINCLOTH: Leather might have worked for cavemen, but what I tested felt like a lobster bib. Leave it in the museum.

HIP BRIEF: Slim-fitting pants can make bulkier underwear uncomfortable. This minimalist pair keeps a low profile.

BOXERS: Sure, your junk will swing. But a button-fly pair ensures that the party doesn't spill out into the street.

Rule 9
NEW BRANDS ARE NEW FRIENDS

Habits can be hard to break, even when they don't involve 64 ounces of piping-hot caffeine.

Consider how you walk through your chosen clothing store: You probably head toward the same old reliable brands. Check out these off-the-radar alternatives the next time you hit your favorite department stores.

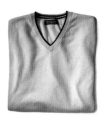

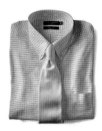

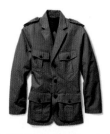

The staple: Banana Republic is the go-to for comfy cashmere V-necks and cotton cardigans.
The splash: Named after the founders of Bloomingdale's, the Joseph & Lyman label is similarly well designed.

The staple: Preppy haven J.Crew is always a reliable source for cool cotton jackets.
The splash: Macy's house brand INC has comparably clean lines and a contemporary feel to its outerwear.

The staple: For traditional shirts and ties, Brooks Brothers is your mecca.
The splash: French label Daniel Cremieux (available at Dillard's) offers a similar range of classics.

Rule 10
COLOR WILL CATCH HER EYE

"Pairing colors is like assembling notes in a melody," says Angela Wright, a British color expert. "There are underlying mathematical relationships, and you have to hit the right notes for the combination to work."

Here's a matching method that considers a color's hue, saturation, and brightness.

A Taiwanese study found that you should shoot for a high color contrast between skin and fabric. So dark skin should be matched with light-toned clothing colors, and paler skin looks best when it's paired with deep, grayish tones.

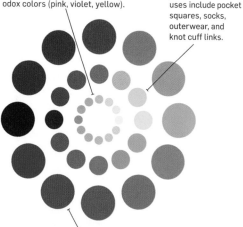

Inner band of color: Most of your dress shirts should fall among these tones, which riff on the safe, classic white button-down with hints of unorthodox colors (pink, violet, yellow).

Middle band of color: Your exclamation point. Judicious uses include pocket squares, socks, outerwear, and knot cuff links.

Outer band of color: Use these bolder colors in moderation—for ties and sweaters or as stripes and checks on dress shirts. They'll work fluidly with the shades in the first band.

Rule 11
YOUR BEST CAN ELEVATE THE REST

Museum curators know that a marquee piece--a van Gogh, Monet, or Klimt, say--brings added luster and attention to the other works hanging in the room. Sure, there's the name value, but the aesthetics add extra punch, too.

That's the kind of principle you'd do well to apply to your clothing by using high-cost, high-quality items alongside more functional pieces. Here's how.

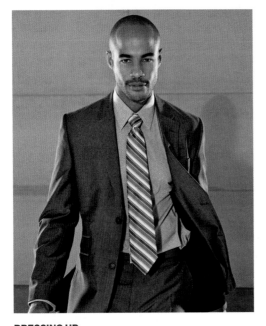

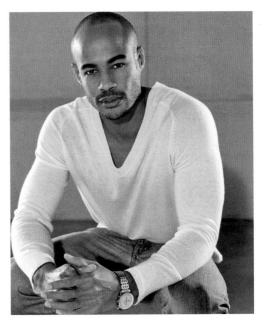

DRESSING UP

Pick the right suit. A high-quality suit delivers niceties lacking in lower-end outfits. The stitching, fabric, and cut are telltale signs of your ability to spot a good sartorial investment, and they'll distract the eye if you choose to save some money when you shop for accessories.

Then save on a shirt. Most basic dress shirts are made with cotton, so it can be hard to tell them apart, especially when they're worn under a suit. Look for brands such as Express.

KICKING BACK

Save on jeans. Lower-end jeans can look just as good as more expensive brands. For about half the price of a high-end label, scoop up basic jeans from such sources as Gap, J. Crew, H&M, and Uniqlo.

And splurge on a sweater. She'll be more tempted to reach out and touch good cashmere. Cashmere's weave is stronger and more supple, which means less pilling and a long lifetime of groping.

HARD TRUTH **$60,000** PRICE PAID ON EBAY IN 2005 FOR A PAIR OF VINTAGE LEVI'S JEANS FROM THE 1880s

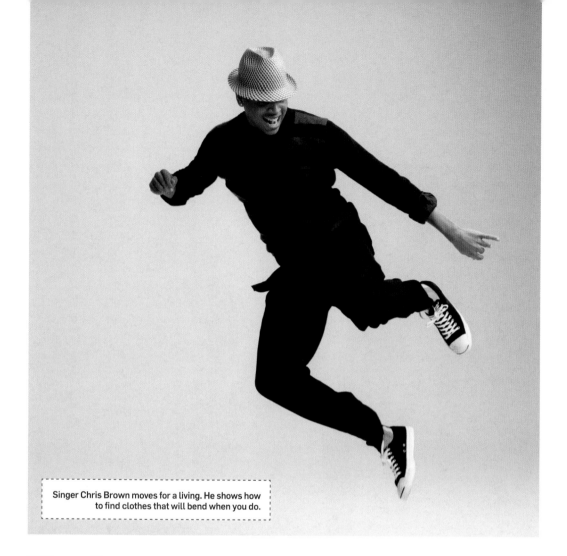

Singer Chris Brown moves for a living. He shows how to find clothes that will bend when you do.

Rule 12
YOUR CLOTHES SHOULD MOVE YOU

Chris Brown's mother likes to joke that as soon as her son could walk, he never stopped moving. It's not much of an exaggeration. When Brown performed at the MTV Video Music Awards, he was busting fresher moves than Usher and getting more air than LeBron James.

"It has a lot to do with youth, as well as trying to be over the top," the R&B sensation says of his acrobatic stage presence.

"I don't want to be in the same lane with everyone else."

While kids his age were learning to drive, Brown was putting together a double-platinum debut album that spawned four top-10 hits. A few years later, the Virginia native's perpetual motion continues, with two movies in his rearview and a host of music awards and nominations decorating his mantel. You might not know it, but

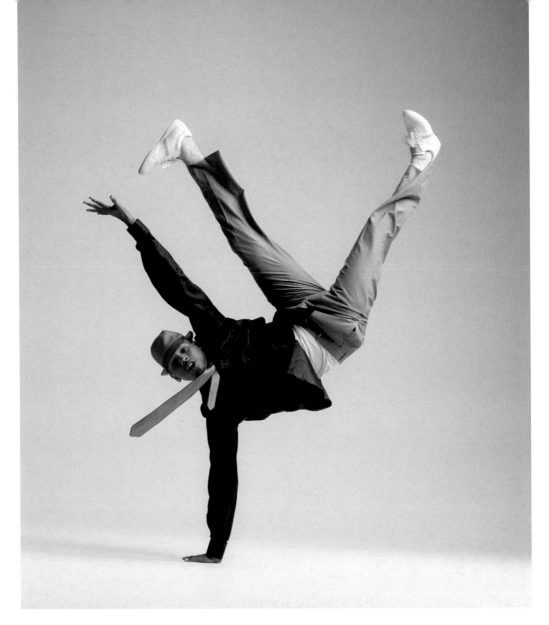

you've probably even found yourself humming the infectious refrain from "Kiss Kiss," the lead single from his sophomore album, *Exclusive*.

Adrenaline informs Brown's personal style as much as his musical approach. Most days the rubber-limbed teen wears sweatpants and his favorite pair of sneakers so he's equally ready to break into a basketball game or song. When Brown dresses up, the same rules apply: Mobility outpaces tradition.

"I like wearing sneakers with my suits because I'm comfortable, and it separates me from everybody." Our take: The shoes aren't the only thing separating him from the pack.

"I'm not much of a flashy person, but when the time is right, I can do it," Brown says.

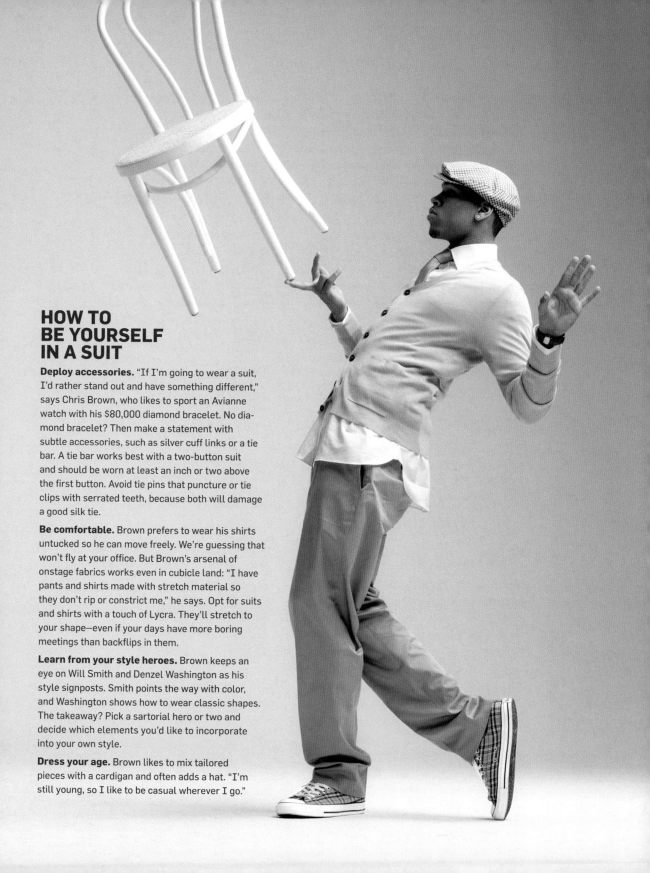

HOW TO
BE YOURSELF
IN A SUIT

Deploy accessories. "If I'm going to wear a suit, I'd rather stand out and have something different," says Chris Brown, who likes to sport an Avianne watch with his $80,000 diamond bracelet. No diamond bracelet? Then make a statement with subtle accessories, such as silver cuff links or a tie bar. A tie bar works best with a two-button suit and should be worn at least an inch or two above the first button. Avoid tie pins that puncture or tie clips with serrated teeth, because both will damage a good silk tie.

Be comfortable. Brown prefers to wear his shirts untucked so he can move freely. We're guessing that won't fly at your office. But Brown's arsenal of onstage fabrics works even in cubicle land: "I have pants and shirts made with stretch material so they don't rip or constrict me," he says. Opt for suits and shirts with a touch of Lycra. They'll stretch to your shape—even if your days have more boring meetings than backflips in them.

Learn from your style heroes. Brown keeps an eye on Will Smith and Denzel Washington as his style signposts. Smith points the way with color, and Washington shows how to wear classic shapes. The takeaway? Pick a sartorial hero or two and decide which elements you'd like to incorporate into your own style.

Dress your age. Brown likes to mix tailored pieces with a cardigan and often adds a hat. "I'm still young, so I like to be casual wherever I go."

Rule 13
LOOK GOOD, NATURALLY

Million-dollar labs can't compete with nature.

"Even with technological advances, some of the most effective products rely on natural ingredients," says Vivian Bucay, MD, a dermatologist in San Antonio. "Science refines and combines them." Here are six products containing natural ingredients worth adding to your grooming arsenal.

PAYOT HOMME SOOTHING AFTER SHAVE CARE
($40, 800-790-9908)

Key ingredient: Hematite

"This mineral helps deflect light away from lines and wrinkles," says Brian C. Keller, PharmD, a dermatopharmacology consultant and former researcher at the University of California at San Francisco.

Tip: Splash cool water on your shaved face to close pores and prevent them from clogging.

LAB SERIES AGE RESCUE EYE THERAPY
($26, labseries.com)

Key ingredient: Grape-seed extract

Grape seeds contain powerful phenols called proanthocyanidins, which have an antioxidant power 20 times greater than that of vitamin E and 50 times greater than that of vitamin C. "They aid the skin's elasticity and flexibility," says Dr. Keller.

Tip: Use your pinkie instead of your index finger to apply the product.

MD SKINCARE SPF 25 LIP BALM
($18, mdskincare.com)

Key ingredient: Blueberries

"Blueberry extracts are better than those of any other fruit for soaking up oxygen molecules that damage skin cells," says Dr. Keller. Australian researchers found that similar extracts decreased a type of skin inflammation in rats by 54 percent.

Tip: Apply this balm 20 minutes before heading out. SPF lip balm is most useful to prevent chapped lips, not to treat them.

BILLY JEALOUSY ABOUT FACE ANTI-AGING SERUM
($50, billyjealousy.com)

Key ingredient: Echinacea extract

German researchers examined 4,500 patients with a range of skin complications and found that 86 percent of the patients showed improvement after treatment with an echinacea extract.

Tip: Massage 3 drops of the serum into your face before bed. Shaving in the morning will evict old skin cells.

YON-KA FOR MEN SHAVING GEL
($28, 800-391-5333)

Key ingredient: Licorice

Lathering up with a licorice-extract foam offers postshave benefits. A University of Iowa study found that licorice lessened skin irritation and redness by 25 percent, compared with oil and water-based lotions.

Tip: Shave 15 minutes after you wake up. Your face swells at night, creating unruly whiskers. As the swelling subsides, your follicles align for an easier shave.

SONYA DAKAR TRIPLE ACTION ORGANIC SCRUB
($50, sonyadakar.com)

Key ingredient: Flaxseed

"Flax has high levels of linolenic, linoleic, and oleic fatty acids, making it very useful in skin-care products," says Dr. Keller. "They moisturize and fortify the skin." The finely ground seeds also help unclog pores, dislodging blemish-causing bacteria.

Tip: This is rough stuff; use no more than a dime-sized amount up to three times a week.

Rule 14

MATCH YOUR JEANS TO YOUR GENES

Jeans, more than any other style of pants, conform to your shape. In fact, three out of four women surveyed by *Men's Health* complained that men don't wear jeans that fit them properly. Follow our pointers on the denim style best suited to your body type to do denim right.

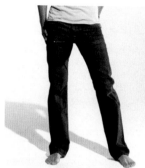

If you're: **LONG AND LEAN**

Try: **STRAIGHT LEG JEANS**

"The great thing about a lanky guy is that he can wear slim-cut jeans without it seeming too skinny or punk-rockish," says Allison Cornia, co-owner of Riveted A Jeans Store, a denim boutique in Seattle.

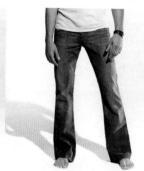

If you're: **BUFF AND BURLY**

Try: **BOOT CUT JEANS**

A classic or boot cut will show off all that hard work. Skinny jeans are too snug, but pants cut too wide can make you look blocky. Avoid distressed touches on burly areas, says Cornia.

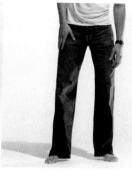

If you're: **HUSKY**

Try: **RELAXED JEANS**

A relaxed style will de-emphasize your heft. "If you have a belly, lower-waist jeans that fit under your pooch are a little more flattering," Cornia says. Stay away from light-colored jeans.

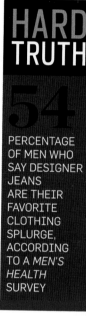

Rule 15

TAKE A PAGE FROM THE PROFESSIONALS

Hints about how to be stylish are everywhere--even at Barnes & Noble. Next time you're surfing for a free table in the café, pick up one of these tomes.

Ralph Lauren
by Ralph Lauren: Lauren's clothes and home products hint at the robust outdoor lives of our forefathers while delivering modern creature comforts. This hefty book is part memoir, part business bio.

Rebel Style: Cinematic Heroes of the 1950s
by G. Bruce Boyer: This short, sharp salute to the actors whose roles exalted outlaw fashion includes Marlon Brando, James Dean, Montgomery Clift, and Paul Newman.

The Elegant Man: How to Construct the Ideal Wardrobe
by Riccardo Villarosa: A reference manual bursting with details, this classic how-to guide explains everything from tying a Windsor knot to matching fabrics with patterns.

The Modern Gentleman: A Guide to Essential Manners, Savvy & Vice
by Phineas Mollod and Jason Tesauro: A gentleman knows more than just which fork to use while hunting endive.

Danny, the Champion of the World
by Roald Dahl: Style can be found in the simplest of gestures. If you have a kid between the ages of 5 and 10, read this at bedtime, side by side, cuddled up.

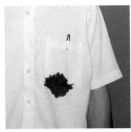

Rule 16
STAINLESS IS PAINLESS

Stains happen in an instant. Shouldn't they disappear that quickly, as well?

We destroyed a brand-new white shirt with the worst stains a guy is likely to face, and then struck back with three instant stain removers, five detergent-enhancing stain fighters, and plain old cold water. Here's a quick guide to making the mess a distant memory.

THE STAIN	QUICK FIX	SPRAY AND WAIT
BARBECUE SAUCE	Tide to Go: This stain-remover pen instantly erased almost every trace. $4, *walgreens.com*	Spray 'n Wash Dual Power: Upon close inspection, even the faintest hint of sauce was gone. $6, *drugstore.com*
BLUE INK	Shout Wipes: A few quick rubs, and there was no ink on our test shirt. $3, *drugstore.com*	Don't spray, don't wait! Attend to stray pen marks immediately—otherwise the ink stains will become a permanent part of the design.
RED WINE	OxiClean Spray-A-Way: Hits large stains hard and prevents them from spreading. $5, *greatcleaners.com*	Cold water: Water works; after one round in the washer, the wine was history. Free!
BACON GREASE	No quick fix: Grease splatters are unfazed by instant stain removers. A round in the washer is your best bet.	Shout Advanced Gel: This spray was the only remover that didn't leave a trace. $4, WalMart

Rule 17
BE A SUCCESS FROM THE GROUND UP

Nick Valenti has seen more foot faults than the senior line judge at Wimbledon. He's a 30-year veteran of B. Nelson Shoes, his family's Manhattan-based repair shop for high-end footwear. Let him spot your shoe missteps before your girlfriend—or your boss—notices. And trust us, they're watching closely.

What to know: An all-leather shoe—including the upper, sole, heel base, and lining—is generally a mark of quality. Good shoes incorporate very few synthetic materials.

The wider the stitch, the more likely it is to break at some point. Tight, interlocking stitches strengthen and reduce the vulnerability of your shoe's seams, says Valenti.

When you buy: Take your shoes for a test drive on a hardwood, tile, or marble floor before you buy; the thick carpeting of the shoe store won't give you an accurate reading of fit and comfort.

Don't be a slave to shoe size. "I tell customers to throw out the number," says Valenti. "Different companies have different scaling methods, and there's no standard."

Make them last: Use sole guards. A piece of rubber applied by a cobbler can offset everyday wear and tear. Cedar shoe trees absorb perspiration—the enemy of your shoes' longevity.

Waterproof your shoes regularly. Polish them after every three or four wearings with a wax or a cream polish, to keep the leather supple and prevent the surface from cracking.

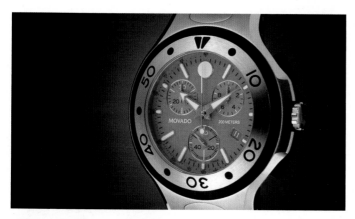

Rule 18
ALWAYS, ALWAYS BE RIGHT ON TIME

The moon has an air of mystery because it appears and disappears in the night sky. Your watch does the same thing; it darts out of your sleeve, is glimpsed for a moment, then vanishes again. It's a subtle clue to who you are, what you like, what you value.

"It combines artistry, craftsmanship, and technology," says Andrew Block, an executive vice president of watch retailer Tourneau.

Punctuality is a fluid construct. Be prompt for anything requiring a judge, a priest, or an usher, but use this schedule for everything else.

First date: Be there 2 to 3 minutes late. Picking her up exactly at 8 p.m. isn't polite, it's neurotic. She'll need an extra minute or two to get ready anyway, and you'll avoid the glares of her roommates or cats.

Your job: Be there 30 minutes early. An a.m. power session gives you momentum, says Karen Leland, the author of *Watercooler Wisdom*. "You take care of the low-hanging fruit and look ambitious."

An interview: Be there 15 minutes early. "More than 20 minutes early says you're too eager," says Barbara Pachter, author of *New Rules @ Work*, "and it'll be awkward as other candidates parade by."

Cocktail party: Be there 60 minutes early (close friend); 10 minutes late per party hour (casual friend). Showing up early scores quality time.

Rule 19
MAKE A CONVINCING CASE

The bag a man carries conveys not just his cargo, but also his character. Yours should communicate that you're a man of action and ideas—with the tools to match—and that you're experienced enough to know what you can get by without.

A svelte sidearm like the Banana Republic case (pictured here) will force you to downsize to just the essentials. This one has room for a 16-inch laptop, an important file folder or two, your favorite paperback, and an MP3 player. Bulk is rarely beautiful after all. ■

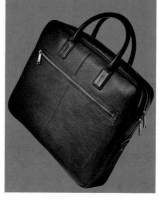

Shave Off Years

TURN BACK TIME WITHOUT GOING UNDER THE KNIFE

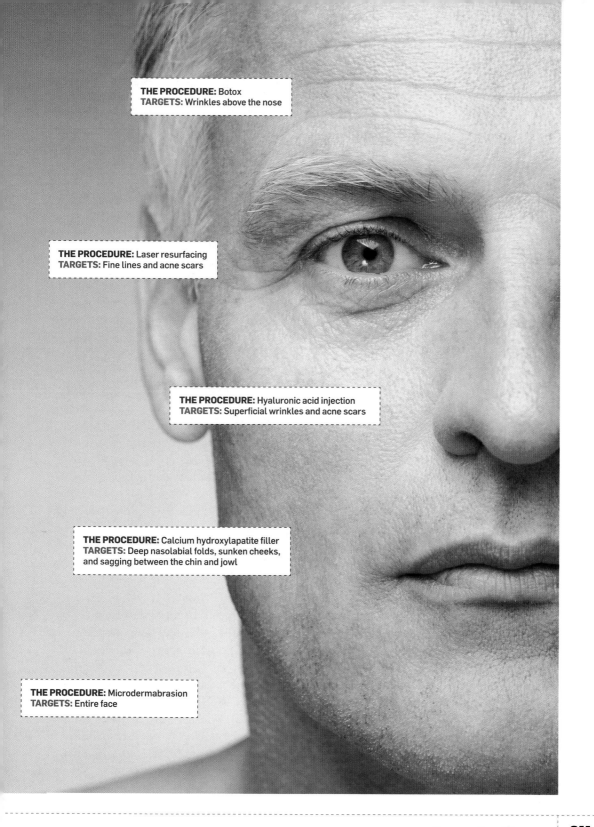

THE PROCEDURE: Botox
TARGETS: Wrinkles above the nose

THE PROCEDURE: Laser resurfacing
TARGETS: Fine lines and acne scars

THE PROCEDURE: Hyaluronic acid injection
TARGETS: Superficial wrinkles and acne scars

THE PROCEDURE: Calcium hydroxylapatite filler
TARGETS: Deep nasolabial folds, sunken cheeks, and sagging between the chin and jowl

THE PROCEDURE: Microdermabrasion
TARGETS: Entire face

When Kenny Rogers appeared on *American Idol*, it wasn't his performance that made headlines. It was his face.

He had the trampoline-taut look of a man fresh from an episode of *Plastic Surgeons Gone Wild*. And if celebs with serious money can't get decent cosmetic work—think Steve Martin's creepy doll eyes and Elton John's moppet hair—what does that say about our own prospects?

For subtler facial improvements, those in the know are skipping the operating room and opting for nonsurgical treatments instead. According to a recent survey by the American Academy of Facial Plastic and Reconstructive Surgery, the number of men undergoing nonsurgical facial plastic surgery increased 91 percent in the past 7 years. Why? "A facelift involves a long recovery time, and often-times the change is more dramatic than guys want," says Peter Hilger, MD, director of facial plastic surgery at the University of Minnesota and president of the American Academy of Facial Plastic and Reconstructive Surgery.

Just because these procedures are "minimally invasive," however, doesn't mean you ought to trust just anybody to top off your mug. Many treatments still require a deft touch. To ensure your nip doesn't leave you royally tucked, find a few board-certified plastic surgeons in your area (search plasticsurgery.org), and then interview them and get at least two or three opinions.

Ask to see pictures of results; you're looking for patients who appear refreshed, not dry roasted. We spoke with Arthur W. Perry, MD, who is a clinical associate at the University of Pennsylvania and the author of *Straight Talk About Cosmetic Surgery*, for his no-nonsense take on the four best treatments.

The procedure: Botox

TARGETS: Wrinkles above the nose

HOW: Since it was FDA approved for cosmetic use more than 10 years ago, it has gone from being whispered about in doctors' offices to being offered in salons. In 2007 alone, 4 million Americans injected the stuff. Its popularity stems from its instant, though temporary, wrinkle-eliminating effect. When injected, it interrupts the communication between nerves and muscles, thus relaxing the facial muscles.

COST: About $500 per treatment

LASTS: 2 to 6 months

DR. PERRY SAYS: "Very effective, with results in a week. But if you decide to get it around your mouth, be prepared to drool and have a speech impediment."

The procedure: Laser resurfacing

TARGETS: Fine lines and acne scars

HOW: An intense light beam blasts away skin layer by layer, vaporizing damage and wrinkles and promoting collagen production. The deeper you go, the better the results but the longer the recovery time. The light CO_2 treatment is the most superficial, with recovery time of less than a week. The deepest treatments cause oozing and redness, so unless you can take a sabbatical, you'll want to stick to lighter treatments.

COST: About $2,200

LASTS: A few months to a few years, depending on the treatment

DR. PERRY SAYS: "It definitely tightens the skin. After the procedure, 1 square inch of a cheek shrinks to seven-eighths of an inch."

The procedure: Hyaluronic acid injection

TARGETS: Superficial wrinkles and acne scars

HOW: This gel-like filler (sold under the brand names Perlane, Restylane, and Juvéderm) is injected to plump up areas with less volume than others. Like collagen, it is biodegradable, but unlike collagen, it is made from nonanimal material, so there is minimal risk of an allergic reaction.

COST: About $600

LASTS: Six to 12 months

DR. PERRY SAYS: "Hyaluronic acid is very good at filling superficial wrinkles, but I wouldn't go near the eyes with it. If the material gets into the retinal artery, it can cause immediate and permanent blindness."

The procedure: Calcium hydroxylapatite filler

TARGETS: Deep nasolabial folds, sunken cheeks, and sagging between the chin and jowl

HOW: When this calcium-based gel (brand name Radiesse) is injected properly, it's not only a filler and plumper but also a strengthener. The stress of the injection causes the fibroblasts (skin cells) to form new collagen and tissue. Calcium hydroxylapatite can also be used to smooth out ridges in the nose because it can create new bone when it comes into contact with existing bone.

COST: About $800

HOW LONG IT LASTS: 2 years

DR. PERRY SAYS: "Very effective. It acts like the rebar in concrete. You can use this to stave off a facelift for a few years." ∎

Avoid a Chemical Reaction

HERE'S THE DIRTY TRUTH ABOUT WHAT'S LURKING IN YOUR BATHROOM

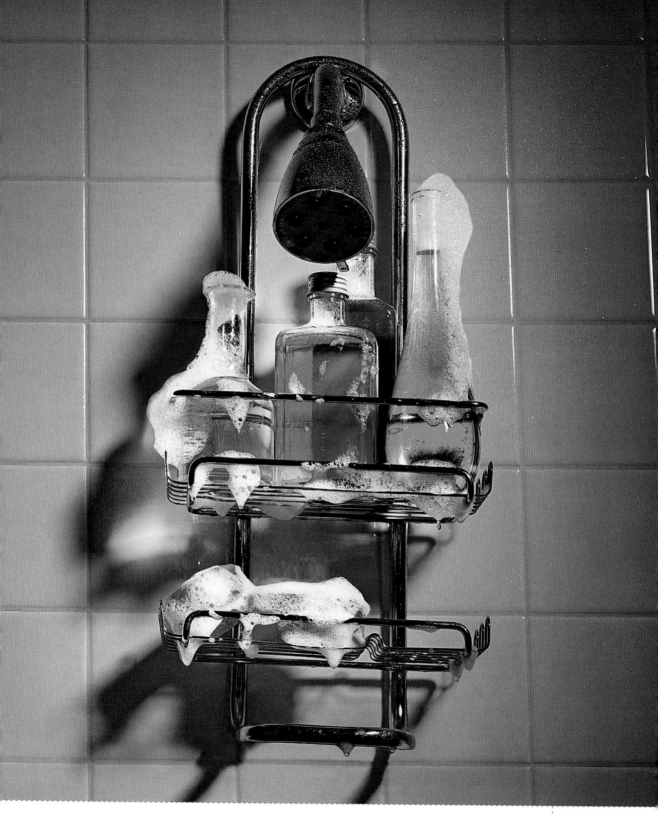

Nearly 90 percent of the chemicals in the products you slather onto your skin—the body's largest organ—have never undergone any testing for toxicity.

That's because the Food and Drug Administration doesn't regulate the safety of ingredients used in cosmetic products. They defer to an industry-funded panel, called the Cosmetics Ingredient Review, which comprises just seven individuals, including a nutritional scientist and . . . a veterinarian. To date, they have examined a mere 11 percent of the ingredients you use to groom yourself, according to the Environmental Working Group (EWG), a nonprofit research organization based in Washington, D.C.

Scientists and toxicologists at EWG recently compared all the ingredients in nearly 25,000 grooming products (information is available online at cosmeticdatabase.com) with lists of potential chemical hazards compiled by 50 scientific regulatory institutions worldwide. Their findings?

"Sixty percent of products on the U.S. market contain chemicals that are potential endocrine disrupters," says Jane Houlihan, vice president of research at EWG, "and a third have ingredients that are likely carcinogens." In the last 30 years, the United States has banned only eight ingredients from personal-care products, while the European Union has banned almost 400 ingredients by some estimates.

"Basically, the E.U. decided to figure out what was causing the rising instances of endocrine problems and dropping sperm levels," says Mark Schapiro, author of *Exposed: The Toxic Chemistry of Everyday Products and What's at Stake for American Power* and editorial director of the Center for Investigative Reporting in Berkeley, California. What they found was a long list of chemicals linked to endocrine problems, including phthalates, which are widely used in cologne, aftershave, hair spray, and moisturizer. A study at the University of California at San Francisco has linked prenatal phthalate exposure to reproductive abnormalities and birth defects, and phthalates were recently banned from use in children's toys in California because they were found to decrease testosterone levels.

So how is it that America, once a leader in environmental protection, allows potentially toxic and mutagenic chemicals into everyday products? According to Schapiro, it has to do with how our government approaches safety.

"The E.U. operates by the precautionary principle," he says, "where if there's enough evidence pointing to the toxicity of a substance, they can ban it rather than wait for the final bit of evidence. The United States, on the other hand, takes no action until there is final scientific data, which is almost impossible and often too late to gather. We saw this before with the global-warming debate."

About 600 U.S. companies have voluntarily pledged to reformulate globally to meet E.U. standards. Until they all do, you can protect yourself by adhering to the better-safe-than-sorry approach and steer clear of a few key potential carcinogens and endocrine disrupters. Following is our list of the five most ubiquitous toxins to avoid, according to the EWG and Gary Ginsberg, PhD, coauthor of *What's Toxic, What's Not* and assistant professor and senior toxicologist at the University of Connecticut School of Community Medicine.

Toxin: 1,4 dioxane

A byproduct of surfactants (the ingredients responsible for producing suds and foam). It usually hides under the name sodium laureth sulfate, but it is found in 56 distinct ingredients, including polyethylene glycol, or PEG.

HEALTH CONCERNS: The Environmental Protection Agency lists it as a probable human carcinogen.

Toxin: Phthalates (pronounced "thal-ates")

Plasticizing agents that make skin products cling to your body and last longer. They hide under the ingredient fragrance, a catch-all term for as many as 7,000 ingredients that are not required to be listed on labels due to trade-secret laws.

HEALTH CONCERNS: Endocrine disrupters are linked to liver and kidney damage, obe-sity, and damaged sperm in men. In utero exposure has been linked to reproductive abnormalities.

Toxin: Formaldehyde

A by-product of diazolidinyl urea that is used as an antimicrobial and a preservative. It's the same stuff that can be found in embalming fluid and cigarette smoke, and it's found on labels under half a dozen different names, including formalin and methyl aldehyde.

HEALTH CONCERNS: It's a known immune-system toxicant and respiratory irritant, and a probable human carcinogen, according to the National Toxicology Program.

Chemical: Hydroquinone

A chemical lightening agent used in hair dyes and skin creams. It is also used in photography developing fluid and has been detected in diesel engine exhaust. It's listed on labels as an "active ingredient."

HEALTH CONCERNS: This is a known skin irritant, immune-system toxicant, and neurotoxin, and it's a possible carcinogen.

Chemical: Parabens

Used as preservatives and antibacterial agents. Identified on labels as any ingredient with the suffix paraben (e.g., butylparaben).

HEALTH CONCERNS: These are possible endocrine disrupters and carcinogens and may impair fertility. ∎

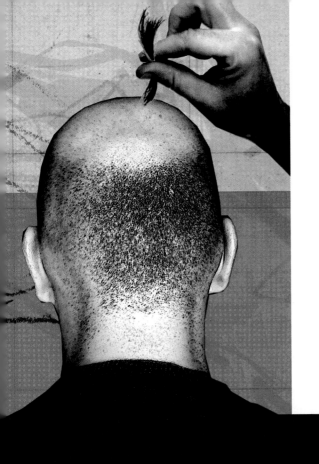

Log on to the forum at hairlosstalk.com, and you'll find men with screen names such as Sheddy Kreuger, Diffusion Guy, and DamnThis venting about going bald. Their anger is understandable.

Don't Get Scalped

THERE ARE NOW MORE TREATMENTS THAN EVER FOR BALDING—SOME EVEN WORK

For the 2,000 years between Julius Caesar's comb-over and Ted Danson's toupee, men have fought a losing battle against the body's hormonal war on its own hair.

The outlook has improved slightly in recent decades with Rogaine and Propecia, the first and only FDA-approved drugs to treat baldness. Used consistently, they can stop or delay balding and sometimes regrow hair. But they're treatments, not cures. The next decade, however, a permanent cure for baldness will move from the lab to clinical trials.

"The cure will come from gene therapy, and it's coming at a rapid clip," predicts Douglas Altchek, MD, a professor of dermatology at New York's Mount Sinai School of Medicine.

If your bathroom mirror shows that you can't wait for a cure, try Propecia and Rogaine. "Start both medications as soon as your hair begins to thin for the best results," advises Robert Bernstein, MD, a clinical professor of dermatology at Columbia University. We asked the experts how the latest baldness treatments measure up.

PHARMACOTHERAPY
Finasteride and Minoxidil

Rogaine's active ingredient, minoxidil, improves blood flow to the scalp, and Propecia's finasteride blocks dihydrotestosterone (DHT), which is a hormone that causes hair loss. Many men triple-treat by using both Propecia and Rogaine—they call it "fin and foam" (finasteride and foaming minoxidil)—plus Nizoral A-D, an antifungal medication used to fight dandruff that has been shown in studies to regrow hair.

OFF-LABEL THERAPY
Dutasteride

Sold as Avodart to men with enlarged prostates, this drug is more powerful than finasteride because it blocks both types of the enzyme that synthesizes DHT.

"The reproductive side effects—decreased libido and ejaculation disorders—may be persistent, so I don't usually recommend this medication for younger patients," says Dr. Bernstein.

SURGERY
Hair Transplant

The leading method today is follicular unit transplantation. It involves moving clumps of up to four hairs from the back and sides of the head to balding areas.

"Hair transplants are most appropriate for people who have not responded to medical treatments," says Dr. Bernstein.

NATUROPATHY
Saw Palmetto and Pumpkin-Seed Oil

Saw palmetto extract has been shown in several small studies to shrink the prostate, working like finasteride to block DHT. Likewise, pumpkin-seed oil is believed to help break down DHT in the liver.

"Men reluctant to try drugs are good candidates for these natural treatments," says Dr. Altchek, "but there is a tremendous placebo effect." ∎

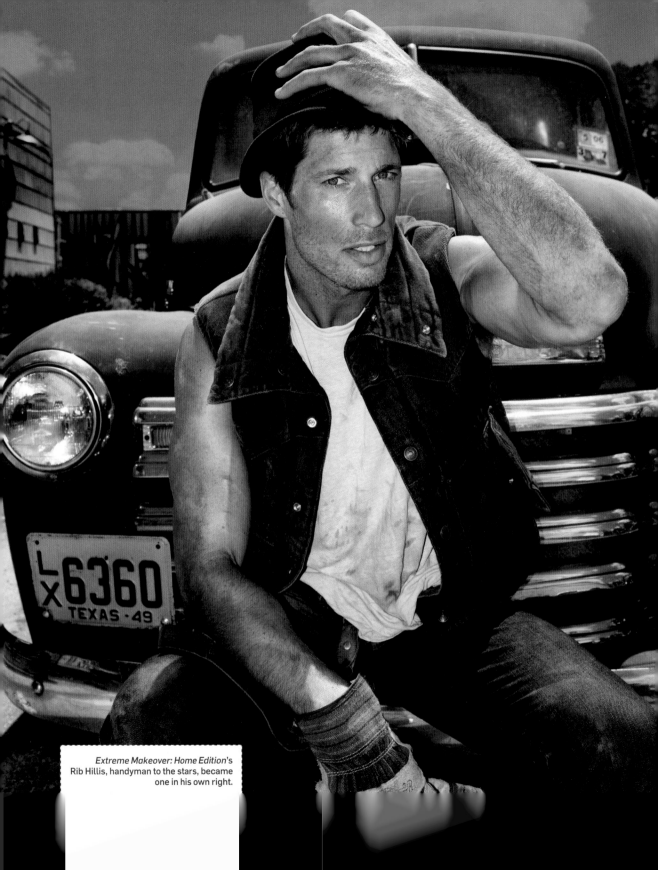

Extreme Makeover: Home Edition's Rib Hillis, handyman to the stars, became one in his own right.

Flaunt Your Jeans

HERE'S HOW TO MAKE THE MOST OF THIS WARDROBE WORKHORSE

It doesn't matter if you're a hip-hop superstar with a $700 set of handmade Japanese denims riding low on your waist, or a cowboy flinging hay bales in your faded blues—chances are you hung that pair on your hips for the same reasons we all do.

Just like us, our jeans are armor strong, yet flexible when it counts. They're hardworking. They wear well—with dignity, proudly displaying their battle scars. And like us, our jeans are always ready for action, whether we're on a first date, a night out, or a game of two-hand touch in the backyard.

Here we'll help you stand tall in front of the harrowing selections of styles, washes, brands, and prices you'll find in stores today. We'll show you how to slash through the marketing jargon to find a pair that precisely fits your build. We'll help you figure out which pair of $300 jeans might actually be worth the price. And we'll even show you how a little TLC can make that favorite pair last just a few years longer. After all, if jeans are our second skin, shouldn't we all know a lot more about them?

DENIM DONE RIGHT

Simple swaps can turn jeans from a sartorial afterthought into the anchor of any look. Here's how to wear your blues well, no matter what the occasion.

THE WEEKEND

Your downtime denim should shield you against rainy-day-project snares, but should also snag the attention of that woman trolling the paint-chip array at Home Depot.

The upgrade: Weekends are for relaxing, not letting it all hang out. More than half of all women we surveyed said wearing baggy jeans is the biggest denim blunder men can make. The key to finding the right fit is matching the shape of your legs to the funnel-like taper of the jeans. Every brand is different (see "Find the Right Fit" on page 224), but you can calibrate your stems by slipping into a straight leg fit first. Too snug? Try a relaxed fit, best for guys with athletic builds (read: you rack up a few 45-pound plates for squats). If you're swimming in the straight legs, try a slim fit.

Watch out for: Details. Distressed or faded finishes are forbidden during the work week, but lighter rinses and natural-looking whiskering are making a return. Finish the look by layering T-shirts, sweaters, and outerwear to match your pants.

Check out: Howe, Lucky Brand, Chaps, Armani Exchange, Diesel

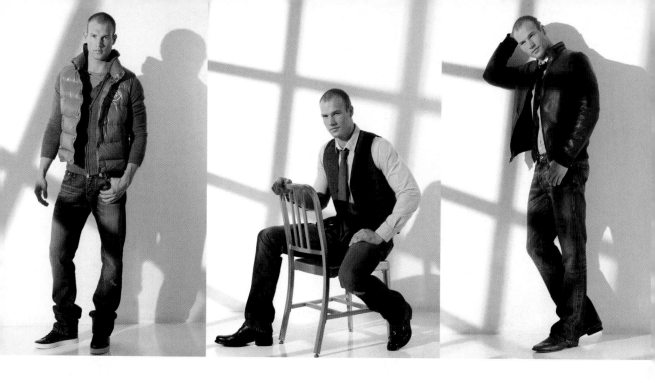

ON THE JOB

Dress codes have relaxed, not retreated. Your goal: finding denim that signals your rising-star status.

The upgrade: Add a style accent to your work wear and you'll show your corporate compass is pointed squarely at the corner office. A well-tailored vest or sport coat or a dress shirt and tie with nice brogues send the right signals. And save your frayed, worn jeans for your next fishing trip. Good work jeans are dark, unadorned, and practically devoid of detail—that means too-ornate back pockets are out. Pay attention to the condition of your jeans, too.

Watch out for: The back hem, which can fall underfoot if it isn't tailored correctly and will telegraph your sloppy sartorial care. The fit of the jeans matters, too. Aim for something that splits the difference between too loose (boot cut) and shrink-wrapped (slim fit). Your coworkers don't want to see your Calvins, nor do they want to suspect you of banana smuggling.

Check out: 7 for All Mankind, Stone Island Denims, Spurr, Agave, Earnest Sewn

A NIGHT OUT

Unless you're inhaling caviar or taking in an opera, sleek, stylish jeans are your go-to garb once the sun drops below the horizon.

The upgrade: James Dean and Marlon Brando pulled off pairing a simple T-shirt with their jeans, but it takes a more refined look to capture the fairer sex these days. More than 34 percent of all the women we surveyed said that guys don't dress up enough—particularly when they're wearing denim.

Know the context: If you're hitting a pizza joint before taking in a flick, anything goes. But if you're planning on throwing back $14 martinis at a downtown bar, opt for darker, slimmer jeans. Straight leg, slim straight, or boot cut are safe options, and offer a more form-fitting silhouette.

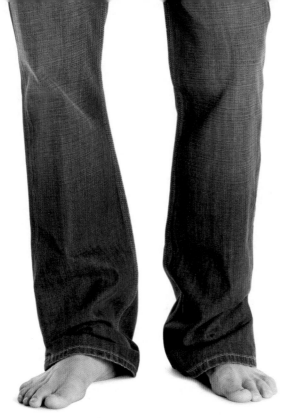
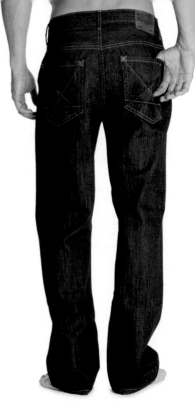

Find the Right Fit

All jeans are not created equal. Consult this guide to find your perfect pair.

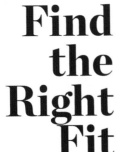

ATHLETIC CUT

A denim hybrid, this contemporary cut blends the legroom of a relaxed fit, the flared hem of a boot cut, and the snug seat of a straight leg. It's an emerging style that can be difficult to track down, but Lucky Brand, Kasil, and Chip & Pepper all cut pairs to these specs.

If your build is . . . **ATHLETIC**, buy in bulk. This style is tailor-made for your physique. . . . **STOCKY**, this cut is a terrific alternative to a relaxed fit, providing more shape and contour to your frame while still offering sufficient legroom and comfort. . . . **AVERAGE**, wear these as a comfy alternative to relaxed-fit jeans. . . . **THIN**, look elsewhere. Lean legs are lost in the roomy cut beneath the knee, reinforcing a skinny shape rather than shadowing it.

RELAXED FIT

These laid-back slacks are cut fuller from the thigh to the hem, allowing ample legroom for maximum comfort. A word of warning, however: Some renditions of this style can be too roomy, creating a sloppy appearance.

If your build is . . . **STOCKY**, breathe easy. Relaxed-fit jeans cut bigger guys some slack, creating interior real estate so legs can flex and move. Look for styles with larger back pockets, which will make you look like you have less junk in your trunk. . . . **ATHLETIC**, wear these for a more comfortable fit. Muscular quads can have a hard time wiggling into some jeans, but an especially forgiving trim in the thighs absorbs them with ease. . . . **AVERAGE OR THIN**, avoid this cut. The width in the legs can be difficult to fill for the typical guy, creating a style that's almost too laid-back.

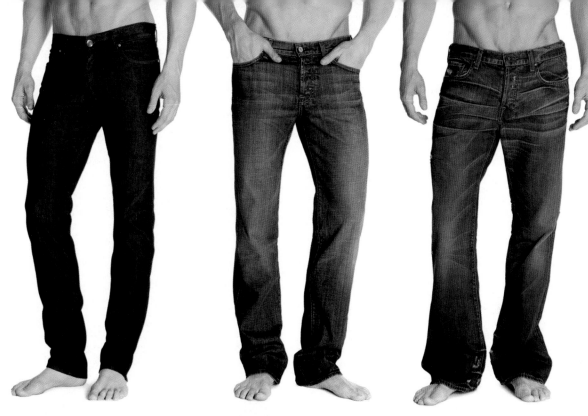

SKINNY JEANS

Calf-clinging denim was the domain of vintage Western icons Roy Rogers and Gene Autry long before Mick Jagger shimmied into a pair. In the past 3 years, this style has been reborn as an indie-rock staple. They come in slightly longer lengths than other cuts, because they're meant to be worn bunched at the ankle. The extra fabric is kept above the shoe line, though, since the narrow bottoms keep the hem from falling underfoot.

If your build is . . . **THIN**, dive in. But don't go overboard; a snug fit shouldn't put your moving parts on display, so look for styles with a small amount of stretch, which will create the illusion of a slightly larger frame. . . . **AVERAGE**, go with your gut. The fabric on these jeans can be forgiving, but they can be a tight squeeze for belly-heavy builds. . . . **ATHLETIC OR STOCKY**, skip these. The cut can make larger legs look like a pair of anacondas.

STRAIGHT LEG

A simple, straightforward design means these classic jeans play a more reserved role in sculpting your appearance. They're equally adaptable on the formality front, capable of being both dressed up and dressed down. The jeans are intended to be straight from hip to foot, which can be difficult to judge in a mirror, but if you leave a couple of inches of wiggle room from the thigh down, they'll fall right into place.

If your build is . . . **ATHLETIC OR AVERAGE**, stock up. This everyman's jean is just snug enough to show off your sculpted lower half, but not so much that you'll look like a beanpole. . . . **THIN**, go with a straight-leg, low-rise fit to ensure that the style sits comfortably on your hips and leaves a few extra inches of leg-room. . . . **STOCKY**, proceed with caution. Bulkier frames are more prone than other body types to be done in by the otherwise natural cut.

BOOT CUT

The enlarged hem on this style accommodates and flatters sturdier footwear like work boots. From the knee to the waist, however, the cut is more traditional, creating a fitted silhouette that sits at or slightly below the waist and remains slightly loose in the leg.

If your build is . . . **ATHLETIC OR AVERAGE**, consider this your go-to style. The cut is especially suited for taller men, because the enlarged hem balances out a stretched frame. . . . **THIN**, rejoice: A leaner build benefits from a boosted emphasis in the seat. Need even more support in the rear? Look for rear flap pockets to round out your exterior. . . . **STOCKY**, steer clear, unless you carry your weight above the waist, in which case the roomier legs can create a straight line from hip to feet.

I AM MY JEANS

Real guys talk about why they love the blues

THE COWBOY

"Bull riders don't dress for fashion. Wearing a pair of Wranglers means one less thing I have to worry about during a ride. A bull once hooked the seat of my jeans. The denim ripped, but I walked out of the arena a lucky man."—Luke Snyder, who competed in the PBR World Finals in Las Vegas in 2007.

THE ROCKER

"Not everybody can look good in a pair of leather pants. Sometimes what's trendy can look cheap in a minute. Instead of seeing the fads in the clothing, you need to see what looks good on you. In the right jeans, you can be possessed by the spirit of rock 'n' roll. You become electrified."—Jesse "Boots Electric" Hughes is one half of the Eagles of Death Metal. He custom fits and designs his own jeans. Listen to his album *Heart On.*

THE TRUCKER

"No one can destroy a pair of jeans like me. I've caught them on fire, snagged and slashed them on sharp metal, and rolled into countless puddles of battery acid and oil. When was the last time your tow-truck operator pulled up in khakis?"—Bill Gratzianna, owner of O'Hare Towing Service in Chicago and the subject of Speed TV's *Wrecked.*

Blue Basics

David Lim, founder and designer of Kasil Jeans, explains how to clean your favorite denim

EVERYDAY JEANS

- Wear your jeans at least two or three times between washings.
- Turn jeans inside out before laundering. Use cold water and mild soap.
- Hang dry. Do not use a clothes dryer; heat will fade and shrink denim.
- To maintain the original color of your jeans, dry-clean them.

SELVAGE OR RAW DENIM

- Don't wash raw and selvage jeans until they feel comfortable and broken in, which can take anywhere from 1 to 3 years.
- Do not wash these in an automatic machine or you'll damage the integrity of the garment and lose much of the pigment. Instead, turn them inside out and hand wash in a tub or sink.
- Use mild soap, and twirl the denim in the water a couple of times instead of scrubbing. Rinse.
- Don't ring them out to dry. Lay them flat or hang them above the tub.
- When in doubt, dry-clean them, but as infrequently as possible.

YOUR ROSTER OF JEANS

Men need six good pairs of denim in their arsenal, says Sean Hornbeak, men's director of J Brand and owner of Denim Revival in L.A. Here is a simple guide.

THE FRANCHISE PLAYER: 1 Pair
A clean, darker wash, such as Japanese selvage, will ensure this pair is easy to dress up with a suit jacket or a dress shirt. Consider these your winning pair on a date.
Price range: $300+

THE UTILITY INFIELDERS: 2 Pairs
These pairs can be a little more casual, but should still be able to go from work to a night out. Branch out into a slightly distressed, lighter wash or break away from blue and try a gray pair. Both work well with a fitted cotton T-shirt.
Price range: $180 to $200

THE MAINSTAYS: 3 Pairs
Durability and wearability are your driving forces here, so pick up some Wranglers or basic Levi's 501s—the old-school kind you break in yourself—or demote a pair of jeans from higher in the pyramid.
Price range: $30 to $60

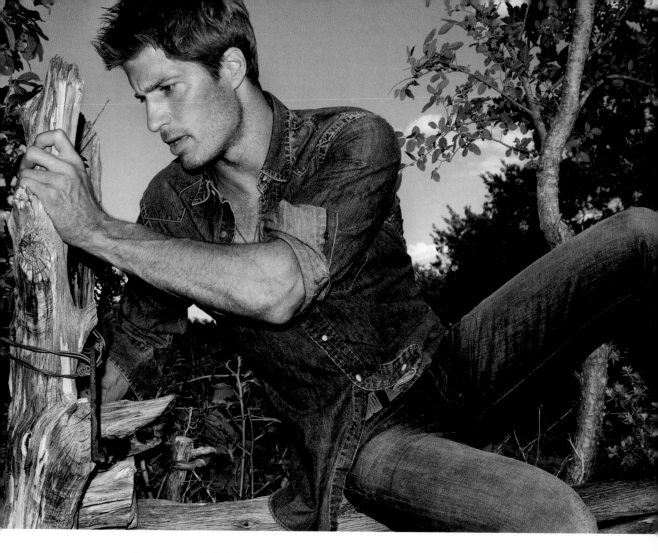

WORKING MAN'S BLUES

Rib Hillis parlayed a handyman gig into his big break as a carpenter on *Extreme Makeover: Home Edition*. Here, he explains how his second skin keeps him covered.

If you want to be a successful handyman, move to Hollywood. That's what Rib Hillis learned a few years ago hanging pictures and tightening doorknobs for Hollywood A-listers. When you're used to sending a page to fetch your latte, are you really going to fix the drip in the sink yourself? Hillis, a struggling actor, used the

fix-it gig to bridge the gap between acting jobs. It put food on the table for his newborn twins and allowed him to set his own schedule. And instead of schlepping egg-white quiches to midlevel producers like most other aspiring actors, Hillis was fixing the world, one home at a time. Then he caught a break. Call it casting or call it fate, but Hillis didn't have to ditch his tool belt to join the cast of ABC's *Extreme Makeover: Home Edition*.

"If you stand still for too long, you can

"I like to wear my jeans in. I'm not one of those guys who buys his jeans already distressed. I WOULD RATHER DESTROY THEM MYSELF."

become built into the wall," says Hillis, 37. "It's amazing what we can do in a week." Hillis's job on the show is to craft specialty rooms. Once, he built a dog haven with drinkable toilets and running water, and installed a B-17 bomber flight simulator in a child's bedroom. This fall, the team will focus on rebuilding homes for firefighters and police officers.

"I actually think our show is the only true reality show out there because it's real, not a fabricated scenario," says Hillis. "We're giving people new houses and a new lease on life. It's real, when all these other shows aren't. It's incredible."

That realism extends to the often brutal week of construction, a whirlwind of activity during which temperatures can drop to freezing. There's no heated wardrobe van for Hillis. His uniform? A pair of his own jeans worn with a cotton tee or a Western shirt. His go-to denim, from Armani Exchange, has a bit of stretch thanks to a touch of Lycra, which helps them hug his athletic legs and gives him the freedom to hoist a piece of plywood into place or drop to the ground to rough out an electrical outlet.

"I'll work in these all day long for 12 hours in the show, so they have to be comfortable," Hillis says. He points to a patch on his jeans, earned after they got caught on a nail while he was carrying a door. Clearly, he sees it as a badge of honor. "My jeans get beat up a lot. They tell a story,"

he says. "The imperfections impart character—my character. These aren't made in the factory. The real wear marks reveal who I am."

Here are a few jeans tips from Hillis.

Measure everything twice. "Baggy pants and protruding boxers are a liability for me," says Hillis, who needs to be nimble on set. A precise fit will keep you from snagging and create a more flattering silhouette. Each brand has its own idea of sizing—often very different from the waist measurement on the tag—so it's best to try on a few sizes in different styles until you find the one that works best.

Stick to the foundations. Blue jeans shouldn't stray too far from their humble origins. Overly embellished or branded jeans attract the wrong kind of attention. "They should be that thing that makes you look great, but you can't put your finger on exactly why," says Hillis, who prefers an understated pair of jeans with a plain pocket and a medium indigo wash. Avoid ornate pockets and unnaturally colored washes (yellow, red, rust-colored) with short half-lives. If you'd be embarrassed to run into your boss wearing a certain pair of jeans, leave them on the shelf.

Put your own mark on them. Rather than buying jeans with mass-produced distressing, Hillis likes to wear his jeans in slowly, letting them acquire natural wear created by his job and his activities.

DENIM DIRECTORY

We've pared down thousands of brands to this tear-and-save list of essentials. Start your search here for the perfect pair of jeans.

Acne Jeans

Key details: This high-end Swedish brand is known for simple cuts and the bright red stitching on its six stylish fits. It's the go-to brand for skinny jeans.
Where: Acne Studio NYC; Barneys New York; and specialty retailers Opening Ceremony, Steven Alan, and Oak; acnejeans.com

Agave

Key details: This company's attention to detail is evident in everything from the Supima cotton used to make the U.S.- and Japanese-woven fabric to the hand finishing, all fashioned in California. Agave offers seven fits (most have 35-inch inseams); these jeans are a popular choice for guys who want high-quality, straightforward denim.
Where: Nordstrom, Barneys New York, and specialty retailers; agavejean.com

AG Adriano Goldschmied

Key details: Denim veteran Adriano Goldschmied emphasizes fit and fabric and avoids trendy details. AG jeans feature classic styles that recall the best denim of 10, 15, or 20 years ago.
Where: Barneys New York, Bloomingdale's, Scoop, Saks Fifth Avenue, Anthropologie, and other specialty retailers; agjeans.com

Armani Exchange

Key details: The Italian fashion label offers youthful, trend-driven styles in six fits. Athletic guys should try the low-rise straight leg or the low-rise relaxed fit.
Where: Armani Exchange stores nationwide; armaniexchange.com

Bread Denim

Key details: These casual California cuts start with American denim and end with finished details like authentic whiskering and vintage washes, resulting in an all-around "real guy's" jean.
Where: Bloomingdale's, Nordstrom, Fred Segal, and Lisa Kline; breaddenim.com

Calvin Klein Jeans

Key details: CK pioneered designer denim in the 1980s. Decades later, the brand remains known for its streamlined fits, which are available in six physique-accentuating shapes.
Where: Macy's, Dillard's, Lord & Taylor, Carson Pirie Scott, and Belk; calvinklein.com

Chaps Denim

Key details: Chaps owns no-fuss styles like classic, straight leg, carpenter, and boot cut. Use as your armor for weekend DIY projects.
Where: Kohl's, Belk, Stage, Peebles; chaps.com; (866) 246-8389

C-IN2 Industries

Key details: C-IN2's denim isn't the typical five-pocket fare. This company, known for its underwear, is debuting a line of jeans for the fashion-forward. Customize with two styles and seven washes of denim.
Where: c-in2.com; (212) 254-3604

DDCLab

Key details: Most jeans make for bog-like conditions during hot days, but DDCLab's breathable fabric ensures you can opt for denim regardless of the temperature.
Where: DDCLab Stores; ddclab.com; (877) 385-8085

D&G

Key details: This Italian luxury brand designs high-end denim, with signature details like elaborate pocket logos. Its low-rise, narrow-silhouette style will showcase your profile.
Where: D&G Boutiques; (800) 979-3038

Diesel

Key details: This denim pioneer champions 30 fits of five-pocket denim in countless washes. Diesel's style forges trends. Stand out, subtly, with its trimmed pockets and sleek fit.
Where: Diesel stores, Bloomingdale's, Neiman Marcus, Nordstrom, Saks Fifth Avenue, and specialty stores; diesel.com

DKNY Jeans

Key details: This New York brand crafts denim to fit from slim to relaxed, at approachable prices. They are a mainstay of the guy who wants to look contemporary without being too cutting edge.
Where: Macy's, Bon-Ton, and Dillard's; dknyjeans.com; (800) 777-4524

Earnest Sewn

Key details: Designer Scott Morrison obsesses over classic American denim, resulting in versatile jeans you can wear to work and to whatever follows.
Where: Barneys New York, Bloomingdale's, Scoop, Ron Herman, and Fred Segal; earnestsewn.com

Edun

Key details: This socially conscious brand, founded by U2's Bono and his wife, Ali Hewson, gives back and uses organic materials from the developing world.
Where: Nordstrom and Barneys New York; edunonline.com

Genetic Denim

Key details: These mad-scientist jeans boil down to two fits. The Dominant Gene is a high-rise, button-fly pair, and is more laid back and casual. The Recessive Gene is a tailored boot leg, which is more classic and refined. Each style sports an embroidered double helix on the back pocket.
Where: Saks Fifth Avenue; specialty retailers Kitson Men, Oliver, and Pittsburgh Jeans Company; geneticdenim.com

Gilded Age

Key details: This brand uses organic yarns and selvage fabric to create Earth-conscious, casual-Friday garb that still commands respect.
Where: Barneys New York; Bergdorf Goodman; and specialty retailers Scoop, Fred Segal, Ron Herman, and others; gildedage.net

G-Star

Key details: Amsterdam-based G-Star spins traditional denim by injecting their jeans with motocross-inspired styles, innovative washes, and a sophisticated urban look.
Where: G-Star stores, Bloomingdale's, Nordstrom; g-star.com

Guess? Inc.

Key details: This classic denim pioneer has carved out a relevant place in the contemporary denim scene with a new organic line. We like the Rebel and Falcon styles best.
Where: Guess? retail stores, Macy's, Bloomingdale's, and specialty stores; guess.com; (800) 224-8377

Habitual

Key details: The Maltese cross design on the back pocket suggests courage, honor, truth, and bravery. Consider it your casual coat-of-arms.
Where: Nordstrom, Saks Fifth Avenue, Bergdorf Goodman, and revolveclothing.com; habitual.com

Howe

Key details: Rock these for the indie-band look. Howe specializes in slim-fit, low-rise jeans that stretch instead of suffocate.
Where: Lisa Kline, The Closet, Fusion Home Fashion, Citizen Clothing, French Corner; hauseofhowe.com

Hugo Boss

Key details: The German powerhouse with four distinct denim brands under its cover features sophisticated looks for men who want to make a lasting impression.
Where: Bloomingdale's, Saks Fifth Avenue, and Nordstrom; hugoboss.com

J Brand Denim Co.

Key details: J Brand pays special attention to hand-crafted detailing, such as chain-stitch hems and hidden rivets. Every component, from the cuffs to the buttons, is made in the United States.
Where: Barneys New York, Bergdorf Goodman, Scoop, Ron Herman, American Rag, and E Street Denim; *jbrandjeans.com*

James Jeans

Key details: Like a cut of fine steak, dry-aging develops the texture of this brand's straight legs and boot cuts.
Where: Specialty retailers and online at *zappos.com* and *bluefly.com*; *jamesjean.us*

Joe's Jeans

Key details: Allow your personality to dictate your jeans, not the opposite. Joe's offers up options based on persona, from the relaxed-fitting Rebel to the slim-cut Rocker.
Where: Nordstrom, Bloomingdale's, Macy's, and Fred Segal; *joesjeans.com*

John Varvatos Star USA

Key details: This manufacturer is big on comfort and light on frills. These no-nonsense jeans come in blue, gray, brown, tan, and green.
Where: Barneys New York, Fred Segal, Bill Hallman, Mario's, and Ron Herman. *johnvarvatos.com*; (212) 965-0700

Kasil

Key details: This brand culls premium fabrics from the United States, Italy, and Japan to create jeans that grab attention with their tailored fit.
Where: Nordstrom and specialty retailers American Rag, Gerry's, Ron Herman, and others; *kasiljean.com*

Lacoste

Key details: The brand known for its colorful polos serves two styles of denim: the classic casual fit and a slimmer straight leg with a low rise.
Where: Lacoste boutiques nationwide; *lacoste.com*; (800)452-2678

Lee Jeans

Key details: Hard-to-fit guys looking for affordability and durability should flock to Lee for its heavyweight ring-spun denim offered in generous sizes.
Where: JCPenney, Kohl's, Sears, Goody's, and other department stores; *lee.com*; (800) 453-3348

Level Jeans

Key details: Level's denim survives trends yet still manages to look contemporary, not old-fashioned.
Where: Macy's West, Fred Segal, and specialty retailers. *leveljeansusa.com*

Levi's Capital E

Key details: This iconic American brand has evolved since its first pair was sold in 1873. This premium, hand-crafted line--founded in 1996--offers higher-end fabrics and styles made by hand and cut from 100 percent organic cotton.
Where: Barneys New York, American Rag, and Fred Segal

Levi's Vintage Clothing

Key details: This line taps into denim history by bringing back exact replicas of original jeanswear from the more than 150-year-old design archives in San Francisco. You'll pay more for these, but you'll have a pair of jeans unlike any other.
Where: Barneys New York, American Rag, and Fred Segal

Levi's Red Tab

Key details: The Levi's Red Tab device--the ribbon detail found inserted into the right rear pocket of nearly every pair of Levi's jeans--was first introduced in 1936. Find it in its original button-fly straight leg, the 501 jean, and the 517 boot cut.
Where: Levi's Store locations and *levi.com*

Loomstate

Key details: This brand was one of the first to plant a 100 percent certified-organic-cotton flag and continues to rely on socially and environmentally sustainable production methods.
Where: Barneys CO-OP, American Rag, and Flying A; *loomstate.org*

Lucky Brand

Key details: This California-based jeans company made its name through its bounty of styles, each hand-detailed with hidden messages and unique finishes.
Where: Lucky Brand stores nationwide, Bloomingdale's, and Macy's; *luckybrandjeans.com*; (800) 964-5777

Nautica Jeans Co.

Key details: Nautica focuses on quality and straightforward denim, and shies away from showy details popular with other designer brands.
Where: Macy's, Dillard's, Carson Pirie Scott, Bon-Ton, and Belk; *nautica.com*

Nobody

Key details: This Aussie brand pulls selvage denim from Japan and transforms it into hand-customized, high-fashion fits.
Where: Specialty retailers American Rag, Louis Boston, Oak, LFT, and others; *nobody.com.au*

Notify

Key details: Add nuance to your wardrobe with this French brand's lineup of innovative washes, like lacquered denim.
Where: Saks Fifth Avenue and Jeffrey New York; *notifyjeans.com*

Nudie Jeans

Key details: Ask a roadie: Jeans are to be worn hard. This label buys denim unwashed and encourages you to keep them that way for as long as possible.
Where: Barneys New York, Atrium, American Rag, and *revolveclothing.com*; *nudiejeans.com*

Polo Denim

Key details: Buy Polo's authentic, preppy fits for an all-American look.
Where: Saks Fifth Avenue, Bloomingdale's, Macy's, Atrium, and E Street Denim

PPD Jeans

Key details: PPD's curved-back yoke tailoring will focus her eye on your backside and torso.

Where: American Rag, Barneys New York, E Street Denim, and Nordstrom; *paigeusa.com*

Prps

Key details: "Prps" stands for "purpose," and the brand lives up to its name. The manufacturer harvests cotton in Africa and then constructs its jeans in Japan on vintage Levis' shuttle looms.
Where: Ron Herman, Fred Segal, American Rag, Barneys New York, Scoop, and Atrium; *prpsgoods.com*; (212) 966-0464

Rag & Bone

Key details: The buzz around this New York denim brand has grown since it debuted its Brit-influenced sportswear back in 2002. The denim remains true to its roots, with styles assembled with Japanese fabric, pure indigo washes, and American craftsmanship.
Where: Rag & Bone store, Barneys New York locations, and smaller specialty retailers; *rag-bone.com*

Replay

Key details: Toss the sweats and make this your new loungewear. This Italian-based premium denim label focuses on a relaxed approach to fashion and uses unorthodox buckles and style embellishments.
Where: Replay stores and better specialty and department stores

Rogan

Key details: Founder Rogan Gregory forged "it" brands Loomstate and Edun. Here he shapes untraditional constructions in hip, downtown collections.
Where: Barneys New York; *rogannyc.com*

7 for All Mankind

Key details: One of the early leaders in the '90s denim boom, 7 for All Mankind still masters the everyman jean with a twist.
Where: 7 for All Mankind retail stores, Neiman Marcus, Bloomingdale's, Saks Fifth Avenue, Nordstrom, Barneys New York, Intermix, and Scoop; *7forallmankind.com*

In Defense of $300 Jeans

Is a pair of pants really worth a night out in Vegas, a five-star dinner, or even a month's rent?

At first glance, the Caitac wet-processing denim facility near Los Angeles seems more like an alien crash site than the last stop for many of the country's premium jeans. But this is where $300 denim comes to life.

Spending $300 on jeans sounds crazy until you talk with Jeff Shafer, the owner and designer of the California-based premium-denim label Agave. Agave is one of a dozen high-end brands that use Caitac to finish (or sometimes rough up) jeans that can cost as much as $250.

According to a market analysis by the NPD Group, men's premium denim sales rose 45 percent in 2007 in the United States, accounting for more than half of the $5 billion men spent on new jeans. But as Shafer explains, the Caitac finishing plant is only the last stop in a whirlwind tour of the globe for his jeans, each step of which adds heft to the price tag.

High-end denim is born rich. The fiber of choice for these brands, Supima cotton, makes up only 3 percent of the world's cotton production, and because it's stronger and finer than the strains popular in the United States, it's also more expensive to produce and process. The good stuff slips right through American saw-ginning machines, so it's shipped to Switzerland, where roller gins spin it into yarn. That spun yarn is then moved to Japan or Italy for dyeing and then woven into fabric on modern shuttle looms—or vintage American shuttle looms that were shed by manufacturers

"AMERICA is where denim was BORN."

in the 1950s and are now prized as rare commodities overseas.

Finally, the fabric makes it back to the United States for cutting and sewing before its Caitac send-off. Both steps could be done overseas, but Shafer says he's willing to absorb the additional $30 of production costs for each pair to come to life under his watch.

"We might have lost the looms, but we still have the history and the heritage," Shafer says. "You don't buy champagne from China. You don't buy tequila from Turkey. America is where denim was born." ∎

EXERCISE SCIENCE

RAISE SOME HAIR

According to a recent study in the *Journal of Dermatological Science*, an amino acid called L-carnitine, which transports fatty acids into mitochondria (cells' metabolic furnaces), works like Miracle-Gro for your hair, increasing the metabolic activity of the cells, which helps hair grow strong and healthy. According to the study, it can actually increase the number of hairs on your head. One brand to try is Revita shampoo. It works best when it's used daily and left on the scalp for 5 to 10 minutes before rinsing (divineskin.com).

SCORE IN THE RED ZONE

You don't have to be Shaq-sized to intimidate opponents. Wearing red can give you a psychological advantage on the playing field, according to a new study in the *Journal of Sports Sciences*. Researchers at the University of Chichester, in England, found that soccer goalkeepers rated opposing players dressed in red uniforms as more aggressive—and more skilled—than those decked out in other colors.

One possible explanation: Our faces turn crimson when we're combative, so we might unconsciously associate red with an impending attack, says study author Iain Greenlees, PhD.

For a mental edge, lock eyes with your opponent. Players who stared down goalkeepers made them less confident in their abilities, say British researchers.

CLEAR YOUR COMPLEXION

What you put in your mouth might end up on your face. Eating refined carbohydrates fuels acne breakouts, states a new study in the *American Journal of Clinical Nutrition*. When 47 pimple-prone men cut refined carbs from their diets, nearly half saw their skin clear up in just 1 week. Study author Neil Mann, PhD, says that sugary foods cause a spike in blood sugar and a corresponding increase in insulin.

"And high insulin levels spur the cells in our oil ducts to multiply, which results in blockages and breakouts," he says.

WASH THAT GRAY RIGHT OUT OF YOUR HAIR

Is your hair hung over?

Instead of buying Just for Men, try cutting your alcohol intake to put the color back into your gray hair. In a new study in the *Archives of Dermatology*, people with drinking problems had twice as much prematurely gray hair as those who didn't overimbibe.

Alcohol halts the production of melanocytes, stem cells that give hair its pigment, says Stuart Reece, MD, the study author, who adds that downing just three drinks a day might be toxic to hair color over time. Already gray? Quaff less and your melanocytes may recover enough of their function to restore the pigment to your pate.

BREAK YOUR SLUMP

Slouch in your office chair and you won't just look like a slacker—you may become one. How you sit can help make or break your work performance, say Colorado College researchers, who found that male students with the best sitting posture scored significantly higher on a logic exam than those who slouched.

An upright posture makes people feel dominant and suc-

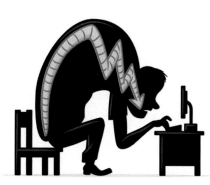

cessful, which in turn improves their ability to relax and focus on problems, says Tomi-Ann Roberts, PhD, the lead study author. To fine-tune your posture, sit and tie a string from an upper shirt button to your belt buckle so that the string is taut when you sit tall. If the string goes slack, you're slouching.

As a bonus: Tilting your office chair's seat 15 degrees forward can ease back pain and improve your posture.

CHECK YOUR SCALP

Head to a barber before your next trip to the dermatologist: A deadly form of skin cancer might be hiding under your hair.

When scientists at the University of North Carolina reviewed more than 50,000 cases of melanoma, they found that patients with cancer on their scalps were 84 percent more likely to die of the disease than those with melanoma elsewhere on their bodies. That could be because the skin on your head is densely packed with blood vessels that can quickly spread cancer cells.

"So help your doctor by getting a haircut to make your scalp easier to scan," says study author Nancy Thomas, MD, PhD. And between screenings, cover your cranium with a wide-brimmed hat when you're out: Hair is not an effective sunscreen. ■

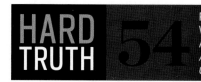

HARD TRUTH 54 PERCENTAGE OF ADULTS WHO HAVE ACNE, ACCORDING TO THE *AMERICAN JOURNAL OF CLINICAL NUTRITION*

TRAINING TIPS

Q: I sweat through my shirts within minutes. What's the best antiperspirant?

A: Fear not the high-five. Sweat experts from the University of Miami's Miller School of Medicine recommend rolling on Certain Dri four or five times a week. This superstrength antiperspirant contains 12 percent aluminum chloride, which has been clinically proved to reduce sweating by up to 45 percent, compared with standard antiperspirants that achieve only a 20 percent reduction.

The key is to apply Certain Dri at night, says Leslie Baumann, MD, the director of the University of Miami cosmetic group. She explains that because you sweat less when you sleep, an evening application gives the aluminum chloride time to enter your sweat ducts and form gel-like plugs. In the morning, wash your underarms to remove any residual Certain Dri (if it's left on, it could cause skin irritation) and then use a few swipes of Mitchum Clear Gel Sport antiperspirant, which contains a form of aluminum chloride that's almost as powerful (and provides deodorant protection, too).

Q: My antiperspirant turns the armpits of my white undershirts yellow. Why? Are there any that won't?

A: Antiperspirants work by plugging your moisture-producing eccrine glands with aluminum or zirconium salts. The problem is that when you smear the stuff onto your pits, it mixes with what's already on your skin.

"The salts chemically react with proteins secreted by the apocrine glands, resulting in that yellow stain," says John Labows, PhD, an organic chemist and the former director of technology at Colgate-Palmolive. To minimize discoloration, Dr. Labows says to make just one pass with your antiperspirant and then wait for it to dry completely before slipping on your shirt. Staining is more likely to occur when the antiperspirant is wet. (Even stick antiperspirants contain some moisture.)

And those pee-colored tees you already

own? The Soap and Detergent Association recommends either using a prewash stain remover, or soaking the shirts in white vinegar (for old stains) or ammonia (for new ones). Then wash them with a product containing enzymes or oxygenated bleach in the hottest water that's safe for the fabric.

Q: **Are there any benefits to using caffeinated soap?**

A: Recent studies suggest that caffeine can both protect the skin from UV rays and stimulate the body after entering the bloodstream through hair follicles, says Bruce Katz, MD, a clinical professor of dermatology at the Mount Sinai School of Medicine in New York and director of the Cosmetic Surgery & Laser Clinic at Mount Sinai Medical Center.

Unfortunately, you'll reap neither benefit from caffeinated soap. The stimulating ingredient doesn't stay on the skin long enough to work its magic; it gets washed down the drain right along with all the other suds and chemicals. If you want the benefits of caffeine, get it the old-fashioned way: Drink a steaming cup of joe.

Q: **What's the best way to reduce dark circles under my eyes?**

A: Sleep with an extra pillow under your head, and, if your nose is blocked, pop a decongestant before you hit the sack, says Haideh Hirmand, MD, an assistant clinical professor of plastic surgery at Weill Cornell Medical College, in New York City.

Fatigue isn't the most common cause of raccoon eyes, nasal congestion is: It triggers the dilation of the veins in your lower eyelids. Taking a decongestant will help. Gravity is another common trigger, because it can cause fluid to pool under the eyelids while you sleep.

If home remedies don't cut it, visit your dermatologist or plastic surgeon, who will likely recommend laser treatments or chemical peels to tighten sagging skin. A plastic surgeon can also contour or remove fat, skin, and muscle from your upper and lower lids through a procedure called blepharoplasty. If the problem is excess pigmentation—the result of genetics—ask your doctor about prescription lightening creams.

Q: **Is it true that men should avoid tea tree oils?**

A: The answer is a simple yes, and no. You should avoid drinking tea tree oil herbal teas.

But on the other hand, used externally, tea tree oil can be very helpful for the skin, scalp, and hair.

Q: **Is it ever a good idea to get a base tan?**

A: Let's be clear: No tan is a good tan. Any change in your skin color caused by sun exposure is evidence that your epidermis has been damaged by ultraviolet rays. And as for the theory that gradually tanning over several weeks will somehow safeguard you from sunburn, it's nothing more than a mirage.

"Having a base color may offer some protection, but it will not protect you from a sunburn," says Joely Kaufman, MD, an assistant professor of dermatology at the University of Miami. "You will absolutely still need to apply a sunscreen with at least a 30 SPF." If you're determined to look the part of a sun bum, Dr. Kaufman recommends combining a squirt of Anthony Logistics Self Tanner for Men ($30, anthony.com) with a palmful of an antioxidant-fortified UVA- and UVB-protecting sunblock, such as Menscience Tio2 ($31, menscience.com).

Q: Why is my skin so oily, no matter what I try?

A: "It's usually a genetic predisposition. Some people just have oily skin. But you'll produce more oil in a hot, muggy environment than you will in a dry, cool one, " says John F. Romano, MD, a dermatologist in private practice, clinical assistant professor of dermatology at New York Hospital–Cornell Medical Center, and an attending physician at St. Vincent's Hospital and Medical Center in New York City.

Q: Should I floss before I brush my teeth, or after?

A: Floss first. David Kim, DDS, DMSc, an assistant professor at the Harvard school of dental medicine, says this will not only lessen the chance that you'll skip this vital ritual altogether, but it will also help ensure that whatever flotsam is stirred up by flossing doesn't stay in your mouth.

"With this sequence, you can disrupt plaque and dislodge food particles from between your teeth, which you'll then be able to sweep out more thoroughly with brushing," he says.

As for which floss to use, go with whatever type you find easiest to slip between your teeth. A new study published in the *Journal of Periodontology* compared different kinds of flosses, including unwaxed, woven, and shred-resistant, and found almost no difference in their ease of use or overall effectiveness.

Q: Can stress make my hair turn gray?

A: Just as stress can screw up other parts of your body, it can also leach the color from your locks, specifically by disrupting hair cells called melanocytes.

"It's believed that stress hormones such as cortisol can affect the melanocytes in their ability to survive and produce pigment," says Charles Crutchfield III, MD, a clinical associate professor of dermatology at the University of Minnesota.

To help rein in runaway tension, grab some yogurt and peanuts. Scientists in Slovakia found that men who supplemented their diets with 3 grams each of the amino acids lysine and arginine had a drop in their stress hormones after 90 minutes. An 8-ounce yogurt and a handful of peanuts will get you halfway to those 3 grams.

Q: What's the best swimsuit for a grown-up man?

A: Beware of Speedos, knee-length shorts, and that mankini thing that Borat squeaked into, says Eric Villency, the president of the design studio Maurice Villency and a contributor to NBC's

Today. It's a jungle out there on the beach, and style mistakes can get you noticed in all the wrong ways.

Oceanside fashion faux pas are easy to avoid, however, if you apply the same rules that you would to other dressing choices. Steer clear of extremes in color and size, and then follow these tenets.

Find your length. Tall guys look good in long shorts (20- to 22-inch outseam). Men with bellies should stick to boxer-short styles (14- to 16-inch outseam) in dark colors, which draw attention away from the midsection. Shorter gents should consider modified board shorts (18- to 20-inch outseam) in solid colors, which can give the illusion of height.

Stick to the originals. Two of our favorite brands are Birdwell Beach Britches and Vilebrequin. Birdwells are the original nylon board shorts, predating OP, Quiksilver, Hurley, Billabong, and all those other hot surf companies that like to splash neon skulls and crossbones over your backside. The family-owned company crafts its lifeguard-style board shorts in Santa Ana, California, and the suits are quick-drying, tough, practical, and the embodiment of timeless style.

Pattern your personality. Most people look best in solid colors, but some personas demand flair, and Vilebrequin provides it. Founded in St. Tropez, France, Vilebrequin produces shorts with bold, sophisticated patterns (think: Fauvism meets Keith Haring), mesh liners, and a waterproof wallet that fits into the pockets. The company also makes identical shorts for toddlers, so your boy can dress like a grown-up, too.

Q: How do I buy a leather jacket that will never go out of style?

A: It's similar to the difference between ordering a martini, and, say, a chocolate-tini, says Villency. Choose a leather jacket that doesn't stray too far from the genesis of the form—a rugged brown coat for aviators, or a black jacket for motorcycle riders—but that's also modern and not junked up with patches or zippers. You don't want your buddies asking why you look like an extra from *The Matrix*. What Villency really likes about leather is that there's a wabi-sabi thing going on (that's the Japanese idea that imperfections can make something beautiful). A great leather jacket is something you can wear for 20 years, and it will become more weathered and look better and better.

Sure, buttery-soft napa leather is beautiful, but we suggest going with something tougher that will age better and last longer. Cowhide is the most durable, but lambskin is close behind and is often smoother. If you fold over the sleeve, you should see imperfections in the grain, tiny dents on the surface, and slight variations in texture. Choose a weight you can wear for three seasons. In general, the highest-quality jackets are made in America and Italy. Belstaff is a strong brand and was a personal favorite of Steve McQueen. ■

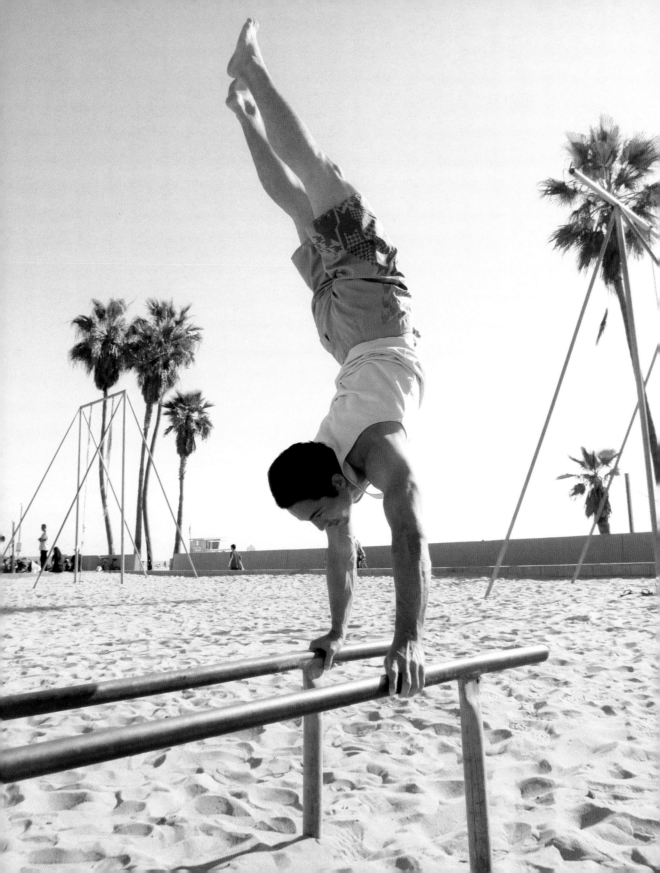

5

Live Long, Live Better

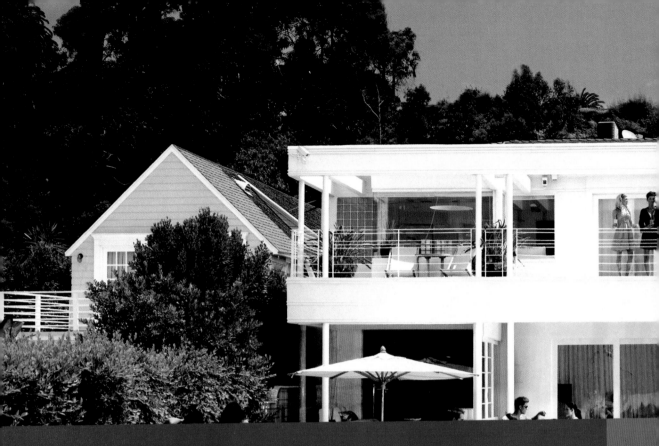

Be as Healthy as the Wealthy

THE RICH ARE DIFFERENT FROM US— THEY LIVE LONGER. HERE'S WHY

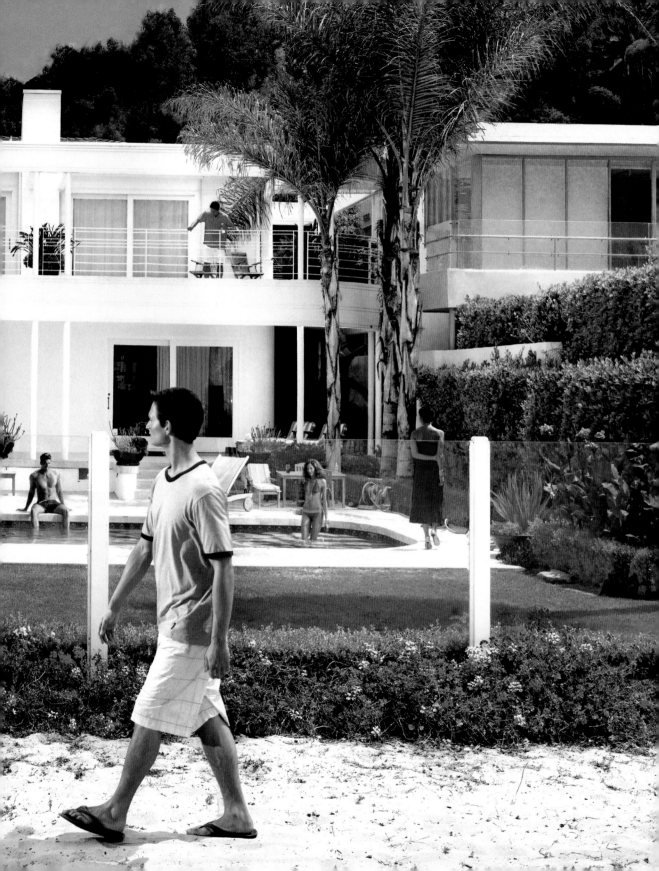

Join us, if you would, on a street corner in southeastern Washington, D.C. It's not a great neighborhood. There's a little liquor store that does a brisk business selling "40s" of King Cobra. Other signs of economic life include "TRY OUR VALUE MEAL" and "WE BUY GOLD."

As if the residents had any of that lying around.

Now let's hop a train at the nearest Metro stop and ride out to affluent suburbia. Our destination is Montgomery County, Maryland. Our tour guide: the pioneering British epidemiologist Michael Marmot, PhD, who wrote about this journey in his provocative book *The Status Syndrome*. For every mile we travel on this Metro route, the life expectancy of the citizenry rises about 9 months. That's right: There's a difference of 12 years between the poor (and mostly African American) people at the beginning of our journey, and the relatively rich (and mostly white) people at the end.

Yes, the rich really are different. They have better health. Not only do they enjoy greater longevity, but their days are less burdened by disease. Don't be fooled by the old idea that more money creates more problems. When it comes to health, the poor are much more likely to suffer physical and mental indignities—everything from asthma and accidents to chronic conditions such as diabetes, high blood pressure, and heart disease. The lower your

position in the economic hierarchy, the more susceptible you are to virtually every major disease affecting men.

The differences are shocking. Take mortality, for example. Harvard University researchers crunched more than 40 years of U.S. Census data to reveal that the gap in premature death rates between the poorest and the richest Americans has nearly doubled since 1980. In fact, people who earned less than $36,000 a year in 2000 faced a 64 percent higher risk of early death than those in households bringing in more than $101,000 annually. Get the raise, or die.

"Social class is simply the best predictor of health," says Nancy E. Adler, PhD, a professor of medical psychology at the University of California at San Francisco. "If you could know only one thing about a person and predict that person's health and longevity, you'd ask about social class. It's even more important than family history."

In cases where someone has bothered asking poor people about their health, research confirms the trend: The poorer you are, the less healthy you're likely to feel. That's the finding of a recent Columbia University study. And results of the CDC's National Health Interview Survey make the case even stronger. In 2006, nearly nine times as many lower-income adults (whose families earned less than $35,000 a year) reported being in fair or poor health as affluent adults (whose families pulled in $75,000-plus). Wealth and health go hand in hand.

Here's Dr. Marmot's way of thinking about it: Our society is a gigantic Titanic. First-class passengers on that ship disproportionately survived. In second class, fewer did. Third-class passengers . . . yikes. Many died before their time. And many of their modern counterparts still do.

The connections between status and health are hugely complex and only partly understood. It's not just a problem in the United States: The Titanic sinks for every nation. No matter where you are, money and status make it easier for you to live in a restful place, go out for a Saturday morning jog, and buy lean protein instead of fast food. It's more likely you'll enjoy a wide circle of friends, more job opportunities, and more control over your schedule. And there's more social pressure to stay away from blood-sucking vices like alcohol, tobacco, and drugs.

If socioeconomic status tells us so much about health, why didn't we know this? In the past, many researchers felt obliged to avoid questions about socioeconomic status when they designed public-health surveys. As a result, they had very little data until about a decade ago. Then the field exploded.

WHY "POOR" GOES WITH "POOR HEALTH"

A few minutes on a street corner in a marginal neighborhood can tell you everything you need to know about what the nation's poor are up against.

A LOT OF FOLKS IN THE SAME PREDICAMENT: Racism and other social biases tend to restrict the poor to certain neighborhoods. This limits their educational and employment opportunities—for generations. The urban infrastructure, physical environment, and quality of life crumble around them, exposing them to health risks and hampering their access to quality health care.

THE CORNER STORE WITH THE MARLBORO SIGN IN THE WINDOW: In this case, the gun really is smoking. According to CDC data, a disproportionate number of smokers in the United States are poor. The tobacco companies do their part by marketing heavily in poor neighborhoods. And government cuts in funds for stop-smoking programs are undermining their effectiveness.

A RAP AS THE BAD PART OF TOWN: The poor (specifically, nonwhite) have less access to decent health care, and discrimination can compound their health problems. A 2003 University of Michigan analysis of 53 studies found that feeling racial or ethnic bias can cause physiological and psychological stress, and systematic exposure to discrimination might have long-term effects.

A COUPLE OF SHADY-LOOKING GUYS HANGING OUT ON THE CORNER: An analysis of data from Britain's Whitehall II study revealed that people who reported a greater fear of crime were nearly twice as likely to suffer from depression as those who reported less fear. They also exercised less and were less social. Why? If you're worried about the local hoods, you won't leave the house as often.

A LOT OF MEN HANGING OUT BECAUSE THEY CAN'T FIND WORK: Anything less than breadwinner status can translate, in a man's own eyes, into loser status. Among studies in a 2003 review, one noted that men in Harlem who were unemployed or underemployed were more likely to smoke and have high blood pressure than men who worked full-time.

Dr. Adler recalls the study that got her hooked. It was one of Dr. Marmot's, a landmark British study that scientists refer to by its shorthand, Whitehall I. Whitehall is the wide street in London where many key government departments are located, and the name is synonymous with the British civil service. In 1967, Marmot's team began a huge survey of 18,000 male civil servants. The men were grouped into quadrants based on office hier-archy, with administrators who set policy at the top, followed by executives, clerical workers, and finally office messengers at the bottom. All the workers had safe office jobs and high job security. The most surprising finding of the study was that not much about the disparity in health outcomes could be explained away by nasty habits or access to care. And in a follow-up study 25 years later in the 1990s, the men at the bottom were found to be not only unhealthier as a group, but three times as likely to die an early death as the men at the top.

Those results started Dr. Adler thinking. What is it about higher social class that matters? How does class affect the body?

With that, she switched her field from adolescent risk behavior to class and health. (As she notes, "I switched taboos from sex to money.") She got the MacArthur Foundation interested. In 1997 she gathered a dozen like-minded researchers together into the MacArthur Research Network on Socioeconomic Status and Health, and became its chairwoman. Since that time, network members have used nearly $9 million in grant money to swap ideas, start pilot studies, and tack their questions onto larger, longitudinal studies. Their collective research provides much

of the scientific basis for the information you're reading here.

Can you take enough action to save yourself from the ill effects of social class? The researchers can't say for sure. But they'll encourage you to try your damnedest. After all, small lifestyle changes accomplish a lot. A whole lot. They're simple, they're easy, they're appallingly obvious— and they have a stunning impact on longevity and health.

The latest proof comes from a 2008 Cambridge study published in the journal *Public Library of Science Medicine*, which examined 20,244 men and women, ages 45 to 79, living in the same English county. The researchers gathered baseline data in the mid-'90s, asking the participants if they en-gaged in any combination of four common healthy habits: exercise, moderate alcohol use, daily fruit and vegetable intake, and abstention from tobacco. Eleven years later, they followed up to see who died in the interim.

Result: The people who engaged in none of the healthy behaviors were four times as likely to have died as those who engaged in all four, regardless of social class. Practicing four simple healthy habits, concluded the researchers, "was equivalent to being 14 years younger in chronological age."

Be mindful about one or two things you can't do anything about—your parents, for instance. You can't choose your mother's social class. And low birth weight, which is more common on lower rungs of the ladder, increases the risk of slow cognitive development in early life and heart disease decades later. Socioeconomic status even affects physical strength and function. In one British study, men born in 1946 were contacted at age 53 and presented with a few challenges, including this one: Close your eyes and stand on one leg for 30 seconds. Sound easy? Less than half of the men were able to do this for longer than 5 seconds. Disproportionately, their fathers were working-class blokes.

One last caveat: Money changes everything, but the trend has a limit. Not a single scientific study has shown that being ridiculously rich will make you ridiculously healthy. Wealth didn't save Donald Trump's hair, for instance. And once you pass a family threshold of about $125K per year, further health gains seem beyond reach. Extra money at that point simply translates into

a desire for more stuff, which leads to the need for more money. A golden treadmill, yes, but a treadmill all the same.

With less money and status, all aspects of a healthy lifestyle are harder to achieve—but not impossible. In essence, you can live the good life by acting rich. You don't even have to wear an ascot. The following lifestyle changes will help you hit your marks.

MAKE YOUR MARK

If you can't be rich, settle for famous.

In a very cool study conducted at the

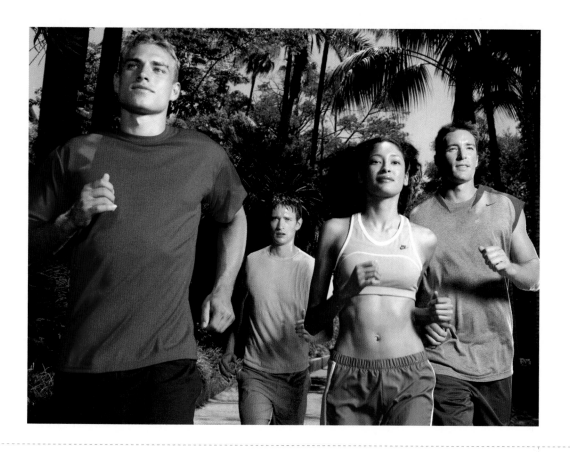

University of Toronto, researchers analyzed 72 years' worth of Academy Award winners. They looked up the age at death of actors who won Oscars, and compared that with (1) costars of those Oscar winners and (2) actors who were nominated for but never won Oscars.

Amazingly, the Oscar winners lived 4 years longer than their costars and fellow nominees. Stars who won multiple Oscars enjoyed an extra 2-year survival boost. That longevity isn't due to a difference in wealth. It's due purely to status.

Researchers are finding out that status is not measured by bread alone. Yes, there's the objective ladder of socioeconomic status, which ranks people by annual income, net worth, and educational level. But there's also a ladder of subjective social status, on which people rank themselves according to how much respect they are given by members of their peer group or community. And both ladders are valid indicators. Your health is predicted by a combination of the two, says Dr. Adler, who pioneered the idea of measuring subjective social status. In one of her studies, the subjective ladder did a better job of predicting heart rate, body-fat distribution, and stress responses than the objective measures of socioeconomic status did.

Her advice: "If you can pick your niche and succeed in that, that's probably going to be good for your health."

HANG WITH THE THIN MAN

You know all about the obesity epidemic sweeping America: Two-thirds of U.S. adults are overweight. Yes, obesity is bad for you; it leads to type 2 diabetes. And yes, spreading wide is widespread. But like most things, obesity is not spread equally across social classes. The CDC's National Health Interview Survey found the highest 2006 obesity rates in the groups with the lowest income and educational levels.

Let's not blame the victims. It's a sad fact that a proper diet is harder to maintain in poorer neighborhoods, which lack supermarkets and the wide variety of healthy choices they offer, but which have plenty of outlets providing cheap, fattening fast food. And if you're working two jobs, who has time to cook or schedule exercise sessions?

But your neighborhood isn't the only problem. In one of the most bizarre findings of 2007, Harvard researchers reported in the *New England Journal of Medicine* that obesity is "contagious"— that your friends are making you fat.

> "If you could know only one thing about a person and predict that person's health and longevity, YOU'D ASK ABOUT SOCIAL CLASS. It's even more important than family history."

Indeed, your closest friends influence your weight more than your genes or your family members.

The researchers studied 12,067 interconnected people who had participated in the Framingham Heart Study from 1971 to 2003. They organized them by their social networks and found the big "whoa": When a participant's friend became obese, his or her chance of becoming obese increased by 57 percent. (Using data from men only, the risk nearly doubled.) If it's a close friend, your chance of bursting your buttons increases by 171 percent. Too many wing nights, evidently.

ENSURE DOMESTIC TRANQUILITY

Where you live shouldn't predict the state of your health. But it does.

In one study of 3,617 adults, simply living in a city increased the risk of premature death (by 62 percent) when compared with suburban or small-town life.

And of course, living in a disadvantaged neighborhood within that city is really bad for you. A huge Columbia University study (13,000 people in four cities) revealed that white people living in the worst neighborhoods had a 70 to 90 percent higher risk of heart disease than whites living in the nicest neighborhoods.

What's so bad about the big city? The air and water are more polluted, leading to an increase in respiratory diseases. The older housing stock is more likely to contain lead paint. One of Dr. Adler's studies found that children and adults in low-income families had six times as much lead in their blood as people in affluent families did. (Middle-income people had double the affluent families' levels.) Also, there's more fear of crime, which results in chronic stress, social isolation, anxiety, and depression. Crime-fearing participants in Britain's late-1980s sequel to the first Whitehall study, Whitehall II, were nearly twice as likely to be depressed as the less-fearful civil servants.

And then there's the noise. Noise exposure has been linked to poorer long-term memory, higher stress, sleep deprivation, and even heart disease. In 2005, the World Health Organization estimated that long-term exposure to traffic noise in Europe might account for 3 percent of deaths from heart disease and strokes. Noise at night can create chronic stress, even while you're sleeping because you continue to react to sounds; this can raise your levels of stress hormones.

What's true for real estate investing is also true for your health: Better to live in the worst house on a nice block than the nicest house on a bad block. You don't need a mansion to get a good night's sleep.

QUIT SMOKING. NO, REALLY

Back in the day, when Humphrey Bogart lit up on the big screen, everyone smoked. Tobacco use was spread evenly across all social classes.

That's no longer true. The class differences are dramatic: In 1995, 40 percent of men who were not high-school graduates smoked. Only 14 percent of male college grads smoked. And here's the sorry part: Those people on the bottom rungs who try to quit are less successful at it than people at the top. It doesn't

THE BEST HEALTH TIPS IN LIFE ARE FREE

Even without a big, fat trust fund, you're still entitled to good health, and it turns out that some of the stuff that can keep you healthy is free for the taking.

GUYS' NIGHT OUT: Worried about having heart attacks as you get on in years? Then keep having (no-stakes) poker night with the guys, even if you can't play as late as you used to. A Harvard school of public health study found that men in their 70s who had full social calendars also had less than half the blood levels of heart-damage markers compared to less socially integrated peers.

A DEEP BREATH: A study in *Health Psychology* found that healthy young adults with higher levels of hostility had lower lung function. The researchers think that the impairment accumulates gradually over the years to take its toll on health. Take a deep breath and count to 10 the next time the copier jams, and you'll breathe easier—and a lot longer.

SUNSHINE: A recent study led by researchers from the Harvard school of public health found that men who had low levels of vitamin D were twice as likely to have heart attacks as those who received higher levels of the "sunshine vitamin."

SEX: You don't have to take matters into your own hand to reap the benefits of ejaculation. Research from Wilkes University links having sex once or twice a week with higher levels of immunoglobulin A, an antibody that protects against colds and other infections.

SLEEP: Stanford researchers found that, in people who sleep less than 8 hours a day, body-mass index was inversely proportional to sleep duration. In other words, short sleepers were more likely to be fat guys. Short sleep was also associated with lower levels of leptin (a hormone that suppresses appetite) and higher levels of ghrelin (a chemical that stimulates it). It's not like being a werewolf, but stinting on your sleep could turn you into a ravenous beast.

JUMPING JACKS: If you're now worried about raiding the fridge during your sleepless nights, here's a free solution: Researchers at Universidade Federal de São Paulo found that a session of moderate aerobic exercise helped one group of subjects increase total sleep time by 21 percent over groups who did heavy aerobics and moderate strength exercises.

mean they lack willpower; it probably means they're surrounded by more smokers in their daily lives.

"Smoking is responsible for the most preventable deaths," says Dr. Adler. It kills more than 400,000 people every year. And because it has become a low-status behavior, it is a major factor in explaining the different health outcomes of haves and have-nots in this country.

So if by chance you get your hands on a box of good Cuban cigars, don't smoke them. No, no, no! Send them along to us.

FIND A JOB THAT FITS

Even though we live in the 21st century, we still carry around 19th-century images of workplace health. As in the physical hazards. But fewer of us are miners or shipyard workers or mill workers anymore. We don't worry about black lung or brown lung.

What we need to worry about are the postmodern killers: jobs with a deadly combination of high demand and low control, jobs that require high effort and dole out low rewards. As Adler's MacArthur Foundation report, Reaching for a Healthier Life, puts it: "Jobs that are plagued by time pressure, conflicting demands, low control over how and when tasks get done, worker/management conflict, threats of pay cuts or job loss, and conflicts between family obligations and work requirements can create damaging levels of stress that surface in disease."

The biggest proof of that came from the first Whitehall study, which found that a greater incidence of heart disease at the bottom of the bureaucratic pecking order

A greater incidence of HEART DISEASE at the bottom of the bureaucratic pecking order was due mainly to a lack of job control—that is, limited permission to solve problems and make decisions.

was due mainly to a lack of job control— that is, limited permission to solve problems and make decisions. Other diseases associated with low job control cited by both Whitehall studies are type 2 diabetes and alcohol dependence. That's no surprise. Men who have a hard time coping with stress tend to turn to alcohol.

But perhaps the most stunning finding from Whitehall II came from 6,000 civil servants who were asked to agree or disagree with this statement: "I often have the feeling that I am being treated unfairly." Those who agreed moderately or strongly were clustered on the lower rungs of the British civil-service system. And by following this group for 11 years, researchers learned that those who felt the most shabbily treated were 55 percent more likely to have had a heart attack in the interim.

Several small studies in various countries have all confirmed these findings to some extent, says Mark Cullen, MD, a professor of medicine at Yale University who directs the medical school's occupational and environmental medicine program. But he thinks the real issue isn't low control; it's psychological stress. "It's the burden that matters," he says. "How much they want from you, how fast they want it, how perfect it has to be." And in his opinion, the amount of stress you feel from your job has a lot to do with whether the job fits you—that is, whether it matches your personality and style and the other demands in your life. Some people actually like low-control jobs, after all—they just want to punch in and punch out. But if you come home at the end of the day feeling angry, alienated, and exhausted, maybe you need more than a new job; you need a new line of work.

"The biggest problems," says Dr. Cullen, "are with a misfit." If you're a misfit, fix it—or you'll die trying.

CALL YOUR FAVES

Do this: In the next 2 weeks, call people in at least six of these categories:
1. wife; 2. parents; 3. in-laws; 4. children; 5. other family members; 6. neighbors; 7. friends; 8. coworkers; 9. school chums; 10. fellow volunteers; 11. members of your social or recreational group; 12. religious friends from your church, synagogue, mosque, ashram, or cult hideout.

If you run low on minutes, face time is perfectly acceptable. Facebook is not.

Do this, and you won't catch a cold. Okay, that's not a guarantee. Put it this way: If your social ties are so frayed that you regularly call three or fewer people on that list, you're three times as likely to catch a cold as someone with a diverse set of social ties, someone who would regularly call or talk to people in at least six of those categories.

A man who is socially isolated has a relative risk of death between two and five times greater than one with better social connections. Why that is, scientists don't know. Social isolation is deadly, and not just in America. In France, the leading cause of death among middle-aged men and women is cancer. In the 1990s, a Harvard study of social integration and mortality among French subjects found that the men who were most isolated were 3.6 times as likely to die of cancer as their well-connected peers.

And, like everything else, social class might play a role here, too. The higher yours is, the less vulnerable you are to loneliness.

GO BACK TO SCHOOL

"Socioeconomic status" is a big, squishy term with several components: the amount of money you earn, the amount of money you have (two different things), your job's prestige, and your level of education. But when push comes to shove, the most important predictor of health is your education.

The most convincing evidence comes from Sweden. One study based on the country's 1990 census tracked 25- to 65-year-old adults who died in the ensuing 6 years and found that each and every step up the educational ladder conferred added longevity. For example: Among men who were 64 in 1990, about 14 percent of those with the bare minimum of education had died by 1996. But just 6 percent of men with PhDs had died. What was most intriguing was the difference between men with doctorates and the next step down—men who were slightly less schooled, but nonetheless were professionals like lawyers and engineers. The PhDs were surely no richer, but they had a 33 percent lower mortality rate.

The experts come away from these numbers with this conclusion: More education gives you more control over your life. And more control means less stress. So stop watching *Law & Order* re-runs and start thinking about going to night school and earning your law degree, so you can kick perp ass for real, tough guy. ■

Get a Checkup— or Check Out

WHAT ARE YOU SO AFRAID OF? PUT OFF VISITING THE DOCTOR FOR A CHECKUP, AND EVENTUALLY BAD NEWS WILL COME CALLING FOR YOU. HERE'S HOW TO AVOID THE KNOCK

Men in the Crystal family shy away from stethoscopes the way vampires recoil from crosses. Stuart Crystal avoided checkups throughout his 20s. His 30-year-old brother, Jonathan, waved him off when Stuart noticed a strange lump on Jonathan's neck. "The lump kept growing bigger," recalls Stuart, now a retired police officer living in Florida.

Months later, Jonathan saw a doctor, who instantly ordered a biopsy. It was lymphoma, and it had spread. A week later, he was dead. "His doctors said that he might have lived had he acted quickly enough," says Stuart.

Jonathan Crystal should be an exception. Yet a recent survey by the American Academy of Family Physicians reveals that 55 percent of U.S. men haven't seen their MDs in the past year.

"They'll ignore blood in their urine and watch testicular tumors grow to the size of grapefruits because they're afraid to come in," says urologist Sheldon Marks, MD, author of *Prostate and Cancer: A Family Guide to Diagnosis, Treatment, and Survival*.

Even young guys sometimes die horrible deaths because they ignore warning signs. We're here to bust your excuses and show you how to maximize your visit once you go.

NUMB YOUR FEAR OF THE DENTIST'S CHAIR

Most of us equate torture with a whirring dentist's drill. But that's the old-school approach to oral health.

"Air abrasion eliminates the need for anesthetic injections and the dental drill when treating cavities," says Jerry Gordon, DMD, owner of the Dental Comfort Zone in Bensalem, Pennsylvania. "It's like a precise sandblaster, with tiny, harmless particles of aluminum oxide powder propelled against the teeth, removing cavities." Fast-acting local anesthetics reduce pain, and quicker-setting impression materials prevent gagging.

And those who've heard horror stories of daylong root canals can stop grinding their teeth.

"New techniques have greatly reduced the time needed to perform a root canal and also greatly limited the potential for discomfort," says Dr. Gordon. "People are afraid of the unknown," says Dr. Gordon. "Now they can see someone successfully go through the procedure before they come in."

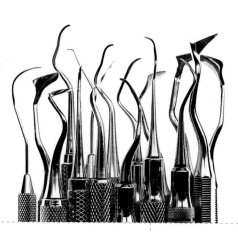

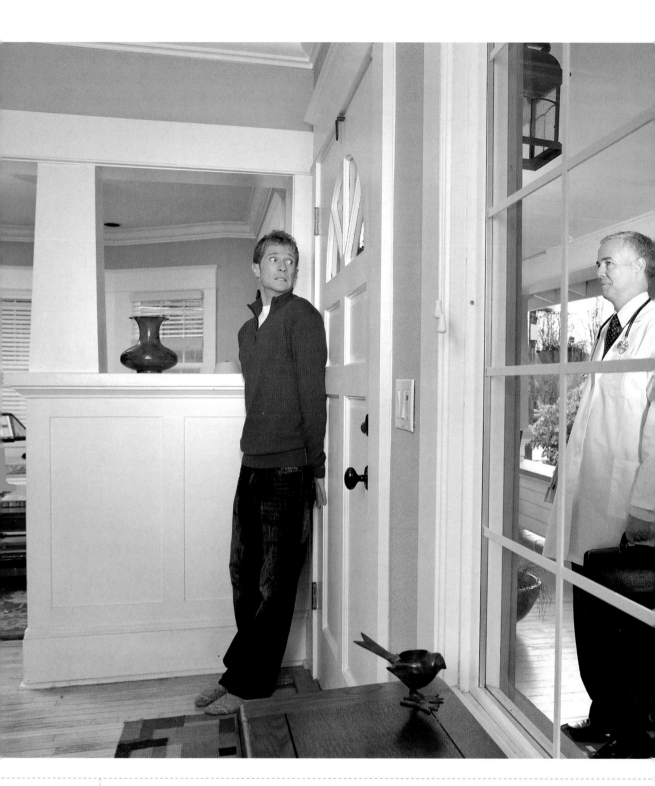

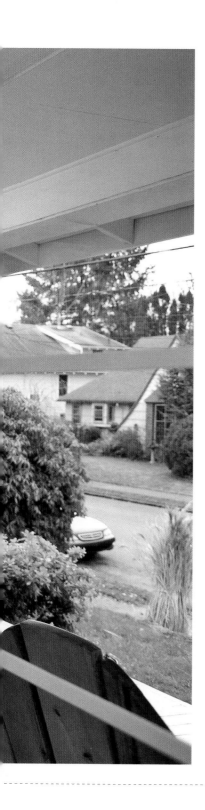

How do you know you're healthy? One-third of all heart-attack victims never have any warning.

"Men often wait until a crisis occurs before they see us," says Rick Kellerman, MD, a family physician in Wichita, Kansas, and board chairman of the American Academy of Family Physicians.

Follow the doctor's orders. To stop dreading exams, find a nearby internist (an MD specializing in internal medicine) you like and respect. Take care of the "like" part by meeting with several physicians in your area before an emergency strikes. See who asks the most questions about your medical history.

Double-check your gut instinct at docboard.org/docfinder.html, a site that lists disciplinary actions and malpractice suits against doctors. All clear? You and your new doctor can decide the frequency of your physicals based on your family history and risk factors, says Dr. Kellerman.

Maximize your visit. The nurse will cuff you as soon as you sit down, but the reading could be misleading. Sitting still for 16 minutes before being tested produces blood-pressure numbers that are more accurate, according to a study in the *American Journal of Hypertension*.

The goal is for your BP to register less than 120/80 millimeters of mercury (mm/hg). If you test out at 115/75 at home but hit 140/90 in an exam, ask for a do-over.

EXCUSE 2: "IT ALL JUST FEELS TOO AWKWARD."

If you think a prostate exam is the height of humiliation, get over it. "Look, as a doctor it's not something I look forward to either," says Dr. Marks. "But I'll do it so you don't die a terrible and preventable death."

An STD is another excuse to shy away from medical scrutiny.

"Men almost always know when they have a sexually transmitted disease," says Dr. Marks. "Usually, there's a painful, burning, itching discharge from the penis. It won't get better without treatment."

Follow the doctor's orders. Remember, a prostate-specific antigen (PSA) blood test is noninvasive. As for digital rectal exams, don't worry about jokes concerning your manhood.

"Outside the office, doctors don't talk about guys' sizes," says Dr. Marks. "The men we do talk about are those who opted for pain and death over 10 seconds of embarrassment."

Regarding STDs, does the idea of stomaching a painful urethral swab have you feeling ill? Chill out. If your faucet has a drip, most docs will simply capture a few drops and send it to the lab. Meanwhile, they'll prescribe a full course of oral antibiotics that covers gonorrhea, chlamydia, and syphilis.

Maximize your visit. Let your doctor know if you take the hair-loss drug Propecia, which can lower your PSA reading by half after a year of use. That doesn't mean your risk of prostate cancer has plunged. In fact, an artificially lower score could be masking underlying trouble, according to a study published in *Lancet Oncology*.

EXCUSE 3: "THIS LOOKS WEIRD, BUT I HOPE IT'LL JUST GO AWAY"

Even something as innocuous as a mole needs to be checked out. Melanoma is a cancer of the skin's pigment-producing cells, and it kills almost 8,000 people each year. What's more, one out of every 58 people will be diagnosed with it in his or her lifetime.

"It's a very aggressive tumor," says John F. Romano, MD, a dermatologist in private practice, a clinical assistant professor of dermatology at New York Hospital–Cornell Medical Center, and an attending physician at St. Vincent's Hospital and Medical Center in New York City.

Still, many men drag their feet. "I've had patients say they saw a mole changing but were afraid to come in because of what we might say," says Dr. Romano. "Bad news becomes a self-fulfilling prophecy."

Follow the doctor's orders. Any mole that suddenly darkens or changes shape should be checked out, especially if you have many moles or a family history of melanoma. Other warning signs: a ragged or blurred border, color shifts across the mole's surface, or a diameter exceeding that of the head of a pencil eraser.

Maximize your visit. Think of your skin as a single organ; cancer can crop up in areas not directly exposed to sun. Point out any suspicious moles, even those normally covered by clothing.

EXCUSE 4: "I CAN'T BEAR THE THOUGHT OF THE DOC PUTTING A SCOPE UP THERE"

"Men aren't used to being probed and examined like women are," says Mark Reichelderfer, MD, the chief of clinical gastroenterology at UW Health in Wisconsin. "But it's a small price to pay to prevent a totally devastating disease."

More than 50,000 people die of colon and rectal cancers each year, and early screening could have prevented many of those deaths.

"One in three people who wait to come in until they're experiencing symptoms—blood in the stool, severe abdominal pain, or a narrower stool—will die," says Dr. Reichelderfer.

Follow the doctor's orders. Everyone knows to see a doc if they're flushing blood down the toilet, but anemia and rectal pain can also signal cancer. Regardless, schedule a colonoscopy every 10 years, starting at age 50. If a family member has had colon cancer, begin screening 10 years before the age at which they were diagnosed.

Maximize your visit. While not as accurate as a traditional colonoscopy, less-invasive virtual procedures are better than no exam at all. A tube is inserted into the colon, but instead of a 30-minute expedition into your bowels, a CT scan captures a 3D image of your innards in 10 to 15 minutes. "We can fly through the colon and look for polyps like a video game," says Dr. Reichelderfer.

EXCUSE 5: "I CAN'T AFFORD A CHECKUP"

Even with insurance, co-pays and deductibles can hurt. If you're having trouble making payments, speak up.

"I've never known a doctor who wouldn't try to help, whether it's by not charging as much or by giving you extra samples of a prescription," says Dr. Marks. If your doc orders a bunch of tests or medications, it's okay to inquire about less-expensive alternatives.

Follow the doctor's orders. Read the bill. "Often, you'll see errors, which are rarely to your benefit," says Dr. Marks. "I've seen men charged for gynecological procedures." If you can't understand the medical jargon, ask your doctor to look over the bill for you.

Maximize your visit. Don't hesitate to ask your doctor for free samples of any medications he's prescribing. Yes, it's playing into Big Pharma's marketing strategy, but it's also a quick way to save money. ■

Check Your Medicine Cabinet

HERE ARE SEVEN DRUGS DOCTORS WOULD NEVER TAKE. IF THEY WON'T USE THESE MEDICATIONS, WHY SHOULD YOU?

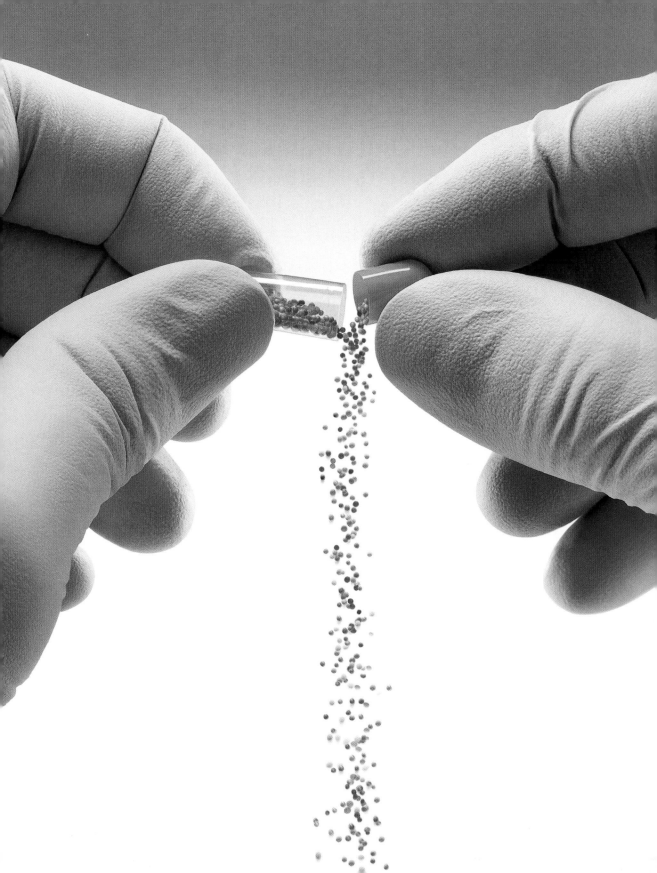

With 3,480 pages of fine print, the Physicians' Desk Reference (aka PDR) is not a quick read. That's because it contains every iota of information on more than 4,000 prescription medications. Heck, the PDR is medication—a humongous sleeping pill.

Doctors count on this compendium to help them make smart prescribing decisions—in other words, to choose drugs that will solve their patients' medical problems without creating new ones. Unfortunately, it seems some doctors rarely pull the *PDR* off the shelf. Or if they do crack it open, they don't stay versed on emerging research that may suddenly make a once-trusted treatment one to avoid. Worst case: You swallow something that has no business being inside your body.

Of course, plenty of MDs do know which prescription and over-the-counter drugs are duds, dangers, or both. So we asked them, "Which medications would you skip?" Their list is your second opinion. If you're on any of these meds, talk to your doctor. Maybe he or she will finally open that big red book with all the dust on it.

ADVAIR

It's asthma medicine that could make your asthma deadly. Advair contains the long-acting beta-agonist (LABA) salmeterol. A 2006 analysis of 19 trials, published in the *Annals of Internal Medicine*, found that regular use of LABAs can increase the severity of an asthma attack. Because salmeterol is more widely prescribed than other LABAs, the danger is greater—the researchers estimate that salmeterol may contribute to as many as 5,000 asthma-related deaths in the United States each year. In 2006, similarly disturbing findings from an earlier salmeterol study prompted the FDA to tag Advair with a "black box" warning—the agency's highest caution level.

Your new strategy: No matter what you may have heard, a LABA, such as the one in Advair, is not the only option, says Philip Rodgers, PharmD, a clinical associate professor at the University of North Carolina school of pharmacy. For instance, if you have mild asthma, an inhaled corticosteroid such as Flovent is often all you need. Still wheezing?

"Patients can also consider an inhaled corticosteroid paired with a leukotriene modifier," says Dr. Rodgers. This combo won't create dangerous inflammation, and according to a Scottish review, it's as effective as a corticosteroid-and-LABA combo.

AVANDIA

Diabetes is destructive enough on its own, but if you try to control it with rosiglitazone—better known by the brand name Avandia—you could be headed for a heart attack. Last September, a *Journal of the American Medical Association (JAMA)* study found that people who took rosiglitazone for at least a year increased their risk of heart failure or a heart attack by 109 percent and 42 percent, respectively, compared with people who took other oral diabetes medications or a placebo.

The reason? While there have been some reports that Avandia use may cause dangerous fluid retention or raise artery-clogging LDL cholesterol, no one is sure if these are the culprits. That's because the results of similar large studies have been mixed. So the FDA has asked Glaxo–SmithKline, the maker of Avandia, to conduct a new long-term study assessing users' heart risks. There's only one problem: The study isn't expected to start until later this year.

Your new strategy: Stick with a proven performer. "I prefer metformin, an older, cheaper, more dependable medication," says Sonal Singh, MD, the lead author of the *JAMA* study. "Avandia is now a last resort." Dr. Singh recommends that you talk to your doctor about cholesterol-lowering medicines, such as statins or the B vitamin niacin. Swallowing high doses (1,000 milligrams) of niacin daily may raise your HDL (good) cholesterol by as much as 24 percent, while at the same time lowering your LDL and triglyceride levels.

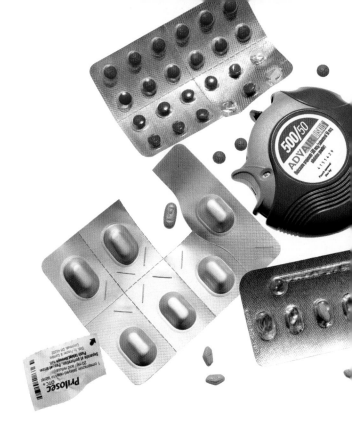

CELEBREX

Once nicknamed "super aspirin," Celebrex is now better known for its side effects than for its pain-relieving prowess. The drug has been linked to increased risks of stomach bleeding, kidney trouble, and liver damage. But according to a 2005 *New England Journal of Medicine* study, the biggest threat is to your heart: People taking 200 mg of Celebrex twice a day more than doubled their risk of dying of cardiovascular disease. Those on 400 milligrams twice a day more than tripled their risk, compared with people taking a placebo.

And yet Celebrex, a COX-2 inhibitor, is still available, even though two other drugs of that class, Bextra and Vioxx, were pulled off the market due to a similar risk of heart damage. The caveat to the consumer? In 2004, the FDA advised doctors to consider alternatives to Celebrex.

Your new strategy: What you don't want to do is stop swallowing Celebrex and begin knocking back ibuprofen, because regular use of high doses of non-steroidal anti-inflammatory drugs (NSAIDs) can lead to gastrointestinal bleeding. A safer swap is acupuncture. A German study found that for people suffering from chronic lower-back pain, twice-weekly acupuncture sessions were twice as effective as conventional treatments with drugs, physical therapy, and exercise. The strategic needling may stimulate central-nervous-system pathways to release the body's own painkillers, including endorphins and enkephalins, says Duke University anesthesiologist Tong-Joo Gan, MD. You can find a certified acupuncturist in your area at medicalacupuncture.org/findadoc/index.html.

KETEK

Most bacteria in the lungs and sinuses don't stand a chance against Ketek, but you might not either. This antibiotic, which has traditionally been prescribed for respiratory-tract infections, carries a higher risk of severe liver side effects than similar antibiotics do.

"Ketek can cause heart-rhythm problems, can lead to liver disease, and could interact poorly with other medications you may be taking," says Dr. Rodgers. "Unfortunately, it's still available, and although many doctors are aware of the risks, some may still prescribe it without caution." In February 2007, the FDA limited the usage of Ketek to the treatment of pneumonia.

Your new strategy: Can't imagine catching pneumonia? The last time the Centers for Disease Control and Prevention calculated the top 10 killers of men, this deadly lung infection (along with the flu) came in seventh. Avoid backing yourself into a corner where you might need Ketek by always signing up for your annual flu shot—if you have pneumonia, it'll reduce your risk of dying of the infection by 40 percent. And if you still end up staring at a scrip for Ketek, Dr. Rodgers recommends asking to be treated with one of several safer alternatives, such as Augmentin or the antibiotics doxycycline or Zithromax.

PRILOSEC AND NEXIUM

Heartburn can be uncomfortable, but heart attacks can be fatal, which is why the FDA has investigated a suspected link between cardiac trouble and the acid-reflux remedies Prilosec and Nexium. In December 2007, the agency concluded that there was no "likely" connection. Translation: The scientific jury is still out. In the meantime, there are other reasons to be concerned. Because Prilosec and Nexium are proton-pump inhibitors, they are both incredibly effective at stopping acid production in the stomach—perhaps too effective.

A lack of acid may raise your risk of pneumonia, because the same stuff that makes your chest feel as if it's burning also kills incoming bacteria and viruses. You may also have an elevated risk of bone loss—in the less acidic environment, certain forms of calcium may not be absorbed effectively during digestion.

"The risk of a fracture has been estimated to be over 40 percent higher in patients who use these drugs long-term, and the risk clearly increases with duration of therapy," says Dr. Rodgers.

Your new strategy: When you feel the fire, first try to extinguish it with Zantac 150 or Pepcid AC. Both of these OTC products work by blocking histamine from stimulating the stomach cells that produce acid. Just know that neither drug is a long-term fix.

"To really cure the problem, lose weight," says Michael Roizen, MD, chief wellness officer at the Cleveland Clinic and coauthor of *YOU: The Owner's Manual*. That's because when you're overweight, excess belly fat puts pressure on and changes the angle of your esophagus, pulling open the valve that's supposed to prevent stomach-acid leaks. This in turn makes it easier for that burning sensation to travel up into your chest.

VISINE ORIGINAL

What possible harm to your peepers could come from these seemingly innocuous eye drops? "Visine gets the red out, but it does so by shrinking blood vessels, just like Afrin shrinks the vessels in your nose," says Thomas Steinemann, MD, a spokesman for the American Academy of Ophthalmology. Overuse of the active ingredient tetrahydrozoline can perpetuate the vessel dilating-and-constricting cycle and may cause even more redness.

Your new strategy: If you still want to rely on Visine, at least make sure you don't use too many drops per dose and you don't use the stuff for more than 3 or 4 days. But you'd really be better off figuring out the underlying cause of the redness and treating that instead. If it's dryness, use preservative-free artificial tears, recommends Dr. Steinemann.

Visine Pure Tears Portables is a good choice for moisture minus side effects. On the other hand, if your eyes are itchy and red because of allergies, pick up OTC antiallergy drops, such as Zaditor. It contains an antihistamine to interrupt the allergic response but no vasoconstrictor to cause rebound redness.

PSEUDOEPHEDRINE

Forget that this decongestant can be turned into methamphetamine. People with heart disease or hypertension should watch out for any legitimate drug that contains pseudoephedrine. See, pseudoephedrine doesn't just constrict the blood vessels in your nose and sinuses; it can also raise blood pressure and heart rate, setting the stage for vascular catastrophe. Over the years, pseudoephedrine has been linked to heart attacks and strokes.

"Pseudoephedrine can also worsen symptoms of benign prostate disease and glaucoma," says Dr. Rodgers.

Your new strategy: Other OTC oral nasal decongestants can contain phenylephrine, which has a safety profile similar to pseudoephedrine's. A 2007 review didn't find enough evidence that phenylephrine was effective. Our advice: Avoid meds altogether and clear your nasal passages with a neti pot, the strangely named system that allows you to flush your sinuses with saline ($15, sinucleanse.com). University of Wisconsin researchers found that people who used a neti pot felt their congestion and head pain improve by as much as 57 percent. Granted, the flushing sensation is odd at first, but give it a chance. Dr. Roizen did: "I do it every day after I brush my teeth," he says. ∎

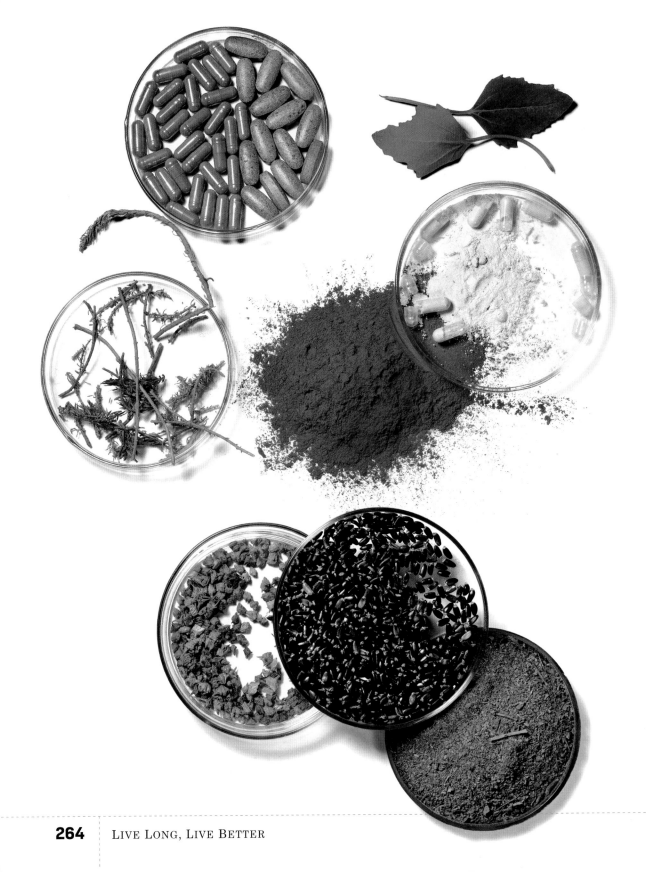

Take an Alternative Route

NATURE'S MEDICINE CABINET IS JAMMED WITH HEALTHY TONICS. HERE'S YOUR GUIDE TO MAKING SURE YOU GRAB WHAT YOU REALLY NEED

If you believe those hypochondria-inducing TV commercials, the pharmaceutical industry can make drugs to cure pretty much anything that ails us.

But drugmakers literally beat the bushes for many of their products. According to one report, nearly 60 percent of the 150 most prescribed drugs in the United States contain at least one plant compound as an active ingredient or are synthesized in a lab to mimic the effects of a botanical chemical.

You should be looking to nature for health tonics, too. But which herbs deliver on their promises, and which ones go up in smoke upon closer inspection? The clerk at the local supplement store probably knows less about these botanical agents than he does about the protein powder he's hawking all day. After all, herbs, like wines, can differ greatly depending on their regions of origin. To cut out the guesswork, we examined the research on every herbal cure out there to determine the best picks in seven key aspects of male wellness.

Read all label warnings carefully before taking any new supplement, and check with a qualified complementary and alternative medicine specialist (nccam.nih.gov) if you're wondering how an herb might affect you. Also, tell your primary-care physician whenever you take any new botanical-based remedy. Finally, remember that these herbs should augment, not replace, a sound diet and plenty of exercise.

AN EXPANDING MIDSECTION

THE REMEDY: Coleus forskohlii root extract
WHY IT WORKS: Unlike the stimulant ephedra (now banned by the FDA), this supplement doesn't hot-wire the central nervous system to ignite fat loss. Its active ingredient, forskolin, increases your supply of hormone-sensitive lipase, an enzyme that allows stored fat to be burned for fuel.

A recent study in *Obesity Research* reported that men taking 250 milligrams of C. forskohlii root extract (with 10 percent forskolin) saw their body-fat percent-

age drop an average of 4 points over 12 weeks. As a bonus, men in the same study increased their testosterone levels.
OUR PICK: Vitamin Shoppe ForsLean ($29 for 120 capsules)

A FAMILY HISTORY OF ALZHEIMER'S DISEASE

THE REMEDY: Huperzia serrata (a.k.a. toothed clubmoss)
WHY IT WORKS: This plant's active ingredient, huperzine A, inhibits production of an enzyme that in turn reduces the amount of an important chemical of the central nervous system called acetylcholine. And acetylcholine just happens to be in short supply in Alzheimer's patients. A review of several Chinese studies found that elderly people with the disease saw their symptoms lessen after they were given huperzine. And preliminary results from a recent clinical trial reveal that 400 (but not 200) micrograms of huperzine a day improved memory in 210 patients with mild to moderate Alzheimer's disease.
OUR PICK: GNC Herbal Plus Huperzine A ($15 for 50 capsules)

A MAN'S ALL-IN-ONE HERBAL SOLUTION
The most bang for your botanical buck might come from ancient Indian medicine

Exotic herbs can be hard to hunt down, and the expense of juggling multiple products can weigh on anyone's wallet. The closest botanical equivalent to a daily multivitamin and mineral supplement may be an offering from the Ayurvedic tradition in India, where people call it "the elixir of life."

"Typically referred to as Maharishi Amrit Kalash mixtures, these preparations combine multiple herbs," says Marc S. Micozzi, MD, the author of *Fundamentals of Complementary and Alternative Medicine*.

"They definitely fit with the apple-a-day philosophy of preventive health," says Steven Dentali, PhD, chief science officer for the American Herbal Products Association. Try spreading a teaspoon or two of Maharishi Ayurveda's Amrit ($55, mapi.com) on toast twice a day.

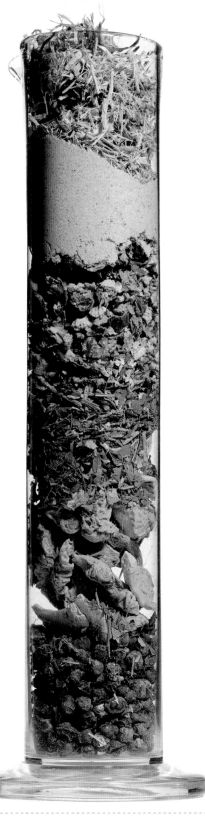

Herbs,
like wines, can
DIFFER GREATLY
depending on
their regions of
origin.

ANGINA

THE REMEDY: Crataegus monogyna (a.k.a. hawthorn extract)

WHY IT WORKS: Germany's herbal-remedy watchdog agency has approved hawthorn leaf and flower extracts as safe and effective for improving heart function in people whose cardiovascular disease has progressed enough to cause them fatigue and angina when they exercise.

"The research on hawthorn for heart disease is very good, even though there's been huge resistance to it from the medical community," says Marc S. Micozzi, MD, the author of *Fundamentals of Complementary and Alternative Medicine*.

OUR PICK: Jarrow Formulas Hawthorn ($14 for 100 capsules)

TOXIC INTRUDERS

THE REMEDY: Silybum marianum (a.k.a. milk-thistle extract)

WHY IT WORKS: Whether you're inhaling secondhand smoke, recovering from a night of boozing it up, or popping ibuprofen, your liver is among the initial lines of defense against toxins. Milk thistle's active ingredient, silybin, modifies existing liver cells to create a protective barrier against these toxins. It also helps form new liver cells. Milk thistle has been shown in various clinical trials to be safe and effective in protecting liver cells from the toxicity of drugs.

OUR PICK: NSI Siliphos Milk Thistle ($40 for 60 capsules)

SLEEPLESS NIGHTS

THE REMEDY: Griffonia simplifica seed extract (a.k.a. 5-HTP)

WHY IT WORKS: 5-hydroxytryptophan (5-HTP) is the chemical that tryptophan must convert to in order to boost serotonin, the sleepy-time hormone. Unlike tryptophan, however, 5-HTP has no trouble crossing the blood-brain barrier, so you'll be sawing wood stat. For nearly half a century, 5-HTP has been used clinically to treat insomnia.

OUR PICK: Natrol 5-HTP ($14 for 45 capsules)

FATIGUE

THE REMEDY: Paullinia cupana (a.k.a. guarana seed extract)

WHY IT WORKS: Sure, caffeine accounts for much of the pop in this elixir from the Amazon. But another active ingredient, theophylline, makes it a high-octane energy booster. In a study published in the *Journal of Sports Medicine and Physical Fitness*, theophylline increased time-to-exhaustion rates in healthy men pedaling hard on a bike.

OUR PICK: Biotest Spike ($20 for 16 tablets)

NAUSEA, UPSET STOMACH

THE REMEDY: Zingiber officinale root extract (a.k.a. ginger)

WHY IT WORKS: Ginger has a history of easing digestive discomfort, nausea, and motion sickness. A study published in the *Journal of Pharmacology and Experimental Therapeutics* found that 1 gram of ginger root, consumed by a healthy adult 30 minutes before slurping a glucose solution, significantly reduced stomach discomfort.

OUR PICK: Solaray Ginger Root Extract 250 milligrams ($10 for 60 capsules) ∎

Take Charge of Your Health

TELL—DON'T ASK—YOUR DOCTOR TO CHECK FOR THESE CRITICAL ABLOOD TEST MARKERS

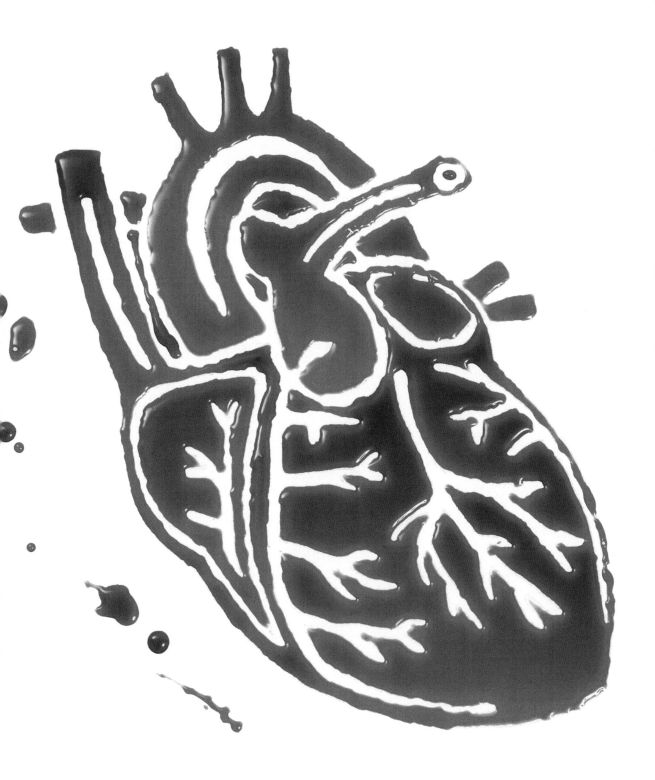

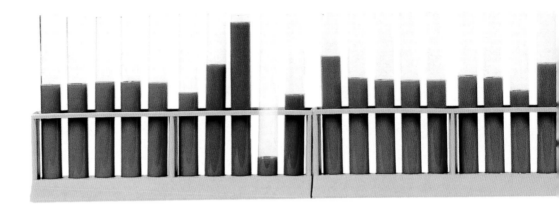

Men spill it, seal friendships with it, and, if they're aging rock guitarists, have it purified at Swiss clinics. But blood also tells a detective story. Just as the amount, color, odor, and feel of the oil on a car's dipstick offer clues about wear and tear on the engine, your blood can reveal critical details about the running condition of your entire body.

Of course, first you need to know what to look for and how to interpret the findings. That's why we've created a guide on how to read the red stuff. Order up all seven of these tests at your next physical, and you'll be doing more than just kicking the tires.

START WITH THE BASICS: THE CBC

"If I had a 30-year-old man coming to me for the first time, I'd order a complete blood count (CBC)," says David Perkins, MD, an internal-medicine physician based in St. Davids, Pennsylvania. Think of the CBC as an array of baseline numbers for key factors such as red (oxygen-carrying) blood cells, white (infection-fighting) blood cells, and platelets (clotting particles).

Within the CBC, a hematocrit score indicates the proportion of red blood cells in your total blood volume, and a hemoglobin measurement assesses the oxygen-carrying protein of red blood cells.

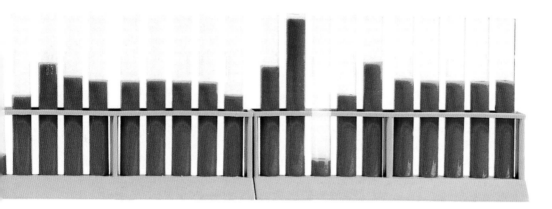

"If you've been following the exercise and nutrition advice recommended in *Men's Health* and are still short of breath while pumping iron, you may have low hematocrit and hemoglobin counts," says John A. Elefteriades, MD, chief of cardiothoracic surgery at Yale University and the coauthor of *Your Heart: An Owner's Guide*. These low numbers may signal anemia, which is a blood disorder that can lead to heart arrhythmia if left untreated.

If your blood is anemic: The good news is that you can treat some types of anemia by taking an iron supplement (best absorbed 30 minutes before breakfast with orange juice or vitamin C). Supplemental vitamin B_{12} or folic acid can also help.

LEARN YOUR SUGAR SCORE

Blood tests are like radar for tracking type 2 diabetes. The standard measure is the fasting glucose test, which is part of what sounds like a congressional subcommittee: the Comprehensive Metabolic Panel. Fasting glucose is a one-off reading, so it's often paired with the A1c test of your average blood-glucose level over the preceding 2 to 3 months.

But if you score high on either of these tests—above 100 milligrams per deciliter (mg/dl) on the fasting test, or above 6 percent on the A1c—you should demand an oral glucose-tolerance test (OGTT).

"Doctors diagnose heart disease with a stress test, not a resting test," says Keith Berkowitz, MD, medical director of the Center for Balanced Health in New York City. "An OGTT does the same for the most basic process in your body—metabolism."

As Dr. Berkowitz points out, the fasting measure can still be in the normal range even if post-meal numbers are elevated. As for the A1c, it can miss some abnormalities because swings from high to low blood sugar sometimes simply average out.

Take an OGTT regardless of your fasting-glucose and A1c scores if you score 140 mg/dl or higher on a random glucose test (one you take without fasting beforehand), your belly's bulging (that is, your body mass index is 30 or higher), or you experience head-snapping slumps after a high-carbohydrate meal. Ditto if you have a family history of diabetes or heart disease.

The test can last 2 to 5 hours, depending on the version you take. If you hit the 2-hour mark of an OGTT with a reading above 140 mg/dl, you're pre-diabetic. If it's above 200 at that point, there's no "pre" about it.

If your blood is too sweet: Shed pounds, if you're one of the 80 to 90 percent of people with type 2 diabetes who are overweight. Slashing carbs from your diet and hitting the treadmill for 15 to 20 minutes a day should do the trick while offering the added benefit of increasing your insulin sensitivity.

KEEP AN EYE ON FATS, TOO

"The fasting lipid profile is where cardiovascular abnormalities are most likely to appear for the average guy," says Dr. Perkins.

Generally, your HDL (good) cholesterol should be between 45 and 50 mg/dl, while your LDL (bad) cholesterol should be below 130 mg/dl. Triglycerides should fall under 150. If you have risk factors for cardiovascular disease—such as past cardiac events, a family history of the disease, hypertension, or you're a smoker—your target LDL may be below 100 mg/dl.

If you're at high risk, ask your physician about an expanded lipid profile test, like the Vertical Auto Profile, which further breaks down the dangerous subtypes of LDL.

If your results don't measure up: If your HDL is too low, tossing walnuts into your yogurt may raise your good cholesterol by 9 percent, according to a study in *Angiology*.

If your triglycerides are high, cut back on starches, breads, pasta, and other carb-loaded offerings. Even if your LDL levels don't go down, you can still halve your chances of dying of a heart attack simply by exercising,

according to a joint study by the Cooper Institute and Canada's Queen's University.

LOOK FOR SIGNS OF INFLAMMATION

The process by which inflamed arteries lead to car-diovascular disease is invisible except for a tracer—an elevated level of C-reactive protein (CRP) in your blood.

"If your CRP as well as your total cholesterol is high, you're at an even greater risk of having a heart attack than you would be with either risk factor by itself," says David Sandmire, MD, a professor of physiology at the University of New England in Biddeford, Maine.

Make sure you feel perfectly healthy the day of your appointment: This highly sensitive test picks up all sorts of inflammation, even from a paper cut. That's a good reason to take it twice, at least a month apart, and average the two scores. Yours should fall under 1 milligram per liter; if it's above 3, your heart-attack risk doubles.

If your score is too high: Smokers, take note: "It's almost certain that CRP levels will decrease after you quit," says David W. Johnson, PhD, an associate professor in the college of osteopathic medicine at the University of New England and coauthor of *Medical Tests That Can Save Your Life*. If your lungs are already a smoke-free zone, raise a glass. A Spanish study found that red wine reduced inflammation markers by 21 percent.

HAVE YOUR PROSTATE CHECKED

More than 180,000 American men will be

diagnosed with prostate cancer in 2008, so pay great attention to tracking your prostate-specific antigen (PSA). Elevation of this marker can signal a problem—at least sometimes.

"PSA testing is not an exact science, because factors external to the prostate can cause the marker to rise," says Dr. Johnson. A high PSA reading might point to a benign enlargement of the prostate or even a bacterial infection known as prostatitis.

That's why the trend can be as important as the static number. "Every year I have a PSA test done along with my physical, and compare the result with that of the year before, to see if further investigation is warranted," says Dr. Johnson. "Once you reach 50 years of age (40 if you're African American), your doctor may recommend a PSA test. Don't hesitate to ask for one if you're in your 30s, however."

Keep your results in range: Eat two Brazil nuts a day, good for 200 micrograms of selenium. National Cancer Institute researchers found that men with the highest selenium levels who also took a multivitamin were 39 percent less likely to develop prostate cancer than those with the lowest levels.

DON'T FORGET YOUR THYROID

Thyroid problems hit men as well as women, and stress and poor sleep are often the culprits.

"Many people don't sleep as well as they should, so the body overcompensates," says Dr. Berkowitz. With an overactive thyroid, there may be signs of a goiter—a swollen area in the neck. Hyperthyroidism, as it's called, can also lead to an increased heart rate, anxiety, sleep problems, and weight loss. Symptoms of an underactive thyroid (hypothyroidism) may include personality changes, hair loss, weight gain, and a cloudy memory.

Both thyroid conditions can lead to more serious, life-threatening illnesses when left untreated. The thyroid-stimulating hormone (TSH) test will determine if you have a problem.

If your results are off the mark: Your doctor might order the more specific free T3 and free T4 follow-up tests. Depending on whether your thyroid is overactive or underactive, a beta-blocker or thyroid-hormone replacement drug may be prescribed.

CHECK ONE FINAL THING

"Aspirin, although a very old and cheap product, is really a wonder drug," says Dr. Elefteriades. That's because aspirin reduces the stickiness of platelets, making them less likely to clump together and block a blood vessel.

But not all men respond to this treatment—and there's a test that identifies the ones who don't. "Aspirin resistance is found in about 20 percent of patients tested," says Eric J. Topol, MD, dean of the Scripps School of Medicine in La Jolla, California. For those men, aspirin is a waste of time and money.

If you're aspirin resistant: Cook with virgin olive oil. Three tablespoons a day can help improve arterial bloodflow, Spanish scientists found. ■

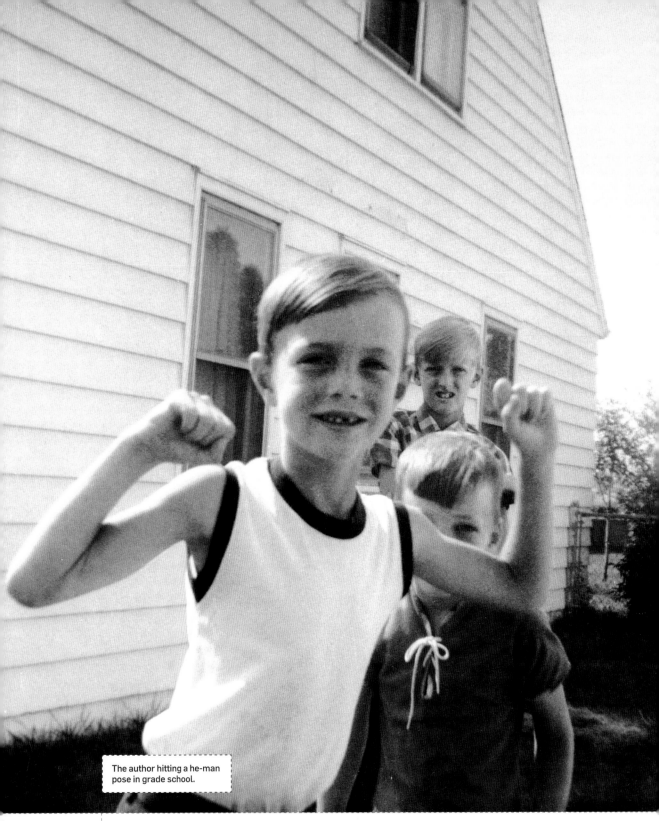

The author hitting a he-man pose in grade school.

Don't Be Derailed by Diabetes

AMERICA'S FASTEST-GROWING DISEASE HAS A SUGAR-COATED SECRET. WRITER JEFF O'CONNELL TELLS HIS FAMILY'S STORY

One of my most enduring childhood images is from a newspaper clipping. Tucker, as he was known, led a team from tiny Merchantville High School in scoring and rebounding during an improbable run to the South Jersey Championship.

New Jersey had its own version of *Hoosiers* in 1952, and for that one season, my father was his team's Jimmy Chitwood.

In February 2008, I arrive at a nursing home in the San Fernando Valley to visit the man in that photograph, a man I've neither seen nor spoken to in 20 years. Entering his room, I barely recognize the gaunt face. Where his right thigh should be sits a corduroy pant leg, gathered up and bobby-pinned. The spindly arm he extends to greet me is splotched with blood bursts. Once 6'3" and 215 pounds, he's now a cadaverous-looking 145. The only cheerful note in the room is a balloon tied to the metal bed frame. His 73rd birthday was last week, apparently. It's a detail I had long since forgotten.

Like a man looking into a foggy mirror, my father strains to recognize me. But if he is staring into his past, I might be peering into my future. I'm 6'6" and weigh 220, with 12 percent body fat and the outline of abs above a 32-inch waist. Yet diabetes has me in its crosshairs as well.

If you think being thin gives you a free pass from this deadly disease, well, it might have a surprise in store for you, too.

COME, SWEET DEATH

The white curtain flanking my father's bed divides him from a man who speaks only Spanish and another who rambles incoherently all day in English. Yet Thomas Joseph O'Connell Jr. has an epidemic's worth of company. According to the Centers for Disease Control and Prevention, one in every four people in the United States is living with either type 2 diabetes (20 million) or its precursor, prediabetes (54 million).

WILL YOU BECOME DIABETIC?
Take our self-test and find out

The American Diabetes Association singles out the fasting glucose test as the preferred way to diagnose type 2 diabetes, citing cost and ease. While useful, this blood-sugar snapshot doesn't reveal the excessive swings that indicate insulin resistance before your fasting level is elevated to diabetes or prediabetes.

For that, you need to take an oral glucose-tolerance test (OGTT), especially if you have a parent or sibling with type 2 diabetes. Being African American, Latino, Native American, or Asian American also elevates your risk. The symptoms of insulin resistance tend to come in clusters, so if you have one indicator, you're likely to have two or three others. However, under the "definitely" category (below), having just a single factor is cause for concern. In this case, contact your physician and schedule a time for an OGTT.

You *might* need an OGTT if . . .
1. You often wake up with a headache.
2. You often wake up in the middle of the night.
3. You had acne, numerous cavities, and hair loss in your teens/early 20s.
4. You feel cranky or forgetful after a high-carb breakfast.

You *probably* need an OGTT if . . .
1. Your blood pressure is 140/90 mm/Hg or higher.
2. Your HDL (good) cholesterol is less than 35 mg/dl (milligrams per deciliter) and/or your triglycerides are higher than 250 mg/dl.
3. You're thirsty or you urinate a lot.
4. You tire easily and/or nap frequently, especially 1 to 2 hours after a meal.
5. You're overweight (BMI 25 to 29.9).
6. You're 45 years old or older.

You *definitely* need an OGTT if . . .
1. Your fasting plasma glucose (FPG) is 100 mg/dl or higher.
2. Your hemoglobin A1C is greater than 6 percent.
3. Any random blood glucose reading is 140 mg/dl or higher.
4. You have any history of cardiovascular disease.
5. You're obese (BMI = 30 or higher).

And the incidence of type 2—the kind of diabetes that people develop over time—has, in the past quarter century, grown 32 percent faster among American men than among American women.

What's worse, type 2 diabetes is showing up in the young in record numbers. "People used to suffer type 2 diabetes in their 60s and heart disease in their 70s," says James O. Hill, PhD, the director of the center for human nutrition at the University of Colorado's health sciences center.

Your pancreas wasn't meant to handle the carb load from a CINNABON AND A BIG GULP ON A regular basis.

"But with teens now developing it, are they going to have heart disease at 25 and need a transplant in their 30s? We've never gone through this before, but based on what we know about what happens once you have type-2 diabetes, the answer is probably yes."

Woe unto them, because raging blood sugar can lead to a litany of ailments, biblical in scope: cardiovascular disease, liver disease, kidney failure (my dad needs dialysis three times a week), stroke, amputations, erectile dysfunction, blindness, and nerve damage—everything, seemingly, but a swarm of locusts. Even cancer has a sweet tooth, recent research suggests.

The total amount of glucose in a typical man's bloodstream is just shy of the amount in a teaspoon of sugar. A man crossing over into diabetes has about ¼ teaspoon more. That seemingly trivial amount can make a huge difference as blood glucose (a.k.a. sugar) plays seesaw with your hormones all day. The game begins whenever you eat carbohydrates—be it the sugar in a soda or the starch in bread and pasta. Your body breaks down these carbs so they can be absorbed into your bloodstream as glucose. The seesaw goes up: elevated blood sugar.

Glucose is important stuff; the cells in your muscles and brain use it for energy. But too much of it coursing through your blood vessels, for too long, is ultimately deadly.

"It's kind of like dynamite," says Mary Vernon, MD, president of the American Society of Bariatric Physicians. "The body realizes it's dangerous, not to be left lying around." That's why people with diabetes are frequent bathroom visitors.

To adjust to a surge of incoming carbs, your pancreas secretes the hormone insulin, which helps glucose enter your cells, where it belongs. (See "How Your Blood Sugar Works" opposite.) This glucose leaving your bloodstream is the downstroke of the seesaw. Problems arise when some of your cells begin to deny access to insulin, and by extension, glucose—a condition called insulin resistance. This situation often goes unnoticed for years, but over time it worsens until the result is chronically high blood sugar and full-blown diabetes.

Here's how it all plays out: Your body tries to clear your bloodstream of excess glucose by signaling your pancreas to squirt out higher and higher amounts of insulin. Eventually, this flood of insulin drives blood sugar sharply lower, which makes you feel hungry and even shaky. So you reach for the quick fix—more carbs—and they send your blood sugar skyrocketing again, triggering the release of still more insulin and perpetuating the cycle. Instead of gently rocking, the seesaw slams down and bounces back up, over and over, for days, years, and decades.

"The constant demand on your pancreas ultimately causes it to burn out, so that it no longer releases insulin," says Dr. Vernon. "That's when blood sugar stays elevated for good."

Of course, this insulin system has worked fine for 99.6 percent of human existence. That's because hunter-gatherers derived no more than 40 percent of their calories from carbohydrates, mostly fruit, according to Colorado State University

HOW YOUR BLOOD SUGAR WORKS

Your body has a finely tuned system for controlling blood sugar. One of the key players is insulin, a powerful hormone that's essential for helping move sugar from your blood into your cells. Here's how the process works—and how it can go wrong.

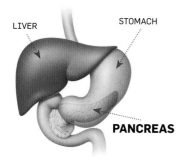

LIVER   STOMACH

PANCREAS

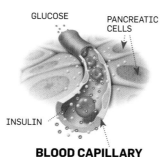

GLUCOSE   PANCREATIC CELLS

INSULIN

BLOOD CAPILLARY

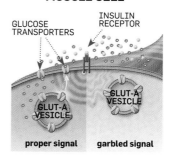

MUSCLE CELL

GLUCOSE TRANSPORTERS   INSULIN RECEPTOR

GLUT-A VESICLE   GLUT-A VESICLE

proper signal   garbled signal

1. THE BASICS

When you eat food that contains carbohydrates, most is absorbed as glucose into your bloodstream. As your blood-glucose level increases, your pancreas reacts by secreting the hormone insulin. Insulin then travels to the capillaries that deliver blood and nutrients to your muscles and brain.

Once it's in the capillaries, insulin is attracted to the insulin receptors that reside on the outer membrane of your muscle and brain cells. Insulin then binds to these receptors.

2. A HEALTHY RESPONSE

In a person with normal blood-sugar responses, the connection of insulin to its receptor sends a signal to a pool (or vesicle) of glucose transporters inside the cell called GLUT-4 proteins.

When the signal is received, these GLUT-4 proteins move out of their vesicle toward the surface of the cell, where they help glucose move across the cell membrane.

This causes blood glucose to decrease and provides your muscle cell with sugar for fuel.

3. WHEN THE SYSTEM GOES BAD

In a person with insulin resistance, the insulin receptor sends out a garbled signal. This leads to what's tantamount to a dropped cellphone call. Some or all of the GLUT-4 proteins never receive the message to move to the surface of the cell. As a result, glucose has no way in. The fewer GLUT-4 proteins on the surface of the cell, the higher your blood sugar remains. Much of this excess blood sugar is diverted to the liver, where it's converted to fat and can lead to increased insulin resistance—and higher blood sugar.

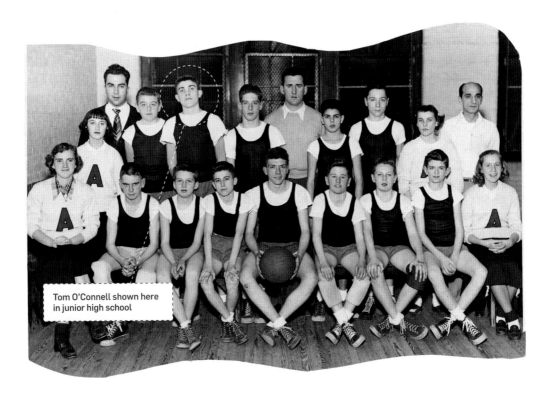

Tom O'Connell shown here in junior high school

scientists. What your pancreas wasn't designed to handle on a regular basis was the carb load from a Cinnabon washed down with a Big Gulp, all part of the 140 pounds of sugar the average American consumes annually.

"The high-blood-glucose response to a high-carb diet is an almost normal response to an abnormal situation," says Ron Raab, past vice president of the International Diabetes Federation. "We've largely created this illness."

AN OMINOUS PREFIX

No single event fractured my relationship with my father. Lacking even the sense of purpose or legitimacy that a blowout argument or fight might have provided,

the dissolution of our bond came after my parents divorced in the mid-1980s. Tom O'Connell had essentially been cast out of my mind for two decades until one of my two brothers told me that he was lying in intensive care in a Los Angeles hospital. He had diabetes and had barely survived two amputations on a leg, above the knee and then farther up. At the time, it didn't cross my mind to make the trip from eastern Pennsylvania to Southern California to say farewell.

I wouldn't be let off that easily, though. A week later I visited my own doctor, who had called me in to review blood work done several weeks earlier for a routine physical. He scanned my numbers and looked up. "Does diabetes run in your family?"

Bad medical news didn't shock me. Both

of my parents survived cancer, and my mother has epilepsy. But I write for *Men's Health*. I've cowritten a book on sports nutrition. I've been the occasional butt of skinny-guy wisecracks in school. Diabetes? Isn't that for grandmothers in wheelchairs?

The doctor slid the lab report in front of me and began explaining the jumble of numbers. One stood out: 116, which quantified the amount of glucose floating in my bloodstream after a 12-hour fast. Under 100 milligrams per deciliter (mg/dl) is good; anything above 126 is diabetes. That meant I was well into prediabetes, a term sugarcoated in more ways than one, since most men eventually lose the prefix.

How the hell did I miss this? I thought. For months, my body had felt like a sputtering car in need of a tune-up. There were the severe headaches I had endured my entire adult life and the naps that left me so groggy it was like emerging from anesthesia. Then I replayed a scene from earlier that year. After months of nearly continuous stress, I woke up one morning feeling like a man who had been lost in a desert for days. I drank a glass of water, and another, and another, all weekend. Gallons, it seemed. Nothing could quench my thirst, a classic symptom of high blood sugar, since you're expelling so much fluid through your urine.

Within minutes of learning the reason for that episode, I would confront another harsh reality: Many physicians really don't have a clue about preventing type-2 diabetes in someone thin like me. My doctor mumbled something about switching from white rice to brown rice and told me to come back in 6 months, even though insulin resistance is a complex metabolic disorder requiring

sophisticated, continuous management.

What's more, the typical advice offered makes you wonder if Americans are being given an antidote against or a prescription for the disease. For example, everyone from my doctor to the American Diabetes Association (ADA) tells people with impaired blood sugar, or prediabetes, to make carbohydrate-rich foods such as breads and grains the foundation of their diets. This

Diabetes drugs are about AS EASY TO DITCH AS CRACK. Most people end up using more medication, not less.

despite a growing body of evidence that points to carb reduction as the best anti-diabetes strategy. After all, there's another term for people who are insulin resistant: glucose intolerant. Meaning they don't respond well to carbohydrates. The higher the dose of carbs, the more problems those carbs cause.

This year, after decades of resistance, the ADA finally acknowledged low-carb dieting as a legitimate response to diabetes. Which goes to show that if you wait for a health organization to issue a position paper before attacking the disease, you might end up reading that paper from a hospital bed.

This isn't the failing of a single physician or organization. It's the breakdown of the U.S. medical system when it comes to nutrition.

"Our medical establishment is set up to treat disease," says Susan M. Kleiner,

PhD, RD, a nutritionist in Mercer Island, Washington. "First-year med students rank nutrition among their top priorities. Yet by graduation, nutrition doesn't even make the list, because it's largely ignored."

In fact, there are still medical schools that don't offer a single nutrition course.

SLASH AND BURN

Perhaps I was scared by news of my father's fate or angry that the disease had cut him down. Maybe I was emboldened by the knowledge that type 2 diabetes comes with instructions for defeating it, even if most doctors don't know them.

Whatever the motivation, I was determined to haul off and floor this condition with one ferocious counterpunch. At least initially, I adopted a very-low-carbohydrate approach—specifically the Atkins diet— based on multiple Duke University studies that show it's effective for both lowering blood sugar and reducing heart-disease risk. It seemed logical: The initial limit of 20 grams of carbohydrates a day would offer my pancreas a reprieve after a lifetime of sugar trauma.

Of course, I didn't know what 20 grams of carbohydrates would mean until I found myself in a supermarket pushing a shopping cart containing nothing but a can of shaving cream, laundry detergent, and a magazine. Everything in sight contained too much sugar for someone on the verge of diabetes, and some of the bachelor-friendly foods I'd relied on most were among the highest in carbs: frozen dinners and pizzas, cereal, cookies and other desserts, and snack foods. Bread, pasta, rice, and potatoes were gone from my list, too.

What remained was what some hunter-gatherers might have recognized as food had they been foraging on the periphery of a supermarket: fresh fruits and vegetables, nuts, eggs, and meat. The biggest adjustment came when I realized all the things I couldn't drink anymore—regular soda, beer, and fruit juices included. What's more, I'd even have to limit milk, because an 8-ounce

EIGHT WAYS TO CONTROL YOUR BLOOD SUGAR

To prevent diabetes, start here.

1 Exercise like it's a prescription. That means at least 20 to 30 minutes every day. It takes only a few days of missed workouts and poor eating to worsen a person's insulin resistance, says Barry Braun, PhD, an associate professor of kinesiology at the University of Massachusetts at Amherst.

2 Sprinkle cinnamon on everything you can. Studies show it can improve insulin sensitivity. This means your body needs less of the hormone insulin to keep your blood-sugar levels in check.

The cheap supermarket stuff works just as well as expensive supplement versions.

3 If you already have high blood glucose, take alpha lipoic acid. This supplement is unexcelled as a blood-sugar nutrient and is a prescription item in Europe. Puritan's Pride Alpha Lipoic Acid is reasonably priced and passed purity tests at consumerlab.com.

4 Skip the sugary sports drinks. University of Massachusetts scientists recently discovered that exercising improved insulin sensitivity by 40 percent when a 500-calorie deficit was created, but produced no improvement when the burned energy was immediately replaced with mostly carbohydrates.

glass contains 13 grams of sugar. A typical meal became steak, fish, or chicken accompanied by steamed vegetables and a glass of red wine, a low-carb godsend.

In addition to following my new diet strategy, I planned to torch any excess sugar by working out briefly but intensively 6 days a week: superset-based weight-lifting sessions one day, cardio intervals the next.

Just how powerful an antidote is exercise? A study published recently in the *American Journal of Physiology—Endocrinology and Metabolism* revealed that insulin resistance in rats decreased more from exercise than from taking metformin, the leading diabetes drug.

Exercise and dieting take effort and discipline, though. And it can be tempting to just take drugs to lower blood sugar and be done with it. After all, the major diabetes organizations have already raised the white flag of surrender and adopted that approach.

A few years ago, "the ADA and the European Association for the Study of Diabetes decided that you really ought to just start people on medicine," says endocrinologist Larry C. Deeb, MD, a past president for medicine and science at the ADA. "Very few people participate in dietary changes and physical activity, so you end up with patients not taking care of their diabetes. My take is, let me give you a prescription. No rule says I can't take you off the medicine later."

Yeah, except diabetes drugs are about as easy to ditch as crack—most people end up using more, not less. It's a vicious circle: The insulin-resistant patient is shepherded onto a high-carbohydrate diet per ADA guidelines, so his blood sugar stays elevated. As a result, his pancreas secretes more insulin—but with less and less effect. So he's given tablets to make his pancreas produce even more insulin. When that's not enough, he must inject the insulin. In contrast, when you exercise daily with few carbohydrates available for fuel, your body needs less insulin.

By my next doctor's appointment, my fasting blood sugar has fallen from 116 to 102, and my triglycerides from a high 289

5 **Invest in a glucose monitor.** It'll allow you to find out how specific meals, foods, and beverages affect your blood sugar. Simply prick your finger 2 hours after a meal. The number shouldn't be above 139 mg/dl, and it shouldn't be below 100 or your fasting number—whichever is lower.

6 **Snack on pumpkin seeds or sunflower seeds.** A small handful won't impact blood sugar, and they're rich in magnesium, which is a mineral that fights insulin resistance, according to a 2006 study from Tufts University researchers.

7 **Eat every 2 to 3 hours.** Eating this often helps prevent drops in blood sugar, which can lead to sugar binges.

8 **Check your meds.** If you're taking a thiazide diuretic for hypertension, ask your doctor about switching to an ACE inhibitor. A 2006 *Hypertension* review of 59 drug trials found a "strong relationship" between low potassium levels caused by diuretics and increased blood glucose.

Up to 15 percent of non-obese people are INSULIN-RESISTANT, putting them at high risk for diabetes.

to a better-than-average 89. (In the insulin resistant, these blood fats tend to rise with blood sugar.) Most impressive is my score on the hemoglobin A1C test, a 3-month running average of blood-sugar levels. The nondiabetic range is 4 percent to 6 percent. After months of exercising and carb slashing, my results fall squarely in the middle: 5 percent. In a word, perfect.

As I turn to leave, the doctor smiles and pats me on the back. "You're proof that diabetes can be addressed with diet and exercise," he says. "Most people don't do that. You're to be commended."

FROM HIGH TO LOW

"Actually, this is really bad."

The voice on the other end of the line belongs to Keith W. Berkowitz, MD. He's the medical director of the Center for Balanced Health in New York City, which specializes in treating patients with serious blood-sugar irregularities. I had faxed the results to his office for a second opinion.

Dr. Berkowitz noticed a mathematical anomaly. While my A1C test was normal, my fasting-glucose score—taken when my blood sugar should have been at its lowest—was still too high. "For those two numbers to exist side by side means your blood sugar has to be in the 60s much of the time," he says. "Your biggest problem is hypoglycemia—low blood sugar." (Hypoglycemia is defined as less than 70 mg/dl; normal

blood sugar, between 70 and 100 mg/dl.) If Dr. Berkowitz was correct, my blood sugar was on a roller-coaster ride, with the perfect A1C averaging two extremes.

Dr. Berkowitz asked me to visit his office in midtown Manhattan, where I would take a stress test for my metabolic system. If fasting glucose is one still image and an A1C is a composite image, the oral glucose-tolerance test (OGTT) is like watching a movie, and it's more revealing as a result. In a study published in the journal *Angiology*, all three tests were given to 144 patients—none of whom had been previously diagnosed with type 2 diabetes or impaired blood sugar. Yet 94 patients yielded OGTT results that revealed one of those conditions. The fasting-glucose test had missed 62 percent of those cases, and the A1C had missed 83 percent.

"The last thing to go up is your fasting glucose," says Dr. Vernon. "The horse is already out of the barn at that point." That means the first signpost doctors are looking for is the last of the indicators to present itself.

My test begins with a lovely brunette in a white lab coat handing me a glass of a syrupy orange drink. It contains roughly the amount of sugar you would ingest from drinking two 12-ounce cans of Coke. Three hours into the test, even the pretty technician's gentle arm grab can't shake me from my stupor. But 20 minutes later, I suddenly become anxious, jittery. At 4 hours I start to feel more like myself again. Mercifully, the test ends.

"Sorry to have put you through all that torture," says a smiling Dr. Berkowitz a week later as he opens a manila folder containing my results. He was right—my condition is called reactive hypoglycemia, and it may be diabetes's most brilliant disguise of all. First my blood sugar shoots up to a prediabetic 165, a spike that by itself presents a significant risk factor for cardiovascular disease, according to a paper published in the *American Heart Journal*. Because my insulin does a poor job of ushering sugar into cells, my pancreas ends up producing 10 times more insulin than it should, according to Dr. Berkowitz.

"That's like using an atomic bomb to take out a small village," he says, except it's my pancreas that will be destroyed over time. The nuke has driven my blood sugar into the 70s an hour later—but my insulin is still blasting away. It drives me down to 59 an hour after that—nap time. Five hours have passed and my blood sugar is still 20 points below where it started.

Granted, my hypoglycemia was induced by a stress test using 75 grams of glucose. But the standard recommendation for people with diabetes (using the American Academy of Family Physicians guidelines) means consuming up to 180 grams of carbohydrates over the course of a day. Split among three squares, as the organization's president, James King, MD, suggests, that's just half an ounce less than an OGTT's worth of carbohydrates at each and every meal. (That's a huge load even with its absorption slowed by some fat and protein.)

"We use the OGTT as a metabolic stress test, and yet the mainstream advice prescribes a diet that produces that amount of carbohydrates at every meal," says Raab. "It just highlights the misunderstanding of how carbohydrates impact diabetes."

No wonder guys are bonking at their desks all afternoon. Your brain produces no energy itself, yet it sucks up 25 percent of the glucose circulating throughout your body while you're up, and about 60 percent at rest. During hypoglycemia, gray mat-ter is literally starving. (That explains my headaches.) You become shaky, anxious, dizzy, sweaty, tired, and unable to concentrate. Your body does whatever's necessary to protect your brain, and that includes breaking down muscle tissue so that it can be converted

DANGEROUS CURVES

Blood-sugar responses to carbs are nearly as individualized as fingerprints, but they do fall within categories. The hours spent with muscle-starving low blood sugar (reactive hypoglycemia) show how a man can be thin and fit yet still at high risk of type 2 diabetes.

CLASSIC TYPE 2 DIABETES
Fasting blood sugar above 126 mg/dl and a 2-hour oral glucose-tolerance test (OGTT) number above 200 both spell diabetes. Insulin injections would likely be prescribed in an attempt to drive down these numbers.

NORMAL BLOOD SUGAR
"Normal blood sugar would be a slow rise and a reasonable drop over several hours," says Keith W. Berkowitz, MD. "But 'normal' is actually becoming less and less typical, given what's in our diets."

REACTIVE HYPOGLYCEMIA
The telltale signs of this condition are (1) blood sugar that drops more than 30 mg/dl within an hour; (2) a half-hour, 1-hour, or 2-hour reading lower than the starting (i.e., fasting) number; and (3) an A1C score lower than it should be based on fasting blood sugar.

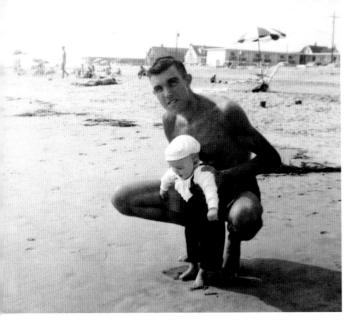

to glucose. Which begins to reveal why someone built like my father or me could be fast-tracking his way to type 2 diabetes. Because our insulin resistance results in frequent periods of low blood sugar, our bodies spend a good chunk of the day eating our own muscle.

As a result, we stay thin instead of gaining weight, as is often the case for people with insulin resistance and type 2 diabetes. In fact, insulin resistance is typically thought to cause weight gain, and vice versa. All of which makes the "thin man's diabetes" that much more perplexing.

"The physiques of people at high risk of diabetes are becoming less stereotypical, making the disease harder to diagnose," says Dr. Berkowitz. His observations are supported by science: "If you look at distributions of large numbers of people, it's striking that not only do the overweight tend to be insulin resistant, but 10 percent to 15 percent of nonobese people are, as well," says Donald W. Bowden, PhD, director of the center for diabetes research

at Wake Forest University school of medicine. Clearly, no one should assume he's immune to this disease.

SUGAR SHOCKED

I'm not the only one whose A1C score has led to serious head scratching of late. In February of 2008, the National Heart, Lung, and Blood Institute halted part of a large study because too many diabetic patients at high risk for heart attacks and strokes were actually dying of them while they were being treated aggressively—in some cases with multiple drugs and insulin injections—to lower their glucose. The goal was to bring them into line with normal, as measured by the A1C. Fifty years of conventional wisdom regarding diabetes says this group should have had the best outcome, not the worst.

It may be the wild ups and downs—replayed several times a day for years or decades—that takes the biggest toll on the body. Yet rather than seeing high and low blood sugar as two sides of the same insulin resistance, most of the diabetes organizations I contacted don't even think about the low side where type 2 diabetes is concerned.

The CDC does acknowledge that reactive hypoglycemia exists, but it has no data for hypoglycemia among men in the United States with diabetes, according to a spokesman. But he goes on to say this: "No data provide sufficient evidence that reactive hypoglycemia leads to diabetes."

"I think reactive hypoglycemia is a big problem," says Dr. Berkowitz. "No, I take that back. It's a huge problem." He tells me what's at stake for me in this battle. "If you don't do what we've been talking about, you will, over time, become diabetic. There's absolutely no question about it." After seeing my father minus his entire right leg, I have no reason to doubt the good doctor.

Dr. Berkowitz says that for a glucose-intolerant person, when to eat is nearly as important as what to eat. It only makes sense: If you want that seesaw to move gently through a small range of motion instead of swooping, you need to tap it more than three times a day, right? So in addition to sticking with my reduced-carb diet, I need to eat before I become hungry and finish my third small meal of the day before most men sit down to lunch. Sure, it's inconvenient at times, but then, not as inconvenient as losing your limbs.

BREAKING THE CHAIN

My father was once a formidable man. He should have wiped out type-2 diabetes like one of the giants he knocked off in that basketball tournament. But how could he? Unless he lives long enough to read this article, he'll die not knowing the name of the metabolic disorder—reactive hypoglycemia—that made him diabetic.

Coincidentally, my second and final visit with him coincides with his evening meal, wheeled into the room by two orderlies. I watch as they gently prick his finger to measure his blood sugar—and then leave behind a meal that includes mashed potatoes and fruit juice. I wonder if they've ever measured him an hour after such a carb-laden meal. Not that it matters now.

Near the end of my research, I'm stunned to learn that my grandfather, Thomas Joseph O'Connell Sr., another thin man, died from type 2 diabetes. One reason

my father got blindsided was that his father had moved on, and one reason I didn't see diabetes coming was that my father and I had parted ways. Consider it one of the unexpected costs of fathers and sons disconnecting: missing what should be obvious signs of family illnesses. Ironically, this disease also reunited us in the end and provided us with our one final bond. As I leave, I realize this isn't just the first time I've seen my father in 20 years. This is probably our last goodbye as well.

The night before my last blood draw for the lab work for this story, I begin my fast at 7 o'clock but still trudge off to the gym at 10 for a cardio blast. I also decide to rise at 6 the next morning; I want to hit the treadmill again for a few minutes of sugar burning before the nurse plunges a needle into my arm. For a year and a half, I've been determined to push that number under 100, no matter what it takes.

The alarm on my cellphone beeps. I roll over, gaze at the ceiling, and change my mind about the gym. What matters are the measurements I've already taken myself. In a year and a half, this disease has made me stronger, fitter, more determined, and more optimistic than I ever was before. In trying to lay claim to my body, diabetes unwittingly gave me a new lease on life instead.

When the lab results come back the following week, along with dramatic improvements in cholesterol and blood pressure, my fasting glucose registers 99. Those two digits say that my blood sugar is normal again. But I know better. Like millions of American men, my body can no longer handle processed carbs in anywhere near the quantities included in the typical American diet. ■

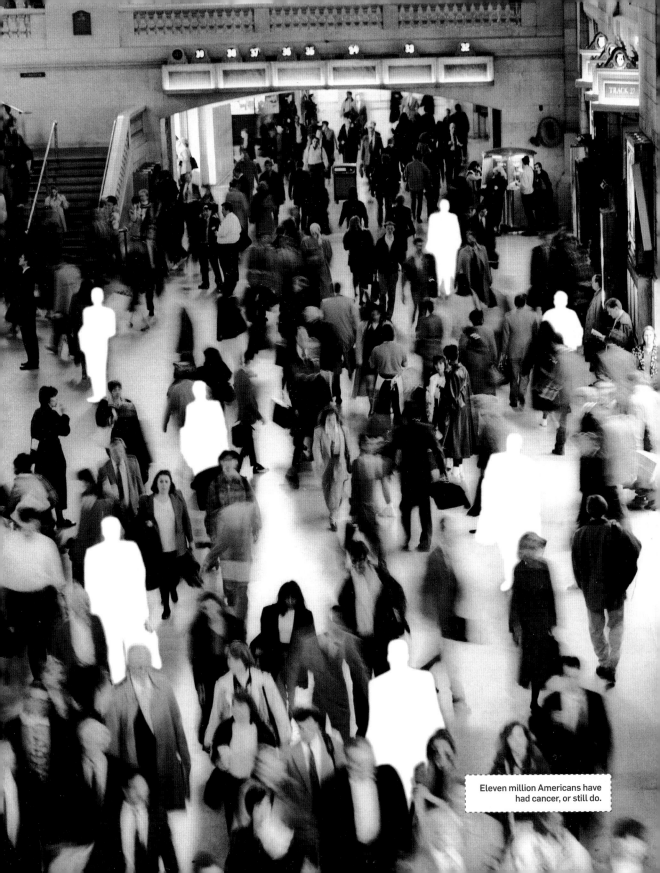

Eleven million Americans have had cancer, or still do.

Cope with the Big "C"

EACH YEAR, 1.4 MILLION AMERICANS ARE TOLD THEY HAVE CANCER. MAYBE YOU KNOW ONE. MAYBE YOU'LL BE ONE. HERE'S HOW TO COPE—AND HOW TO FIGHT

Stand-up comedian Kevin Knox gets paid to go to Las Vegas, play in golf tournaments, and say outrageous things. He also has cancer. Not so funny.

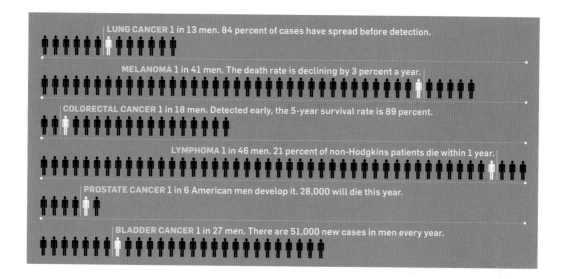

LUNG CANCER 1 in 13 men. 84 percent of cases have spread before detection.

MELANOMA 1 in 41 men. The death rate is declining by 3 percent a year.

COLORECTAL CANCER 1 in 18 men. Detected early, the 5-year survival rate is 89 percent.

LYMPHOMA 1 in 46 men. 21 percent of non-Hodgkins patients die within 1 year.

PROSTATE CANCER 1 in 6 American men develop it. 28,000 will die this year.

BLADDER CANCER 1 in 27 men. There are 51,000 new cases in men every year.

"You've been taken over by an alien that's trying to kill you. You feel betrayed by your body, and you feel devastated," Knox says.

Knox, 53, has stage-four melanoma, and points out, "There's no stage five."

When his doctor delivered the diagnosis, he gave him a year to live. Knox wasn't shocked, and he wasn't accepting it. He'd done some research.

"I was pissed. I knew people could survive, and I felt he was just piling on," Knox recalls. "I said, 'Well, I understand that's your diagnosis, but I don't believe that.' He reiterated that I could believe what I wanted, but it is what it is.

"For him to dismiss me like that was really annoying. I wasn't in denial. I knew I had cancer, but I also knew how I wanted to fight my battle."

He'd been through this before, both personally (a cancerous mole removed 17 years earlier) and with his parents and a sister, all of whom died of cancer while receiving conventional treatments.

So Knox was prepared to follow an uncharted course of natural treatment. His research led to a regimen that included raw and organic foods, certain types of teas, essential oils, exercise, and immunity-building injections and pills.

In February, it will be 5 years since the diagnosis. Knox isn't a zealot for his approach; he says it's up to each person to assess his or her needs. But he does know that the diagnosis can be a beginning, not an end—if you respond intelligently.

Knox is one of 11 million living Americans who have had cancer, or still do. You probably know one of them. Nearly four out of five Americans have a family member or close friend who has been diagnosed, according to the American Cancer Society. And every year in the United States, 1.4 million more are told they have cancer.

Here's what they—and their friends and relatives—should know about receiving that diagnosis and reacting to it.

WARNING SIGNS OF 6 CANCERS THAT STRIKE MEN

PROSTATE

Early signs: Usually there are none. A digital rectal exam can tell if your prostate is hard or irregular, and cancer is suspected with a high PSA (prostate specific antigen) level.

False alarms: Urination problems—frequency, urgency, slow stream, incomplete emptying— can be related to prostate enlargement or narrowing of the urethra.

The test: A biopsy if the PSA is high or its rate of change is high. But a spiked score can also be a sign of infection, which should be treated with antibiotics for 4 weeks. The cancer grows slowly; waiting isn't dangerous, says Christopher Saigal, MD, a urological oncologist at UCLA.

LUNG

Early signs: Frequently, none. But a cough that won't go away—or one that brings up blood—is often evidence the cancer is there. Also, chest pain that's always present and not influenced by movement, says Ezra Cohen, MD, a medical oncologist at University of Chicago Medical Center.

False alarms: Pneumonia. On a chest x-ray, both pneumonia and a tumor look white. The pneumonia will resolve, but you'll need another x-ray 4 to 6 weeks later.

The test: Biopsy.

COLORECTAL

Early signs: Blood in the stool. Never ignore it, even if it's a one-time occurrence. It could be a pre-cancerous polyp leaking blood, and bleeding is the only early warning you'll receive. In more than half of cases, there is no sign, says Greg Enders, MD, PhD, a gastroenterologist at Fox Chase Cancer Center.

False alarms: In men under 50, bleeding is probably from hemorrhoids, diverticulosis, colitis, or an abnormal blood vessel. Still, see a doctor.

The test: A colonoscopy allows the doctor to check for large and small problems and remove polyps in the same procedure.

BLADDER

Early signs: Blood in the urine, which should always be checked, although if you're younger than 60, it's often a sign of kidney stones. Most bladder cancer only affects the lining. If it is caught early, it can be beaten, says Brian Rini, MD, an oncologist at the Cleveland Clinic Taussig Cancer Institute.

False alarms: An overactive bladder or painful urination is more often a sign of an infection.

The tests: A scope through the penis to look at the bladder and a urine test that detects cancer cells.

LYMPHOMA

Early signs: Painless, swollen lymph nodes in your neck, armpit, or groin. Nodes swell with infections, but if they don't subside in a week, have them checked. Also, unexplained weight loss over 1 or 2 months, pain in the node area after drinking alcohol, or generalized itching with swelling (without rash) could be cause for concern, says Cleveland Clinic oncologist John Sweetenham, MD.

False alarms: Nodes can swell because of an infection.

The test: A blood test can occasionally pick up something, but a biopsy of the node is more thorough.

MELANOMA

Early signs: A spot that jumps out at you as irregular or large, or one that has recently changed, either in size, color, or contour, or that comes with symptoms, such as itching, pain, or bleeding, says Hensin Tsao, MD, PhD, a dermatologist at Massachusetts General Hospital.

False alarms: Seborrheic keratosis, which is a brownish, crusty formation that looks like it's stuck to the skin. It's just a benign growth.

The test: Biopsy.

DON'T PANIC

Easier said than done. "Cancer" is a scary, over-whelming word. But it's also a vague word. The doctor giving you the news is probably not a specialist and doesn't know the nuances, says Michael Fisch, MD, the interim chairman of the department of general oncology at the University of Texas M.D. Anderson Cancer Center in Houston.

DO THIS

Breathe deeply. Once you hear the diagnosis, you need to calm down. "You won't die in 5 hours," Knox says. "When you panic, you can't accomplish anything."

Nearly 4 OUT OF 5 AMERICANS have a family member or close friend who has cancer.

Take notes. Before you leave the office, tell the doctor to write down the exact diagnosis. Get a photocopy of the pathology report. It will help when you call for a specialist's appointment, and it will also help in your research. Write down the physician's phone numbers and e-mail addresses. As the news sinks in, you will probably have more questions.

Go online. But focus narrowly on established sites. Cancer.gov (the National Cancer Institute) and cancer.net (the American Society of Clinical Oncology) have unbiased, updated information to help you know what to expect, Dr. Fisch says.

Get a second opinion. Certainty is worth the few hundred dollars it might cost. University medical centers are usually best because doctors who teach tend to stay up-to-date.

"The teacher gets taught as much as the trainee," says Derek Raghavan, MD, PhD, director of the Cleveland Clinic Taussig Cancer Institute. Either ask the doctor who gave you the original diagnosis for a name, or go to web.facs.org/cpm/default.htm, which lists centers that have passed a stringent approval process.

REACH OUT

Resist the impulse to visit a specialist immediately, unless you have pain. "Common tumors are not galloping away on people," Dr. Fisch says.

DO THIS

Assemble a team. In addition to your primary-care physician, you'll want to find a local oncologist, even if you plan on traveling for treatment; a social worker who knows the hospital and insurance systems (your doctor or hospital has names); and an organized friend to help you and act as a firewall.

Make sure your friend is rational. "You want someone who's grounded," Knox says. "As a cancer victim, you have the tendency to become hysterical. You want someone who'll let you be hysterical for a little while—and then talk about your plan." You may freak at unrelated symptoms. "Every ache and pain isn't cancer. You need to be reminded that you're just human," he says.

Find a guide. Eventually you'll want to talk to someone who has been through your kind of cancer, preferably a person who has gone through support-group training, Dr. Raghavan says. Your hospital or the support society for your condition can help.

Release the news. In general, telling people soon is easiest. Yes, it may be hard to say the words out loud—and harder to watch the reactions of friends and family. As for children, kids as young as 3 will know something's up. Not telling them breeds fear and mistrust.

Once you hear the diagnosis, you need to calm down. WHEN YOU PANIC, you can't accomplish anything.

The best place to begin when telling a child about a parent's diagnosis is by asking the child what he or she has already noticed, says Paula Rauch, MD, the director of a program at Massachusetts General Hospital Cancer Center that helps parents.

Break the tension. "People don't want to say goodbye to a friend," Knox says. "I had to break the ice." He says that he'd just walk up and ask, "What's up? You're acting like I robbed your house." Then they'd talk.

VET THE SPECIALISTS

Shiny credentials and a recommendation aren't enough, Dr. Fisch says.

DO THIS

Ask around. First, ask your primary-care physician. The American Society of Clinical Oncology (cancer.net) allows you to search by city, state, and specialty. Ask your candidates how many people they see with this condition each year.

You want someone who's dealing with your disease every week, meaning at least 50 patients, says John Sweetenham, MD, an oncologist at the Cleveland Clinic Taussig Cancer Institute.

Gauge the doctor's commitment. Watch how locked in he or she is. You want to feel that the doc is focused. You should walk out knowing what's happening with a course of treatment or the choices, Dr. Fisch says.

Ask, ask, ask. Some basic questions include: What is it? What proportion of patients are cured? What is my quality of life going to be? What are the alternatives? What can I do to help myself and you? Are there any late effects? (These are side effects that arise a year or so after treatment ends—cardiac trouble, liver problems, or second malignancies, for example.)

Listen. If any answer is, "Let me worry about that," that's a red flag. You need to understand the process, and you need someone who will work with you. "Without that, you're out of control," Knox says.

ASSUME NOTHING

Treatment isn't a straight line. Setbacks are common. And your doctor can't know everything about your condition at day one, Dr. Raghavan says.

DO THIS

Step back. At 2 months, sit down with your doctor and revisit expectations. Ask, Are you satisfied with my progress? Are we still on track? Is there anything I should be doing? Some physicians aren't great communicators, Dr. Raghavan says, in which case you may want to reconsider your choice of a primary-care doctor.

Keep a journal. Note highs and lows and major changes so you can tell your doc.

Don't shrug off symptoms. People on your medical team can help you manage fatigue, pain, nausea, and constipation— if they know about them, Dr. Rauch says. Feeling better can help you spend more quality time with children and loved ones.

REMAIN OPEN

After 6 weeks, your disease isn't a novelty. Still, there will be shifts. "You can map out the first segment, but then you just keep your eyes open," Dr. Fisch says.

DO THIS

Reclaim your life. Return to the things you've strayed from—friends, golf, the gym.

"You become obsessed with what you have to do for the disease, and your everyday life disappears. You have to find that again," Knox says. "You need your health and happiness." It may be hard for you to believe in the early weeks, he adds, but this attitude shift will come.

Help your partner. "You go from being lovers to nurse-patient," Knox says. "You become incredibly needy, but you need to remember it's not all about you." Call a backup to drive you to appointments and give your wife or girlfriend the day off.

Be firm with friends. If you're in no mood for visitors, acknowledge their concern but send them away—nicely.

"You have the right to be caringly assertive," says Steve Thorney, staff chaplain at M.D. Anderson Cancer Center.

Don't judge. Some people will be there at the start and then fade. Others will pitch in after the crowd dies down. Accept this; shed resentment, Dr. Fisch says.

Deal with the impermanence. "After a while, the initial shock wears off. You'll think, It's 2½ weeks and I'm still not dead," Knox says. "But things come in waves. You can have an amazing day—Oh, look at that flower. Then all of a sudden, it could flip.

It could be the slightest thing, a guy eating a cheeseburger, that throws you." Ride out the emotions, and then get back to life. ■

Be Your Own E.R. Doc

WHETHER YOU'RE BLEEDING, BURNED, OR STUNG, HERE'S HOW TO FIX THE INJURY— OR AT LEAST SURVIVE UNTIL THE CAVALRY ARRIVES

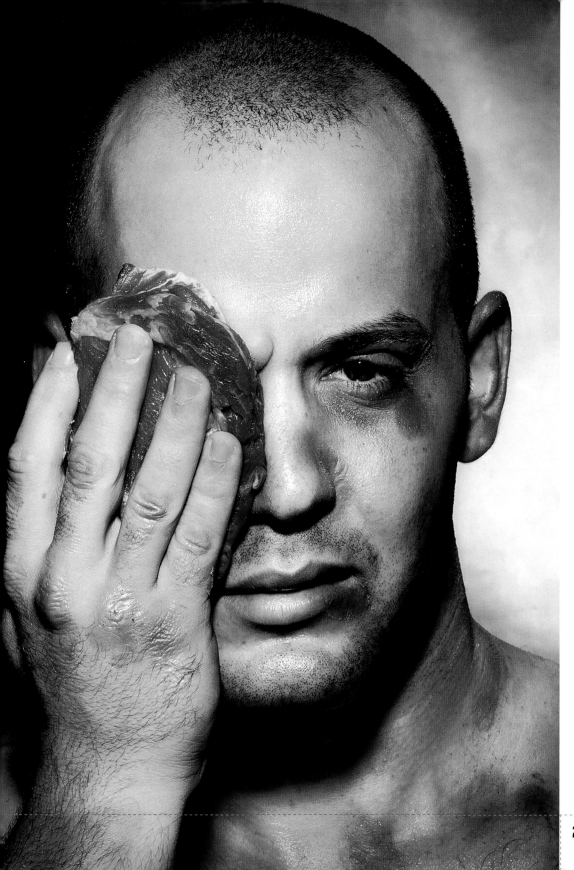

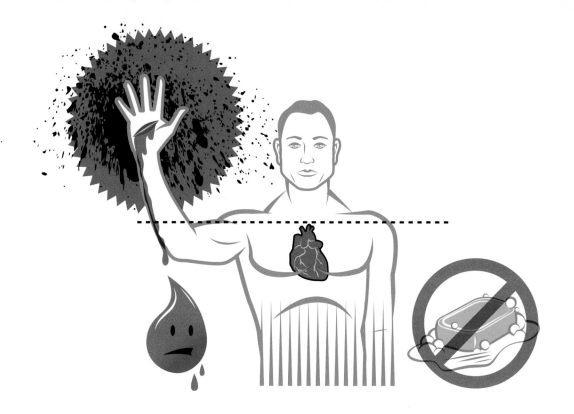

As a 30-year-old engineer living in a Philadelphia suburb, Joe Cammarata's combat experience amounts to playing Street Fighter II on his computer. Yet his medical history makes it sound like characters leaped from the screen to rough him up: a torn rotator cuff and torn Achilles tendon, both from playing baseball; third-degree burns on both legs after a drunken sprint through a frat-party bonfire; a sprained ankle from playing soccer; and, after a memorable roll in the hay, a missing front tooth.

"My reaction has always been to run around screaming," says Cammarata of his stock response to injury, one mimicked by other men. And there's no shortage of screamers: The National Center for Health Statistics says injuries sent nearly 18 million American men to the E.R. in 2005. Most of those scrapes, burns, and cuts occurred at home or on the field or court.

But here's the thing: Men like Joe would recover more quickly if they knew what to do before a paramedic or doctor took over. And armed with some simple yet effective DIY techniques, your only E.R. experience might come as you're sitting on the sofa.

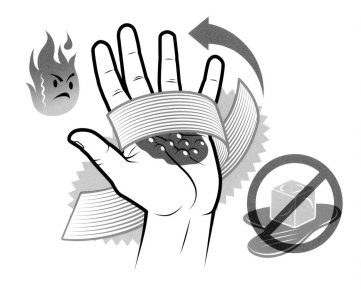

IF YOU'RE CUT...

FIRST THINGS FIRST: Grab a clean napkin or towel or some sterile gauze, place it over the wound, and apply pressure. If the wound is to a limb, raise it above your heart to slow bloodflow to the site and encourage nature's bandage—clotting.

"If the cloth soaks through with blood, keep adding to it," says paramedic Connie Meyer, a board member of the National Association of Emergency Medical Technicians. "If you disturb the clot, it'll start bleeding again."

THE "UH-OH" MOMENT: If the blood is bright red and spurting, an artery has been breached. EMTs often focus on pressure points—key places on the body where an artery is next to bone—and apply direct pressure. Done correctly, this tactic at least slows the bleeding. If you cut your hand, for example, find the brachial artery, located on the inside of your arm just above the elbow. Press it hard with your fingers or palm. If you're severely gashed and can see

inside the wound, pinch the artery shut. Hold on tight until you make it to an E.R.

DIAL 911: If you've lost enough blood to fill a 20-ounce soda bottle or if you start to feel thirsty, cold, or both, you could be going into shock. Phone for help, stat. Then work to control the bleeding—without panicking. Stopping a severe bleed could take as long as 20 minutes, Meyer says.

ROOKIE MISTAKE: Putting soap into a wound. If you slice your finger, run it under the tap for a few seconds. Then cover it with a bandage and watch it the next day. Increasing pain at the site, redness, warmth, and foul-smelling drainage are all signs of infection.

IF YOU'RE BURNED...

FIRST THINGS FIRST: If the affected area is smaller than 3 inches in diameter, run it under cold water for 5 minutes, says Meyer. If the skin isn't blistered or charred—signs of serious burns—pop two ibuprofen or acetaminophen and leave the burn exposed to air. Don't slather on an antiseptic cream right away, says Meyer. "Wait at

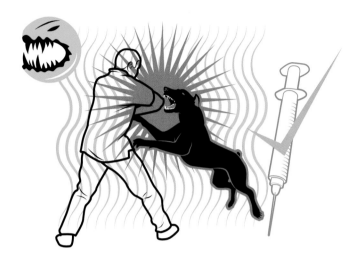

least an hour, or until the skin has cooled." When the burning sensation stops, prevent infection with an antibiotic ointment. Mild soap and water can work in a pinch.

THE "UH-OH" MOMENT: Blistering skin means a second-degree burn. "These are fairly serious, but an area smaller than your palm can be managed at home," says David Ross, DO, an emergency physician at Penrose Hospital in Colorado Springs and a member of the American College of Emergency Physicians. Don't pop the blisters, and skip the cream. Cover unhealed blisters loosely with gauze or an adhesive strip.

DIAL 911: If your skin resembles an over-cooked rib eye, you have third-degree burns. While you're waiting for paramedics, don't submerge the burns in cold water, which could lead to shock and hypothermia. Make sure your skin is no longer in contact with smoldering fabric, and let the experts remove any stuck clothing.

ROOKIE MISTAKE: "Applying ice to any burn interrupts tissue repair," says Charles F. Pattavina, MD, chief of emergency medicine at St. Joseph Hospital in Bangor, Maine. "Use water that's 40°F or warmer."

IF YOU'VE BEEN BITTEN...

FIRST THINGS FIRST: How deep is it? "An abrasion or scratch doesn't usually need a doctor's attention," says Dr. Pattavina. "The risk of infection is much lower than with penetrating wounds." Rinse away germs with cool tap water, cover the site with an adhesive strip, and watch for infection.

THE "UH-OH" MOMENT: If teeth do plunge into your skin, it's a different story. "These are dangerous," says Dr. Pattavina. "Long fangs push bacteria deep into the wound, where they can thrive in an inaccessible, low-oxygen environment." You can try flushing the wound with cool water, but your best bet is an E.R. "Even with irrigation by a doctor, these wounds are prone to infection," says Dr. Pattavina. "They may need a lot of cleansing and antibiotics."

DIAL 911: If man's best friend suddenly turns into a creature from a horror movie, and you can't stop the bleeding or a huge chunk of tissue is missing, call for an ambulance immediately.

ROOKIE MISTAKE: Not keeping up with your tetanus shot. Dr. Ross recommends receiving a booster within 72 hours if you've been bitten and 5 years have elapsed since your last shot.

IF YOU'RE STUNG...

FIRST THINGS FIRST: A bee sting produces an odor that can prompt other bees to attack, so cover your face and neck with a shirt or jacket until you can scramble indoors. Then curb the pain with acetaminophen or ibuprofen.

No matter what your mother slathered on a sting, topical home remedies such as baking powder and mud only cool the skin.

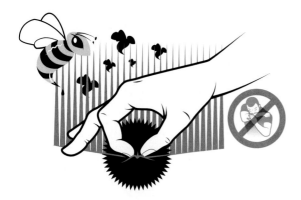

"They don't actually mediate your body's reaction," says P. Kirk Visscher, PhD, an associate entomologist at the University of California at Riverside.

THE "UH-OH" MOMENT: The longer the stinger stays stuck in your skin, the more venom your body receives. So yank the stinger out with your fingers, scrape it off with a fingernail or credit card, or brush it off on your jeans—just remove it ASAP. Seconds matter, says Dr. Visscher, who notes that the squeeze itself won't affect the amount of poison that leaks into your system.

DIAL 911: If you've been stung 20 or more times, develop hives away from the site of the sting, or experience difficulty breathing, you might be having an allergic reaction, which in extreme cases can be fatal if not treated quickly.

ROOKIE MISTAKE: Sucking on the sting to remove the venom, which does nothing more than cause the venom to infuse the tissue further, resulting in a larger, uglier welt.

IF IT'S SPRAINED OR BROKEN...

FIRST THINGS FIRST: Whether it's a sprain or a break, apply ice (alternating 10 minutes on and 10 minutes off) for the first day or so. To make a quick ice pack, place crushed ice in a zip-top bag and then wrap the bag in a thin towel or T-shirt. A bag of frozen peas will work, too.

If you can move the joint or bone without major discomfort and there's no obvious deformity, it's probably not broken, says Dr. Ross. Ice it, elevate it, and grab an ibuprofen or two to dull discomfort.

THE "UH-OH" MOMENT: The huge crunch you heard or the disturbing S shape of your arm leaves little doubt. It's broken. Try to keep the bone immobilized on your way to the E.R., and elevate a broken arm or leg above heart level. This counteracts gravity's pull on blood moving into the arm.

DIAL 911: Call an ambulance immediately if you can see the bone or if there's a hole in the skin—a broken bone may have pierced the skin. Resist the urge to pop pain meds: They could cause complications if you need immediate surgery.

ROOKIE MISTAKE: Jury-rigging a splint or sling. "Splints are necessary only if you're far from help," says Dr. Ross. "A sling does nothing but remind you not to move the injury. If you're thinking sling, see a doctor." ■

EXERCISE SCIENCE

DON'T OVERHEAT

Cigarettes can kill, but what about smoking-cessation drugs? A study on rats in the *Journal of Physiology* suggests that Zyban can spike your risk of exercise-induced heatstroke. Turns out, the drug's active ingredient, bupropion, over-rides cell communication in an area of the brain that regulates body temperature. Bupropion is used to treat cigarette addiction, and also depression.

"It causes a release of feel-good brain chemicals that keep you exercising even when your core temperature hits danger-ous levels," says study coau-thor Romain Meeusen, PhD. If you're taking Zyban, ask your doctor about other drug options.

PREVENT CANCER WITH CARDIO

It's time to take America's sec-ond leading killer of men down

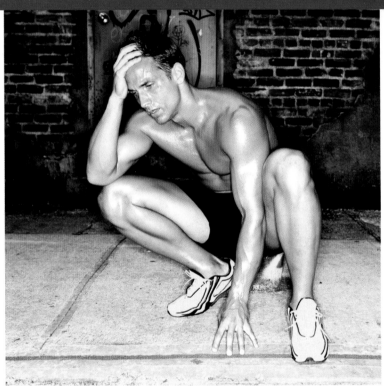

a few notches. Men with the highest fitness levels are three times less likely to die of can-cer compared with those who are least active, according to a University of Buffalo study.

The benefits of staying in good cardiovascular shape

were constant regardless of whether the men were lean or overweight. Moderate exercise appears to help disarm free radicals, the rogue chemicals that cause the DNA damage that leads to cancer, says the study author, Steve Farrell,

PhD. Find out your current fitness level at MensHealth.com/cardiotest.

Swim for just 60 minutes a week, and you'll cut your risk of prostate cancer by 31 percent.

SPRUCE UP YOUR IMMUNE SYSTEM

You might finally have a legitimate reason to hug a tree: A hike in the woods can boost your immunity, say Japanese researchers. They found that men who walked through a forest for a total of 6 hours over 2 days experienced a 46 percent spike in their blood levels of natural killer cells, which are part of your body's SWAT team against invading viruses. Apparently, all trees release airborne chemicals called phytoncides that not only protect their foliage from microbes, but also help to stimulate our own immune systems.

BANISH BACK PAIN

Tylenol may be the best over-the-counter medicine for back pain, according to a study review from the Cochrane Collaboration. After analyzing research on more than 11,000 people, the scientists concluded that acetaminophen was as effective at relieving acute lowerback pain as prescription-

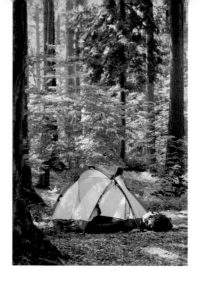

strength ibuprofen—and with fewer side effects.

Just limit your Tylenol to 4,000 milligrams a day, and don't wash it down with alcohol: The combo causes liver problems.

SOOTHE YOUR ACHING KNEES

Tired of popping pills for joint pain? Ask your doctor about Voltaren Gel, which is a newly approved treatment for osteoarthritis. Unlike aspirin, which must be taken orally, the gel is applied to the joint and absorbed there, reducing your risk of stomach ulcers while providing faster relief.

KICK THAT CRICK

Lifting weights might remedy a stiff neck, according to a new study in *Arthritis & Rheumatism*. When 48 adults with nagging neck pain spent 20

minutes three times a week strengthening their upper trapezius muscles, they reported 80 percent less discomfort after 10 weeks. That's because resistance training may help repair damaged muscle tissue. And stronger muscles can bear more strain, preventing further wear and tear, say the study authors.

To work your upper traps, stand with your arms hanging straight down at your sides, hold a weight in each hand, and shrug your shoulders. Do 2 sets of 8 to 10 reps.

COUCH DEPRESSION

The only thing the doctor needs to order for depression is exercise. A new study from Duke University examined the effects of four different treatments on 202 depressed adults: home-based exercise, supervised exercise, sertraline (a depression drug such as Zoloft), and a placebo. They found that exercise is as effective as drug therapy for treating depression. Because antidepressants don't work for everyone—and they carry crazy side effects such as increased suicide risk, impotency, and abdominal bleeding—the Duke doctors think exercise is a viable alternative.

MONITOR YOUR MUSCLES

If you're taking cholesterol-lowering drugs, beware of muscle problems, advises a Loyola University study. That's because statins may lead to myopathy, which is a malady with symptoms that, if untreated, can range from muscle weakness and pain to muscle damage and even death.

"Research suggests this can occur in 1 to 5 percent of people," says study author Sung Ahn, DO. If you have symptoms, see your doctor.

SAVE GAS; GAIN LIFE

Where you park your car may increase your risk of heart disease, according to Danish researchers. When men were asked to park close to buildings, take the elevator instead of the stairs, and walk less in general, their triglyceride levels went up 18 percent in 2 weeks. The explanation is NEAT (non-exercise activity thermogenesis), which consists of all the ways we expend energy without actually exercising.

Take walking out of the NEAT equation and you'll not only gain weight, but also accumulate more triglycerides in your bloodstream, says the study author, Rikke Krogh-Madsen, MD. So look to the men in the study, and then do the opposite: Take the farthest parking spot you find, hoof it up the stairs, and squeeze in extra steps wherever possible.

Hiking through parking lots has a bigger impact on your total calorie burn than gym workouts.

CHILL A LITTLE

While exercise can decrease heart-disease risk, if you're one of the 72 million Americans with high blood pressure, there is a fine line as to how hard you should push yourself. A recent study published in the journal *Hypertension* found that excessive exercise causes structural abnormalities in the hearts of those with high blood pressure—aberrations such as enlarged hearts and decreased pumping ability. Your doctor can tell you how much exercise is too much. ∎

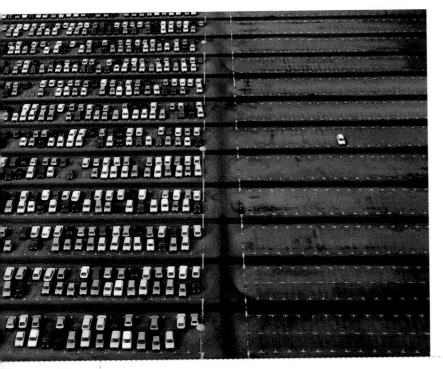

TRAINING TIPS Q&A

Q: What are the best ways to monitor my health at home?

A: First, learn to listen to your body's built-in sickness sensors. Men have a habit of ignoring or minimizing obvious indicators of illness, such as pain, fatigue, and numbness. If you're sufficiently tuned in, then consider the early warning systems shown next. "You want to catch deviations from the norm at the earliest possible time," says Eric Topol, MD, a senior cardiology consultant at the Scripps Clinic in La Jolla, California, "like identifying high blood pressure before it damages your heart, kidney, or brain function." And if in the end a stroke or heart attack still manages to sneak up on you, use that other high-tech health tool: the phone.

CHOLESTEROL
Your goal: Less than 100 mg/dl LDL and 150 mg/dl triglycerides; more than 60 mg/dl HDL
CardioChek, $100. After a quick prick of your finger, the CardioChek's optical sensor analyzes the drop of blood with a test strip and then computes your triglyceride, LDL, HDL, and total cholesterol levels.

TEMPERATURE
Your goal: 98.6°F, plus or minus 1°F
Vicks Comfort-Flex Thermometer, $14. It'll take your temp in 8 seconds flat and flash red when you have a fever. Recheck your temp every 6 to 8 hours to make sure it doesn't approach the 103°F danger zone.

BLOOD PRESSURE
Your goal: Less than 120/80 mm Hg
Omron Deluxe Blood Pressure Monitor, $90. The Omron monitor quickly and accurately measures your blood pressure and pulse, and also stores as many as 60 readings so you can track changes over time.

BODY FAT
Your goal: Less than 15 percent for men under 40, and 18 percent if you're older
Tanita Ironman Segmental Body Monitor, $300. Unlike monitors that calculate the fat percentage of your entire body only, the Ironman allows you to separately measure the dangerous visceral fat in your belly, too.

Q: What's the number one way to improve my cardiovascular fitness?

A: "Alternating short bursts of high-intensity exercise with easy recovery. Intervals also stoke fat burning and boost HDL cholesterol, the good kind," says Michael Fredericson, MD, an associate professor in the department of orthopedic surgery at Stanford University and the head physician for the track, cross-country, swimming, and gymnastics teams.

Q: How do I know when to stop going to the chiropractor?

A: When your pain stops. Chiropractic medicine is best used in the acute phase of lower-back pain. But consider it to be more of a bandage than a treatment that goes on indefinitely.

Q: I was diagnosed with a bulging disk. Which free-weight exercises should I avoid?

A: Disk bulges are common with age. And they don't always have symptoms. Avoid deadlifts and other moves requiring your back to work like a crane, says Nicholas A. DiNubile, MD, an orthopedic surgeon in private practice and a clinical assistant professor of orthopedic surgery at the Hospital of the University of Pennsylvania.

Q: My elbow cracks when I flex it. Do I have arthritis?

A: Some guys' tendons just tend to snap. But if it just started on one side only and hurts or causes swelling, have it examined, says Dr. DiNubile.

Q: Do I need to worry about catching something if I don't use the paper protective covers in public restrooms?

A: The loo is the least of your worries. "There really aren't any significant butt-borne diseases," says Charles Gerba, PhD, a professor of environmental microbiology at the University of Arizona.

In one study of suspected office hot spots, Dr. Gerba and his colleagues found the toilet seat to be the cleanest location, holding a measly 49 bacteria per square inch. (By contrast, an office telephone receiver carries about 25,000 per square inch.)

"The sinks and taps are actually the dirtiest areas of bathrooms—hundreds of germy hands have touched those handles," says Dr. Gerba. He notes that most of the bugs come from what has accumulated on users' hands throughout the day and not necessarily just from using the toilet. So if

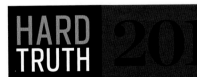

HARD TRUTH **201** BILLIONS OF DOLLARS AMERICANS SPENT TREATING BACK AND NECK PAIN IN 2005, ACCORDING TO THE *JOURNAL OF THE AMERICAN MEDICAL ASSOCIATION*

you really want to limit your disease risk, focus on more effective defenses, such as properly washing your hands and then keeping a clean paper towel between your mitts and everything else as you exit.

Q: Am I being a germophobe when I wipe off the top of a soda can with a napkin?

A: We fully expected to find out that soda cans are swarming with bacterial baddies. After all, who knows where those cans have been? But it turns out that putting mouth to metal won't make you sick.

Cold aluminum simply doesn't offer a hospitably warm, moist environment to the germs that make us sick, especially when refrigeration is involved, says University of Iowa microbiologist Michael Pentella, PhD.

But even if a few hardy bugs do make it to your lips, they'll be eliminated by the acids in the soda, he says. What you should worry about is this: A University of Arizona study found traces of saliva on the buttons of one out of eight vending machines. So either push the button with your elbow or, better yet, stop drinking soda.

Q: Is it okay to hold in a sneeze?

A: The human sneeze was once clocked at 103 mph, so trying to squelch one

by holding your nose is a bad idea.

"All the air has to go somewhere," says Andrew P. Lane, MD, director of the Johns Hopkins Sinus Center in Baltimore. "It's rare, but you can rupture an eardrum, damage membranes in your inner ear, or cause small capillaries in your eyes to burst." Plus, the irritant that caused the blast remains.

Q: Which is better for my heart—peanut oil or olive oil?

A: "Both are good sources of monounsaturated fats, but extra-virgin olive oil also contains healthful compounds from the olive fruit," says Mary Ellen Camire, PhD, a professor of food science in the department of food science and human nutrition at the University of Maine and a foodscience communicator for the Institute of Food Technologists, a not-for-profit scientific organization.

Q: How can I rid myself of an athlete's-foot problem?

A: Apply Lamisil cream to your entire foot, including the spaces between the toes, every day for at least 2 weeks, says Adnan Nasir, MD, PhD, an adjunct clinical assistant professor at the University of North Carolina at Chapel Hill and medical director of dermatology research at Wake Research Associates. ■

HARD TRUTH

4

PERCENTAGE DROP IN LDL AFTER 12 WEEKS OF TAKING STAIRS, NOT THE ELEVATOR, ACCORDING TO THE EUROPEAN SOCIETY OF CARDIOLOGY CONGRESS 2008

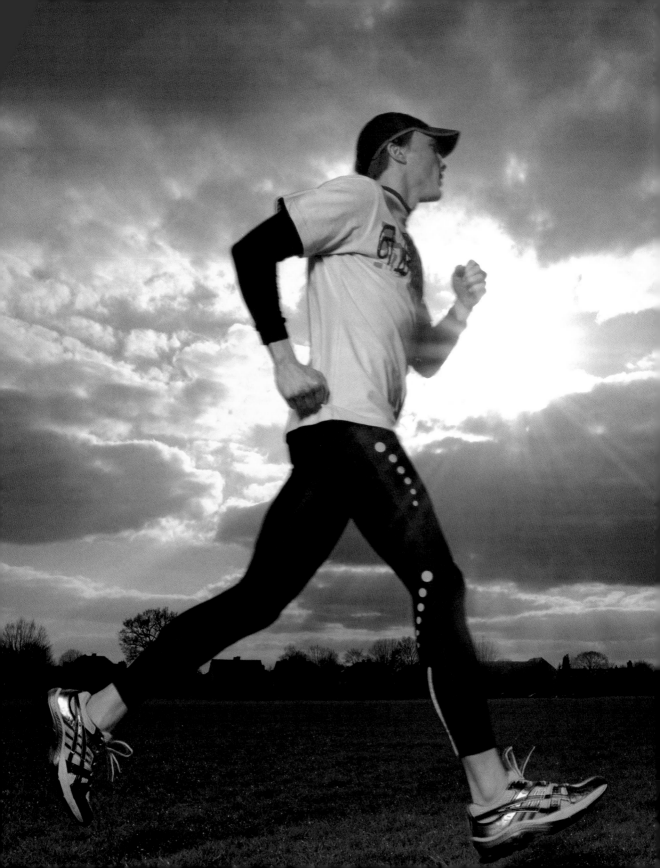

6

Strip Away Stress

Swing into Action

HERE ARE THE FIVE BEST EXERCISES TO BOOST YOUR GOLF DRIVE AND STRENGTHEN YOUR BACK

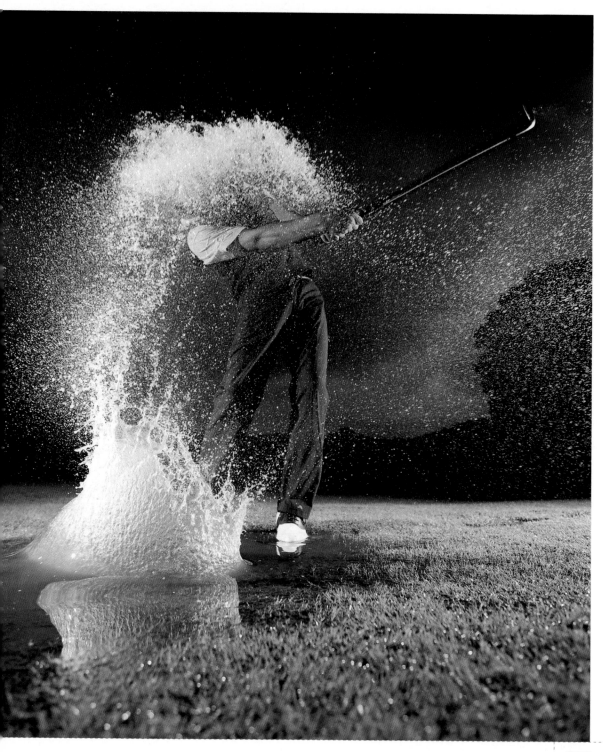

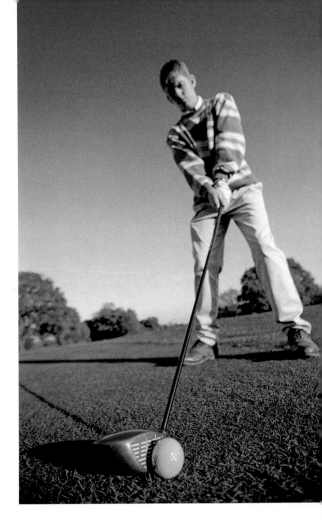

Never mind Phil Mickelson's marshmallow midriff or John Daly's dough-boy pudge. The flabby, unfit golf pro is a vanishing breed on the PGA Tour, where the average player is stronger, leaner, and longer hitting than ever before. Call it the Tiger Woods effect. Pressed to keep up with the world's best (and most chiseled) player, most pros are now treating golf like a contact sport.

"Fitness is transforming the game," says Mark Verstegen, CSCS, the owner of Athletes' Performance in Tempe, Arizona. "Today's pro blasts his tee shot 50 yards farther than players of 15 years ago."

Golfers, in other words, are becoming athletes. But you don't have to be a golf pro to reap the benefits of golf fitness. Weave the following exercises into your weekly routine, and you'll add another 25 yards to your drive and strengthen your core and back, says Verstegen, author of the fitness tome *Core Performance Golf*. "Better still," he says, "you'll play without pain or injuries." ∎

CHEATER'S GOLF
How to sneak your way out of the sand trap and into the hole

A once-simple diversion invented by glengarry-topped Scotsmen strolling the moors with their sticks, golf has come to resemble some high-tech war game. But before you drop a bundle at the pro shop, realize that no amount of graphite or titanium is going to turn a mediocre player into a (Gary) Player. Despite the numerous "breakthroughs" in golf technology, the driving distances of the best professional golfers have increased about 30 yards since 1968. Meanwhile, the average winning score has fallen less than one stroke per round in 40 years. Here are several better—and cheaper—ways to improve your score.

LUBE UP. If you tend to slice or hook—who doesn't?—try spreading some Vaseline on your club face. "It takes away any sort of spin you would normally put on a ball," says Adrian Cho, editor and creator of the "Stixx Review" golf blog. "In turn, it will give you more distance and a little more accuracy."

GET HOT. Before you head off to the links, heat your golf balls—say, by wrapping them in a hand warmer. The hotter they are, the farther the little white orbs will travel off the tee. On a 60°F day, for example, if you were to heat your golf balls to 90°F and use them on drives, you could give yourself about 15 more feet.

POINT OUT TROUBLE SPOTS. Never let a hole pass without mentioning the dangerous woods lining the fairway or that big pond snuggling the green. "By blurting out something such as, 'Damn, that's enough ocean to start a naval academy,' you'll psych even seasoned players into dwelling on it," explains Captain Bruce Warren Ollstein, author of *Combat Golf.* "And if they do clear the hazard, they may end up 30 yards off their intended target."

CHECK HIS BREATHING. If your partner is on a roll, ask him about a particular detail of his swing. The point is to get him to analyze things that have become second nature. A good line: "So tell me, do you inhale or exhale during your backswing?"

SUPPLY COUNTER-INTELLIGENCE. If you hit a ball short and know it's because you didn't connect well on the shot, immediately comment, "Gosh, I really whacked that ball, and it still didn't go anywhere." If you say the opposite of what really occurred, "your opponent will assume it's an extremely slow green or that there's a lot of wind and you didn't use a big enough club off the tee," says Ollstein. If he's putting, he'll hit it harder. If driving, he'll pull out a bigger club, and then send the ball into the woods.

ONE-SIDED DUMBBELL BENCH PRESS
Lie off-center on a bench so that only your left glute and shoulder touch the bench. Hold a dumbbell directly above your chest with your right hand, and grasp the bench behind your head with your left hand. Lower the weight until your elbow is in line with your shoulder, and then return to the starting position. Do 3 sets of 8 to 10 reps per side.

SINGLE-LEG ROMANIAN DEADLIFT
Hold dumbbells in both hands and stand with your feet shoulder-width apart, knees slightly bent, and arms at your sides. Lift your right foot off the floor and bend at the hips, maintaining a straight line from the heel of your right foot to your shoulder as you lower your torso until it's as close to parallel with the floor as you can get. Pause, then return to the starting position. Do 3 sets of 8 to 10 reps per side.

RUSSIAN TWIST
Lie faceup on an exercise ball with your shoulders on the ball, your feet flat on the floor, and your hips in line with your shoulders and knees. Holding a weight plate above your chest with both hands, roll your upper body to the right until your shoulders are perpendicular to the floor (your hips shouldn't move). Twist back to the starting position, then repeat on your left side. Do 3 sets of 8 to 10 reps per side.

FRONT PILLAR BRIDGE
Get into a modified pushup position, supporting your weight with your forearms and the balls of your feet. Lift your left leg into the air; hold for 2 seconds. Place it back on the floor, switch legs, and repeat 10 more times. That's 1 set. Do 3.

PERPENDIC-ULAR THROWS
Stand 4 feet from a wall with your hips perpendicular to it, and hold a medicine ball with one hand under the ball and the other hand behind it. Rotate away from the wall until the ball is behind your hip, and then initiate the throw by driving your back hip toward the wall, followed by your trunk and arms. Catch and repeat. Do 2 sets of 8 to 10 reps per side.

Survive a Marathon

RUNNING A MARATHON PUTS SEVERE AND SOMETIMES DANGEROUS STRESS ON YOUR BODY. WHY DO SO MANY MEN STILL WANT TO DO IT?

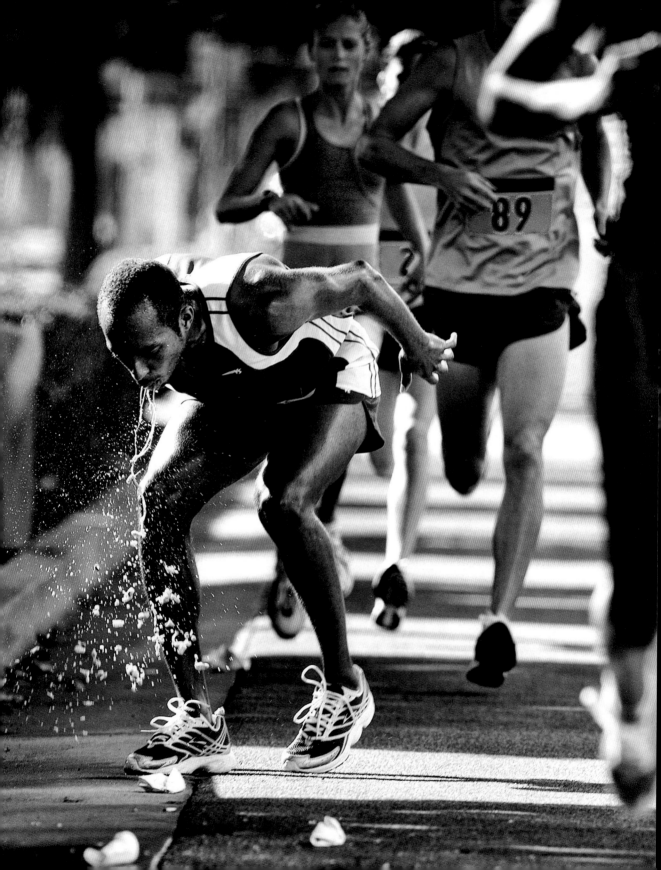

On the first Monday of November 1994, if you happened to be in Ardmore, Pennsylvania—actually, anywhere near 7 East Athens Avenue—at about 8:30 in the morning, you would have heard the following sound coming from an aging red-brick apartment building.

Thud. Arghh. Thud. Arghh . . .

Ax murder? Not exactly. No, this was the sad, solitary sound of writer Tom McGrath, walking down three flights of steps the morning after running the New York City Marathon. As his feet landed on each step, pain spiked into his race-fatigued thighs. By the time McGrath reached the bottom, 48 steps later, he was so exhausted that all he wanted to do was go back to bed. But that would have required climbing back up three flights of steps. McGrath drove to work and slept at his desk instead.

New York '94 was McGrath's third and last marathon. Since then he's downgraded his running efforts to more manageable distances like the half marathon and 10-K. Secretly, he's come to wonder if he didn't do damage to himself in each of the marathons he ran. McGrath doesn't have any scars or permanent injuries (that he knows of), but where pain and exhaustion typically fade from memory, his postmarathon distress is as vivid to him now as it was on that horrific morning after.

Which is why it's kind of strange, you'll have to agree, that lately he's found himself wanting to run another one.

A RITE OF PASSAGE

Over the course of a generation, the marathon has undergone a startling change in status. What was once a loopy stunt attempted by only a few weirdos is now a must-do for many men, the coolest test out there of fitness and health.

Many men actually put running a marathon on their lists of Things a Man Must

MILE MARKERS

15,000 to 28,000:
number of times each foot hits the pavement over 26.2 miles

45:
minimum number of weekly training miles recommended to reduce chances of a cardiac event

6.5X:
increase in levels of cardiac troponin I, a marker of heart-cell damage, in runners after a marathon

Do in His Lifetime, right there alongside reading *War and Peace* and seeing the Grateful Dead (before Jerry Garcia croaked anyway). In 2007, nearly 400,000 runners finished marathons in the United States, up from 300,000 in 2000 and a mere 25,000 in 1976.

On one level, you can file our current marathon mania under "extremely good news," because there's little doubt that training for the race is one of the best ways to improve your health and fitness. Over the years, studies have shown that regular exercise decreases everything from high LDL cholesterol to high blood pressure.

The problem? Lately, evidence has begun to mount that running the race is anything but good for your health. Not only did two high-profile marathon deaths occur in fall 2007 (one in Chicago, the other at the Olympic trials in New York), but recent studies have shown that pushing your body to run 26.2 miles can cause at least minor injury to your heart.

"We didn't find any gross injuries, such as blocked arteries or blood leakage. But we did find some enzymes leaking through the heart membrane, which is consistent with significant stress on the heart," says Malissa Wood, MD, the lead author of a 2006 study in the journal *Circulation*.

Now, hardly anyone is suggesting it's time to pull the plug on America's marathon obsession. A handful of deaths versus hundreds of thousands of happy survivors every year aren't horrible odds. (And a new study found that closing roads for marathons prevents more traffic deaths than the running causes.) Even Dr. Wood remains an active marathoner. But if you're one of those men with "run a marathon" on a current to-do list (or even on a "maybe-do-again" list), the latest news should definitely give you pause. Could the race you're running as a demonstration of your health and fitness actually make you unhealthy? Or, to put a finer point on it: Could this stunt you're attempting to give meaning to your life end your life?

A CAUSE OF DEATH?

The Chicago marathon and Olympic Trials in 2007 weren't the only races marred by casualties in the past couple of years. There have been several others, including the Little Rock Marathon in March 2008, the London Marathon in 2007, and the Tucson, Twin Cities, and Marine Corps Marathons in 2006. (Also in 2006, two runners died at the Los Angeles Marathon.) And that's not counting the races during which runners suffered cardiac arrest but managed to survive.

HARD TRUTH

30

PERCENTAGE OF MARATHONERS WHO SAY THE SPORT HELPED THEIR SEXUAL PERFORMANCE, ACCORDING TO THE SOCIAL ISSUES RESEARCH CENTRE

1 in 50,000:
approximate risk of suffering sudden cardiac death during or within 24 hours of completing a marathon

40:
median age of male finishers in marathons in 2007, up from 34 in 1980

40s and 50s:
Ages in which marathon fatalities are clustered

Recent studies have shown that PUSHING YOUR BODY to run 26.2 miles can cause at least minor injury to your heart.

Any historian of running will tell you there's nothing new about death and the marathon. Legend has it, remember, that the original marathoner, Phidippides—the Greek courier who ran 25 miles to deliver news of victory at the Battle of Marathon—dropped dead immediately after his job was done. At the inaugural Boston Marathon in 1897, authorities were so concerned about fatalities that

they had two attendants on bicycles trailing closely behind each of the runners—all 15 of them.

It's a risk that has persisted through the decades. "There was actually a cardiac arrest at one of the first Boston Marathons I ran, in the 1970s," says Arthur Siegel, MD, director of internal medicine at Harvard's McLean Hospital in Belmont, Massachusetts. In addition to

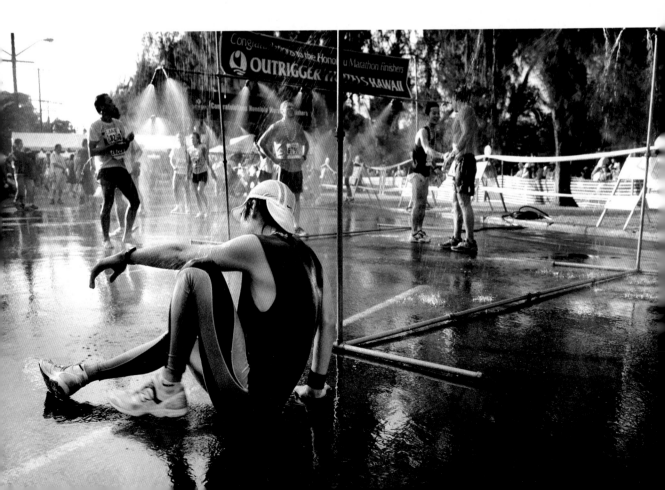

running the Boston race some 20 times, Dr. Siegel has published many studies on the health consequences of marathons. He's an engaging man in his late 60s with white hair and a round belly, for one simple reason: to understand what exactly happens to a man's body when he forces it to run 26.2 miles.

Researchers have identified a number of physical effects of running a marathon, including changes in immune system and kidney function. But Dr. Siegel says the brunt of the damage falls exactly where you'd expect: on your muscles. As the miles pass, skeletal muscles stiffen and leak injury-signaling enzymes into the blood.

Now, a certain inability to walk down steps the next day notwithstanding, this may not seem like such a big deal, particularly given that the damage is self-inflicted. But your body's internal balance is deeply affected. As Dr. Siegel puts it, "Your body doesn't know whether you've run a marathon . . . or been hit by a truck." This is why, as you go deeper into the race, your body reacts to injury by mounting an emergency-repair response. Your adrenal glands and brain produce the stress hormones cortisol and vasopressin; your damaged muscles churn out proteins called cytokines, which trigger your liver to start producing C-reactive protein. The result is what Dr. Siegel calls "an inflammatory storm" throughout your body, one that sets the stage for some potentially adverse consequences.

Early on, marathon researchers weren't sure if the heart was among the muscles being stressed, but in recent years they've confirmed that it most definitely is. In a 2001 study published in the *American*

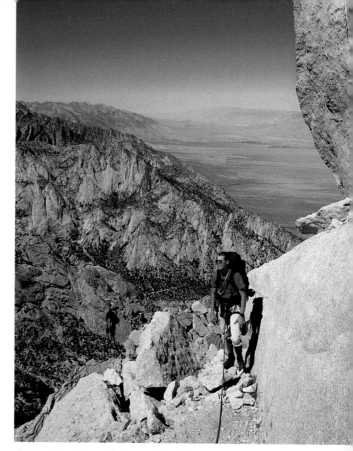

TRY SOMETHING ELSE
Five fitness feats to brag about, with none of the pounding of a marathon.

CLIMB A MOUNTAIN. You can hike California's Mt. Whitney (14,494 feet, a 22-mile round trip) in a day—if you're fit and can handle a predawn start. (760-873-2485)

COMPLETE A TRIATHLON. Try an Olympic-length race (1.5-K swim, 40-K ride, and 10-K run) or sprint (typically about a 750-meter swim, 20-K bike, and 5-K run). Find one in your state at trifind.com.

SKI THE BIRKIE. The American Birkebeiner is the nation's foremost cross-country skiing event. It's a 3-day festival of races held in Hayward, Wisconsin. (birkie.com)

BIKE A HALF-CENTURY. That's 50 miles (get it?). Racing or joining a group ride is terrific low-impact exercise. Races and fun rides of all lengths are sorted by state at bicycling.com. (Click on "events.")

ROW NOWHERE FAST. The C.R.A.S.H.-B. Sprints World Indoor Rowing Championships are "races" on rowing machines (crash-b.org). Find more events at concept2.com.

FOUR SECRETS TO RUNNING FOREVER

A few tours back, Bruce Springsteen performed "Born to Run" at a dirge pace, so it limped along like a death march. It could have been an anthem for many runners who'd racked up long miles, achy knees, touchy tendons, and balky backs.

But it doesn't have to be that way, says Thomas Best, MD, PhD, co–medical director of the Ohio State University sports medicine center. Here's how to overcome skeletal and muscular imbalances and banish injuries for good.

1 **Build a solid foundation.** Strong feet and solid stability muscles in your ankles will keep you moving for the long run. The following two exercises can help stop imbalance injuries before they start, says Michael Smith, a track coach at Kansas State University.

Toe curls: Use your toes to pick up a golf ball or a towel for 3 sets of 10 reps, or until you feel the burn in your arches. Do it in your office or while watching the tube.

Alphabet balance: Stand barefoot on one foot with the other foot poised 12 inches above the ground. With the raised foot, write the alphabet in large letters.

2 **Gain speed by walking.** Add a walking break of 30 seconds to 2 minutes after each mile you run. This prevents muscle fatigue, says Jeff Galloway, an Olympian and the author of *Running Until You're 100*.

"I typically see my runners drop at least 13 minutes from their marathon times because fatigue is so drastically reduced," says Galloway.

3 **Follow the meatheads.** Running breaks down muscles, says William Kraemer, PhD, a professor of kinesiology at the University of Connecticut's human-performance lab.

"Weight lifting spurs muscle and tendon regrowth, giving you stronger joints and muscles." As little as 60 to 90 minutes of strength training each week, over two or three sessions, can offset the destructiveness of running, adds Dr. Kraemer.

4 **Know thyself.** Gait analysis is the best way to eliminate a hurtful hitch in your running form, says Roy Lidtke, DPM, a Des Moines University clinical associate professor of podiatry. Contact a local university's sports medicine department—they may be able to slip you in. Or go to motion-labs.com/index3/4links.html to find a lab in your area.

Journal of Cardiology, Dr. Siegel and his colleagues analyzed the blood of marathoners less than 24 hours after a race and found high levels of inflammatory and coagulation markers that are also associated with heart attacks.

Then came the 2006 *Circulation* study, led by Dr. Wood, which upped the ante. Using ultrasounds and blood tests of 60 marathon finishers, the researchers found that after the race, some runners' hearts experienced difficulty refilling chambers. The researchers also noticed abnormalities in how blood was pumped from the right side of the heart to the lungs.

A SPOT OF GOOD NEWS

Before you go into full freak-out mode, there is some good news. First, proper training seems to go a long way toward protecting you from heart injury during the race. The *Circulation* study found that people who'd averaged at least 45 miles a week in training were significantly less likely to suffer heart damage than those who ran 35 miles a week or less.

That makes sense to Dr. Siegel, who notes that training is an injury-and-repair process: Your body suffers damage when you exert yourself during training but then repairs itself and becomes stronger. So runners who log lots of training miles are able to withstand more punishment during the race than those who train less.

More good news is that even among marathoners who were undertrained, heart damage didn't appear to be permanent. Within a month, all the runners in the study showed relatively normal cardiac function.

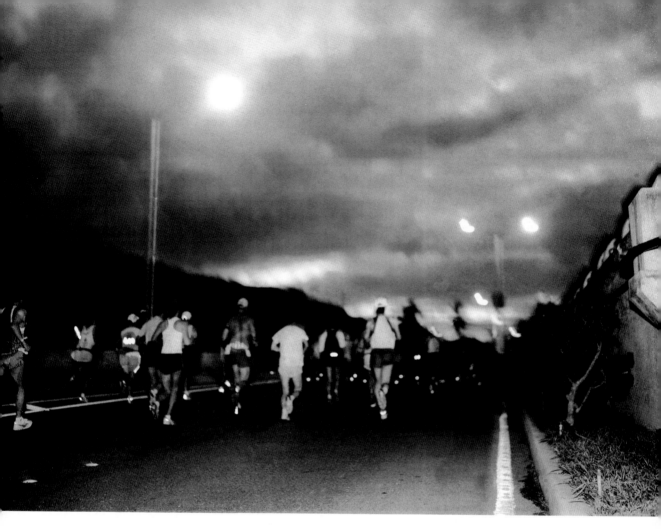

"There is no data to suggest that any long-term aftereffects were caused by the changes," says Dr. Wood.

But blocking out that dose of sunshine is still a very dark cloud: During the race and for several hours afterward, the systemic inflammation significantly increases your risk of a cardiac event, particularly if you're middle-aged and have some silent coronary-artery disease. (Men in their 40s and 50s form the biggest cluster of marathon fatalities.)

Two things happen: First, inflammatory mediators released during muscle injury may make the thin, fibrous plaque that lines your artery walls more likely to rupture; second, this inflammation can lead to an imbalance of coagulation factors, mak-

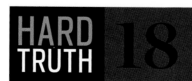

HARD TRUTH 18 PERCENTAGE OF RUNNERS WHO SUSTAIN LOWER-BODY INJURIES DURING A MARATHON, ACCORDING TO THE *SCANDINAVIAN JOURNAL OF MEDICINE & SCIENCE IN SPORTS*

The paradox is that marathoners' training puts them at an OVERALL LOWER RISK of heart trouble.

ing blood more susceptible to clots. The result: a heart attack.

The paradox is that marathoners' training puts them at an overall lower risk of heart trouble. But when you start doing the event for which you've been training, your relative risk increases. To oversimplify: At the starting line, you're Lance Armstrong; at the finish line, you're Louie Anderson.

"Marathon running may be regarded as a dose of exercise that pushes you past the zone of cardioprotective benefit into one of enhanced risk," says Dr. Siegel, who stopped running marathons more than a decade ago, partly because of the risks involved. If you want to be smart, he suggests, do all the training for a marathon . . . and then watch the race from the sidelines.

But, well, what fun is that, right?

The reason most people suffer through all those dreary training miles is for the thrill of the race. Take away that carrot, and many marathoners would be on the couch munching Pringles and watching *American*

EVOLUTION OF THE RUNNING MAN

The human animal realized his destiny when he set off in hot pursuit of dinner, a mate, or dinner for his mate. The result: a host of specific adaptations that make us fit for the long run.

BRAIN
Adaptation: Hippocampus stimulation
Result: Running activates 33 genes in the hippocampus, the brain's center for mood, memory, and learning. Exercise also stimulates the formation of new brain cells and blood vessels.

HEAD
Adaptation: Flat face
Result: Humans lack the protruding snout of apes, so our heads are more balanced over our necks when we're in motion.

NECK
Adaptation: Nuchal ligament
Result: Running down the back of your neck from the base of your skull, this ligament helps stabilize your head and prevents it from pitching back and forth. This feature is found in other mammals built for running, such as dogs. Pigs don't have one, which may explain the development of the ham sandwich.

RESPIRATORY SYSTEM
Adaptation: Mouth breathing
Result: Unlike the panting of many quadrupeds, human mouth breathing permits more airflow with less muscular effort. It also helps expel heat.

SHOULDERS
Adaptation: Low, broad shoulders
Result: Our wide shoulder span increases arm swinging, which counteracts the torque generated by our legs. Otherwise our bodies would rotate and we'd be thrown off balance. Your head moves separately from your shoulders and trunk, so you can look forward as you run.

RUMP
Adaptation: Larger gluteus maximus muscle
Result: Extends the thigh to propel the body, and keeps you from pitching over with forward momentum.

CONQUER THE TRIATHLON

Merely finish? Ha! Use these strategies to crush the three-legged beast.

Completing a triathlon—even a sprint triathlon—isn't as simple as having the endurance to cross the finish line, says Andy Potts, the 2007 USA Triathlon male triathlete of the year. "You need a strategy for each leg so you can set yourself up to race to your strengths."

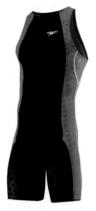

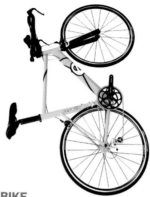

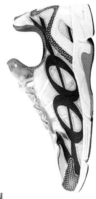

SWIM

• If you're not a strong swimmer, hang back. In a French study, athletes who drafted during the swim decreased their energy expenditure but not their speed, so in the next leg they could bicycle about 5 percent more efficiently.

• Building gradually to race pace in the first 3 to 5 minutes can help you finish faster, says Potts. A 2005 study found that athletes who swam at 80 to 85 percent of their maximum speed improved their overall sprint triathlon times by 1 minute, 45 seconds.

• French researchers found that wetsuits helped reduce swimmers' lactate levels by 47 percent and boost their cycling efficiency by 12 percent. In warm weather, wear the Speedo Fastskin FSII Unitard throughout the event. ($270, speedousa.com)

BIKE

• Quality gear, like the full-aeroframe Cervélo tri bike pictured here, can shave seconds off your time. "But similar gains can be made by simply rehearsing the transitions at full speed as part of your training schedule," Potts says. ($1,650, cervelo.com)

• Carbohydrate depletion kills endurance, but so does dehydration: A 1 to 2 percent loss of body mass can result in a 44 percent drop in performance, say South African researchers. On your bike, drink 3.5 ounces of a sodium-spiked sports drink every 10 minutes.

• In the final 2 or 3 miles, pick an easier gear and crank out a higher cadence (100-plus rpm). A University of Colorado at Boulder study found that a higher biking rpm helped increase stride frequency during the run.

RUN

• Tri-specific shoes like the Zoot Sports Ultra TT drain excess wetness and stay lightweight and have laces that tighten with a tug.($130, zootsports.com) Or equip your sneakers with Yankz! ($8, yankz.com), a lacing system that shaves seconds at the changeover.

• Test your pace in the first 2 or 3 minutes of the run. "Close your mouth and breathe through your nose," says Potts. "If you can't close it, you're going too hard and you need to pull back a little. If you don't, you'll wreck your form and spoil your finish time."

• Good form is crucial for a strong finish, but hard to maintain. "If you're hunched over, you're just plodding yourself along," says Potts. "Stand tall and your hips will propel you, allowing you to run faster and more efficiently."

FORETELL YOUR FINISH

Six weeks before your sprint tri, time a swim. Then 2 weeks before, time a run. Use this equation, developed at West Point, to estimate your finish time.

$$6.61 \times \left(\substack{\text{150-yard} \\ \text{swim in} \\ \text{seconds}} + \substack{\text{2-mile} \\ \text{run in} \\ \text{seconds}} \right) - 695.41 = \substack{\text{Total sprint} \\ \text{time in} \\ \text{seconds per} \\ \text{mile.}}$$

Gladiators. Eliminate the risk, and you inadvertently eliminate an incentive.

McGrath's motivations: He likes to run. He knew he'd be in kick-ass shape. And his buddy McDade was doing it, so he felt some camaraderie and competition. As it turns out, he's pretty typical. A study of motivation in the *Journal of Sport Behavior* found that most runners have multiple reasons for participating in the sport, from

We seem to have an innate need to do things SIMPLY FOR THE SAKE of doing them or to see if we can do them.

improving their health to socializing to competing.

"People might have started with one motivation—say, becoming fit—but when they got into it, they found all these other side benefits," says one of the study authors, Ohio University psychologist Benjamin Ogles, PhD.

While women were most likely to cite weight control and socializing as reasons for running marathons, men were more into achievement and competition, either with themselves or others. It is, we suppose, easy to mock this as typical lunkheaded guy behavior: Me tough guy. Me run marathon. But Dr. Ogles says there

are definite mental health benefits to setting and meeting a challenge.

"Running a marathon brings a great sense of accomplishment," he says. Citing research that dates back decades, he adds, "This need for us to have success at things can be a strong motivational force. Even young kids can be motivated by successful mastery of basic skills—[researchers] talk about the gratification that comes from learning how to walk." Mastering a skill is crucial, he says: "When there are problems with self-mastery, you end up with problems like depression."

To put it another way, we seem to have an innate need to do things simply for the sake of doing them or to see if we can do them. What makes us and half a million other people want to run a marathon, even though we know it might not be good for us? Maybe it's the same things that drive people to climb Mount Everest or drove Leo Tolstoy to write a 1,400-page epic about Russia in the time of the Napoleonic wars.

Because it's there. Because we can.

Which brings us back to the dilemma at hand: Is the satisfaction that comes from running a marathon worth the risk?

Dr. Siegel hopes that studies may someday show that "drugs that undermine inflammation, such as aspirin or statins, may protect runners during the transition from low to high risk during and after races." For now, if you're planning to run a marathon, you should have some respect for what you're getting yourself into. That means training properly—a minimum of 45 miles a week. It also means understanding that there's some risk involved.

RUN AWAY FROM PAIN
Five fast-acting tips to cure potential aches before they hobble you

There's a saying in the running world: Listen to the whispers and they won't turn into screams. Unfortunately, most men live up to another adage: They just don't listen.

"Seven out of 10 runners suffer injuries serious enough to keep them off the road each year," says Sam Murphy, coauthor of *Running Well*. What's worse, more than half of those knocks—be they a twinge in the calf or a "Hey-o!" in the groin—are entirely preventable, even if you're speeding past 40 years old. "They can creep up gradually from overtraining or suddenly from such easily avoidable missteps as buying eye-catching but ill-fitting shoes," says Murphy.

Follow these steps to prevent niggling pains from occurring in the first place, and run pain free forever.

1 FIND YOUR FIT.
Determine your foot type by wetting the soles of your feet and stepping on and off a flattened paper bag. See your entire arch? You overpronate (i.e., your feet roll inward excessively), so you require a motion-control shoe, such as Asics' GEL-Evolution 4 ($110, asics.com). See a thin line on the outside of your arch? You supinate (i.e., your feet don't roll inward enough) so you need a neutral cushioned shoe, such as the Adidas Response Cushion 17 ($80, shopadidas.com). See half an arch? You're a neutral pronator (the biomechanical ideal). Wear whatever you like.

2 WARM UP.
"At 40, the body doesn't circulate blood as efficiently as it did at 20," says Murphy. "A proper warmup will raise your body temp and juice your circulatory system, making your muscles and connective tissues more supple and less likely to tear." Skip your stretch-and-hold routine and do an active warmup with shoulder rolls, side bends, knee raises, ankle circles, tiptoes, and five minutes of light jogging (or sprints if you're preparing for intervals). When you hit the shower, alternate between 30 seconds of hot water and 30 seconds of cold for 3 minutes.

3 BEAT BACK PAIN.
"A common cause of lower-back pain is tight hip flexors," says Murphy. Keep yours loose by sitting on the edge of a bench and pulling one knee to your chest as you roll onto your back. You'll feel the stretch in the hip of your trailing leg. Let that leg hang off the bench without arching your back. Hold for 30 seconds, switch legs, and repeat.

4 BUILD YOUR ABS.
A strong core greatly reduces your risk of leg injuries, including iliotibial band syndrome, which is one of the most common causes of knee pain in runners. Why? If your core is strong, your legs won't have to overcompensate to keep your body stable. In addition to bicycle crunches and planks, do the following exercise to strengthen your pelvic floor. Get on your hands and knees and squeeze the muscles you'd normally use to stop a stream of urine. Next, draw in your lower stomach and hold for 10 seconds. Relax and repeat.

5 VARY YOUR TERRAIN.
Running on pavement exerts a force up to 10 times your body weight on your joints; dirt trails are gentler but increase the risk of sprains; tracks can inflame your Achilles tendon; and treadmills can shorten your stride.

"By varying your terrain, you'll reduce your risk of injury and prevent your muscles from adapting to any one surface," says Murphy. The less they adapt, the more they'll develop, and the faster you'll get.

"People choose all the time to do risky things, like mountain climbing and scuba diving," says Dr. Siegel. "Thrill seekers are well advised to understand the risks involved to limit any adverse consequences. Marathon running is potentially dangerous for susceptible individuals. Phidippides is still out there."

Well, actually, he isn't. He's dead. And that's a message to remember as you lace up your running shoes and start training for an event that, for some reason, you just can't seem to resist. ∎

Sink Every Free Throw

WRITER CHRISTOPHER McDOUGALL TELLS HOW TO TAP INTO YOUR PRIMAL MARKSMAN

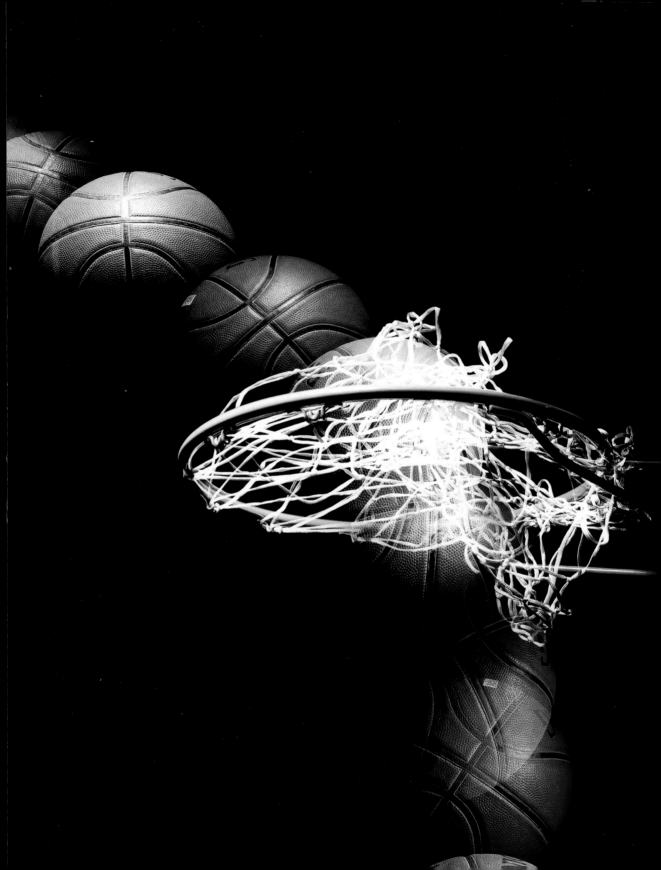

Joe Darrah is holding four tomahawks

in one hand and a king of spades in the other. He pins the playing card to the target—a thick log slice bolted to an old table—and walks back to where I'm standing, 20 feet away.

"What do you need for good aim?" he asks.

"Vision, repetition, concentration," I say. I've done my homework.

He hands me one of the tomahawks. "Close your eyes," he says. "Now don't think. Just throw."

I squeeze my eyes shut, mentally apologize to whatever cat is about to die or whoever owns the window I'm about to shatter, and let fly.

Thwock!

I open my eyes and see the tomahawk sticking a few inches from the card.

"What were those three again?" Darrah asks.

"Vision, repetition, and . . .

Thwock! Thwock! Thwock!

Without looking, Darrah whips around and buries the other three tomahawks into three different targets. The last is dead in the middle of the card.

"So," he says, "explain what we just did."

I can't. I'm not sure if he can, either.

When it comes to instant gratification, nothing beats a bull's-eye. The whole process of taking aim and letting fly can last for as little as an eighth of a second—roughly the amount of time a sensory impulse takes to travel to your brain and cause your muscles to react—and the result of nailing your target is a weird, almost embarrassing sense of personal awesomeness. No matter how lousy your day is going, all you need to do is swish a McWrapper in the trash can, and for a few seconds you're a god. Darrah still enjoys that glow, and he's been sinking sharp steel into hardwood for 45 years.

"You can tell the throw is good as soon as the tomahawk leaves your hand," he says. "At that moment, it's like the whole universe came into alignment just for you."

William H. Calvin, PhD, a professor of neuroscience at the University of Washington and a specialist in the evolution of the human brain, explains that this surge of joy has been programmed into our DNA for 2 million years, ever since primitive man relied on marksmanship for life's two greatest prizes: babes and breakfast. Judging from the behavior of our close genetic cousins, chimpanzees, hunting was how we acquired mates as well as meat: When a male chimp kills a tasty rodent, he's often surrounded by flirting females offering to trade sex for a snack. It's only after the monkey business that he surrenders a little meat.

But unlike chimps, humans are not equipped with lethal jaws and lightning dexterity. Our Stone Age ancestors had only one natural weapon: the ability to turn something lying on the ground into something flying through the air. We had

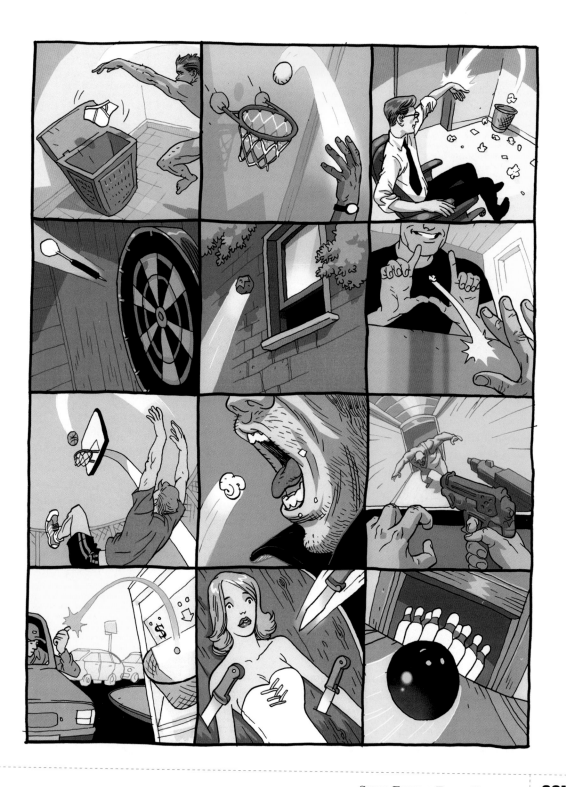

HOW YOUR BRAIN SINKS A BASKET
Here's the mental magic that happens every time you drain one.

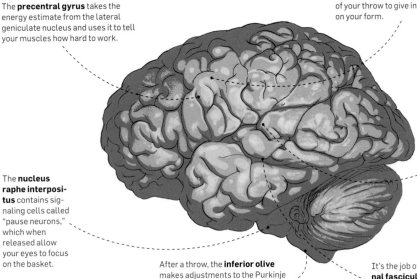

The **precentral gyrus** takes the energy estimate from the lateral geniculate nucleus and uses it to tell your muscles how hard to work.

Using input from receptors in your skin and joints, the **postcentral gyrus** evaluates the release portion of your throw to give instant feedback on your form.

Your brain's **lateral geniculate nucleus** calculates the distance between you and the basket to gauge how much energy you'll need to make the shot.

The **nucleus raphe interpositus** contains signaling cells called "pause neurons," which when released allow your eyes to focus on the basket.

After a throw, the **inferior olive** makes adjustments to the Purkinje cells (neurons that help govern the preciseness of actions), so you improve with practice.

It's the job of the **medial longitudinal fasciculus** to monitor and adjust your visual crosshairs so you remain locked onto the basket even if your head moves.

to be amazing with rocks because we're awful with everything else. Strip us naked, and we humans are the wimps of the wild kingdom. We have no offense or defense, no fangs or claws, no speed, and—compared with the competition—hardly any muscle. All we have on our side is a flair for geometry. We can estimate distance, trajectory, and speed in the blink of an eye and translate that data into precise commands that are then fired off to every muscle from our toes to our fingertips.

"Throwing with accuracy makes demands on the brain that no other activity makes," says Dr. Calvin. "Humans seem to be the only creatures in existence with this capability."

And that's just aiming at stationary targets; think about the complexity of aiming

at and hitting a fleeing animal. Stone Age rabbits weren't just standing around waiting patiently to sacrifice themselves in the name of human evolution. They were darting off in mad bursts of speed, which meant a hunter had to mentally process three different movement sequences—his, the prey's, and the weapon's—to calculate the exact point where rock would meet rabbit.

"That kind of sequential thought requires intellect of a higher order," says Dr. Calvin. Specifically, he's talking about imagination—the ability to project into the future, visualize possibilities, and think in the abstract. That's why Dr. Calvin believes language, literature, medicine, and even love are all rooted in our ancient ability to hit a hare at 20 paces.

"Throwing is about finding order in chaos,"

he says. "The more you're able to think in sequence, the more ideas you're able to string together. You can add more words to your vocabulary, you can combine unrelated concepts, you can plan for the future, and you can keep track of social relationships."

But just because you're hardwired with this circuitry doesn't mean you're maximizing its potential. So the lingering question, the one that put a tomahawk in my hand, is this: If we go back to the fundamentals and master the mysteries of aim, can that help us master everything else?

Dr. Calvin thinks it can. "Evolution doesn't give many chances for extra credit, but throwing is one of them," he says. "Sequential movement, and all that comes with it, is one of the few instincts you can improve through practice."

Darrah was in kindergarten when his dad, a U.S. Army Airborne Ranger, put a Special Forces trench knife in his hand and taught him the rules of chicken. By the time Darrah was a teenager, he was flinging razor-sharp bowie knives around girls in a traveling circus. Now, past age 50, he's a seven-time world champion with both knives and tomahawks, and he's also deadly accurate with the blowgun, bull-whip, and atlatl, an ancient spear-throwing weapon.

Darrah's neighbors in the suburban village of Berwyn, Pennsylvania, are so used to lethal weapons whistling across his front yard that no one pays any attention when we begin to practice with a pile of tomahawks. One of our targets is a custom-built board with five log slices bolted to it in an X configuration, and each slice has a playing card pinned in the middle. The other target is a holdover from a TV show Darrah filmed for ESPN: It's an old door with an eye-level rectangle of bullet-proof glass, so you can acquire a feel for throwing a weapon around a human target by seeing a person's face through the glass.

"Don't think about your arm. When it's cocked behind your head, you can't see it anyway," Darrah says as he begins feeding me 'hawks. "You're just guiding the 'hawk

When it comes to INSTANT GRATIFICATION, nothing beats a bull's-eye.

along its way into the target." Each tomahawk has a 12-inch hardwood handle and a cold-forged steel head sharp enough for a shave. He's handing them to me so quickly I barely have time to windmill one before two more are ready. I'm way too rushed to "think" them into the target, but at least I'm managing to hit logs and not the neighbors.

Then something strange happens. Darrah hands me a 'hawk and then stands back and watches. Now that I finally have a chance to really aim, I take my time and run through all of his pointers. Left foot forward; wide stance; easy overhand motion; tap the car keys in my right pocket on the follow-through to make sure I'm staying straight; and . . .

Clank!

The tomahawk shanks off the edge

"I never think about whether the shot is going in—that's showmanship. I only FOCUS ON THE JOB at hand—that's craftsmanship."

of the target, dropping into the dirt. Joe hands me another. Left foot forward . . .

Clank!

"What am I doing wrong?" I ask.

Darrah smiles. "Here comes the Zen stuff. You're trying to control your throw, and you can't." Don't aim, he says; just look. Don't rehearse; just throw. Don't analyze; just feel. "You have to enter yourself and let the rhythm come. Once you do that," Darrah says, "you can do all kinds of crazy things."

Whatever. They're his tomahawk handles I'm splintering. I grab a handful of 'hawks and start windmilling one after the other, with no aiming, rehearsing, or analyzing.

Three throws later, I split the king of clubs down the middle.

"You want proof this can change your life?" asks Tom Amberry, DPM. "Look at me."

Back in 1992, Dr. Amberry was coming to the end of an extremely successful surgical career. He was known among podiatrists for his "time-and-motion technique," which greatly reduced the duration of certain foot surgeries as well as the number of post-op complications. His innovation was in reversing the usual relationship between speed and precision: Instead of slowing down in an effort to be more careful, he accelerated. The upside to speed, he discovered, was that his body picked up on tiny deviations even before they registered in his brain. That way, Dr. Amberry could tell from any little hitch in his flow if his scalpel was leading him into trouble, much the way Darrah knew on release if his throw was good and could make instantaneous corrections to his next attempt a split second later.

But before Dr. Amberry could speed up his surgeries, he realized that he had to formulate an efficient sequence of actions—in other words, the same kind of sequential thinking that helped our Stone Age ancestors kill prey with surgical precision.

"If I picked up an instrument, I planned my steps so I used it for everything necessary before I put it down," he says. Then after refining those steps into one seamless motion—from initial incisions to closing sutures—he was able to accelerate his actions so that they became automatic and practically self-correcting. In essence, he had turned a skill into a reflex.

Dr. Amberry never heard of Joe Darrah or Professor Calvin, but he became the human link connecting their theories: (1) that great aim is a muscular reflex ("Don't think; just throw") and (2) that the sequential thinking necessary to develop this reflex is the foundation of some remarkable human achievements. Except Dr. Amberry went about it backward: He applied his aim reflex to innovative surgery first, and only later tried it out on raw marksmanship.

When Dr. Amberry retired at age 69, he started playing hoops to stay in shape. And what did he discover? That even though he hadn't touched a basketball in 50 years, he'd been practicing free throws the whole time in the operating room. "It was time and motion all over again," he says. "Foul shots and surgery required the same approach."

After studying the sequence of actions necessary to sink a free throw and then practicing for an entire year, Dr. Amberry sped up his shooting and wowed everyone: He was able to drain his shots for 12 hours straight, entering the *Guinness Book of World Records* for making 2,750 consecutive free throws. Soon, he was humiliating NBA stars in free-throw contests. (Sorry, Kobe, 84 percent doesn't cut it.) Most of the awed spectators focused on Dr. Amberry's form: three dribbles, thumbs in the seams, elbows tight, deep knee bend, no more than a quick glance at the hoop. What they missed was the real show going on inside his head.

"It's craftsmanship over showmanship," Dr. Amberry tells me. He's been jovial and jokey until this point, the master storyteller letting the war stories roll, but as we come to the end of our phone conversation, his tone becomes quiet and firm. "It sounds simple, but it's the key to everything you'll ever do. I never think about whether the shot is going in—that's showmanship. I only focus on the job at hand—that's craftsmanship."

Funny thing, but while Dr. Amberry couldn't convince many NBA players to take his advice ("They'd give me 5 minutes"), hundreds of regular guys listened. That bugged him for a while, until it

HOW TO ACE ANYTHING
From sports to speeches, hit the bull's-eye every time.

STEP 1: Do your homework. For sports, that means a ton of practice; for something more mental, such as a speech, it means research. Either way, the goal is to know your moves or your topic inside and out. "Your mind loves to compartmentalize," says Herbert Benson, MD, a mind/body researcher at Harvard medical school, "so once it knows that you're equipped for the task, it will shift from 'Needs Urgent Attention' to 'Automatic.'"

STEP 2: Turn over the controls. You can't shift to autopilot if your hands are still on the stick. Distract your conscious mind by creating a silent mantra or some ritualized action. For example, bounce the basketball exactly three times before every foul shot. Still can't let go? Focus on a sensation, such as the taste of your last sip of coffee or the sound of the air conditioner.

STEP 3: Stay detached. Once you sense that your performance is peaking, resist the temptation to gloat—even mentally. "When you know you're in the zone, you're out of it," says Dr. Benson. "Back off and ignore the highs and lows of the moment. You're just doing your thing."

STEP 4: Believe in yourself. After the applause has died down, watch what you tell yourself about the feat. Specifically, do not think, I was lucky or I played over my head. Instead, prepare yourself for next time by reinforcing the belief that you can hit your peak whenever you want, which, of course, you can.

dawned on him why amateurs were more interested in perfecting their shots than the pros: They were looking for something more important than a bump in their summer-league roundball stats.

"I've taught guys, and they come back to me later and tell me it's like a mantra," Dr. Amberry says. "They slow down, breathe, look for rhythms in their everyday lives. One man, a professor, tells me he has a lot more confidence in front of his class." ∎

Burn Fat, Not Fuel

CRANKING OUT YOUR COMMUTE IS THE EASIEST WAY TO DODGE PRICE GOUGING AT THE PUMP. BONUS: YOU'LL SHED CALORIES AND SAVE THE EARTH, TOO

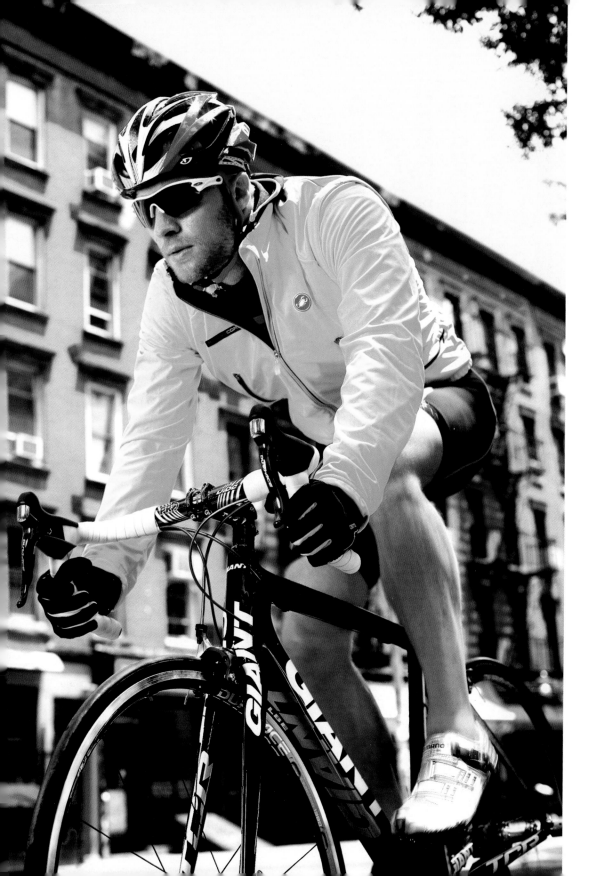

Biking to work

might seem like a lot of trouble, but when's the last time you enjoyed a traffic jam?

"We're so used to the hassles of car commuting that they've become ingrained," says Bill Nesper, who heads the Bicycle Friendly Community program at the D.C.–based League of American Bicyclists. "Once you solve the logistical obstacles of bike commuting—where to shower, where to stow your bike, how to avoid traffic—it becomes routine. You'll end up healthier and happier at your desk because of your commute." Try saying that about a car trip.

We've laid out the ultimate rides and accessories you'll need to smooth over any kind of bike commute. You don't have to do it 5 days a week—some people ride in on Monday, stash the bike, and ride back on Friday. Whatever your schedule, use the weekend, when the streets are less crowded, to plot your best route and find a safe place to lock up your bike.

YOUR COMMUTE:
20+ MILES

The terrain: Paved roads

The bike: The long-distance cruise missile: 1 Giant TCR Advanced SL Team (see photo, page 337)

If you're willing to sit in the saddle for 2 hours or longer every day, you deserve a bike that's fast, yet supple. This pro-level frame is made from a recently declassified, military-grade carbon composite that transfers more power from your pedal stroke while leaving some vertical compliance to suck up road chatter. The oversized tubes add stiffness around the head tube for precise steering. The TCR Advanced SL doesn't come cheap, but thanks to the price of gas, you should be able to justify it after a few years of commuting. $8,000—or 131 tanks (15 gallons each) of 87-octane gas, giant-bicycles.com

NUMBERS BREAKDOWN

Calories burned (*1 day*):
1,804
For an athletically built 5'10", 180 lb man biking at 16 to 19 mph

Gas money saved
(*1 month*):
$163.20
Based on a 40-mile (round-trip) commute 5 days a week, at an average 20 mpg, paying the average U.S. gas price as of June 24, 2008

CO_2 savings (*1 year*):
10,296 pounds
Because your car isn't belching exhaust

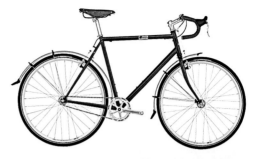

YOUR COMMUTE:
15 MILES

The terrain: Roads and trails

The bike: The cross-country cruiser:

Raleigh One Way

Cross-country bikes blend the aggressive geometry of road bikes with the wider forks and burly tires of mountain bikes. This steel bike has fenders to shun mud, a fixed-gear drivetrain (see the messenger machine, page 340), and cantilever brakes. A vintage-inspired Brooks saddle adds old-school panache. $710 (or 11.4 tanks of gas), raleighusa.com

NUMBERS BREAKDOWN

Calories burned (*1 day*):
1,476

Average speed:
14 to 16 mph
(more calories with hill intervals)

Gas money saved
(*1 month*):
$122.40

CO_2 savings (*1 year*):
7,722 pounds

ESSENTIAL ACCESSORIES:

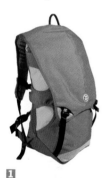

The Castelli Insolito Radiation Jacket ($450, castelli-us.com) has a heat-reflecting inner vest and removable arms, while the lenses of Oakley Polarized Radar Pitch sunglasses ($255, oakley.com) repel sweat. **1** Fill the capacious Famous Wine Bar backpack ($150, crumplerbags.com) with your work clothes, like a wrinkle-free shirt ($80, brooksbrothers.com) and pants ($70, dockers.com). Keep it all in place with a packing folder from Eagle Creek ($25, eaglecreek.com). Stash a week's worth of shirts in a backpack each Monday, and keep a couple of blazers at the office, Nesper suggests.

ESSENTIAL ACCESSORIES:

1 A rear-mounted Brooks Holdall case (Glenbrook model, $135, brooksengland.com) matches the vintage leather on the bike. **2** The Garmin Edge 705 ($500, garmin.com) helps you analyze shortcuts using GPS. **3** Shimano SH-MT21 bike shoes ($60, bike.shimano.com) clip into SPD pedals but won't click-clack on the pavement or at work. **4** The NiteRider MiNewt.X2 headlight ($210, niterider.com) gets you home safely.

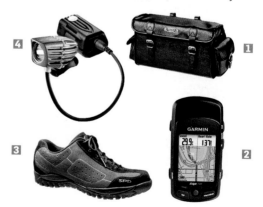

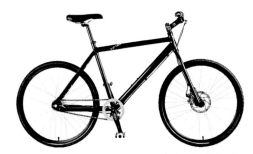

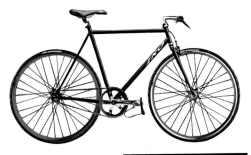

YOUR COMMUTE:
10 MILES

The terrain: Paved roads

The bike: The grab-and-go city commuter: Swobo Otis

Smart engineers simplify complex things. This no-nonsense city ride has a rear hub that houses an internal gearing system (saving your pants cuffs from greasy chain rings and derailleurs) and a coaster brake (which leaves your right hand free for signaling). Plus, the sealed system is less likely to suffer mechanical breakdowns or rust. $720 (or 12 tanks of gas), swobo.com

ESSENTIAL ACCESSORIES:

Door slams, pedestrian jams, and swerving cabs are obstacles for every city biker. **1** Push through herds of clueless tourists with a simple brass bike bell ($8, rivbike.com). **2** Guard your dome with a rakish Lazer Urbanize Nlight helmet ($100, lazer.be), which features slots in the front and back for LED lighting systems. **3** Watch your back with a Topeak Bar'n Mirror ($35, rei.com).

NUMBERS BREAKDOWN

Calories burned (*1 day*):
864

Average speed:
12 to 14 mph

Gas money saved (*1 month*):
$81.60

CO_2 savings (*1 year*):
5,148 pounds

YOUR COMMUTE:
5 MILES

The terrain: The mean streets

The bike: The bare-bones messenger machine: IRO Custom Bike

Fixed-gear bicycles were adopted by messengers, many of whom run without brakes, using backward pressure on the cranks to slow down. "Fixies" have fewer moving parts to break down (or steal). This one has a steel Angus frame, a single front brake, anodized rims, and bullhorn handlebars. Build your own at the IRO Web site. $840 as shown (or 14 tanks of gas), irocycle.com

ESSENTIAL ACCESSORIES:

1 A frame tube pad ($30 and up, biciconcepts.com) cushions your shoulder as you lug your bike up stairs. **2** A pedal kit ($39, mountainracingproducts.com) means power without clipping in. **3** A leather trouser strap ($40, brookssaddles.com) protects your pants leg. **4** Lock up with a Kryptonite Evolution Mini lock and KryptoFlex 1004 Looped Cable ($55, kryptonitelock.com) and you'll be insured against theft up to $2,000.

NUMBERS BREAKDOWN

Calories burned (*1 day*):
410

Average speed:
10 to 12 mph

Gas money saved (*1 month*):
$40.80

CO_2 savings (*1 year*):
2,574 pounds

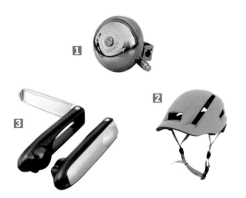

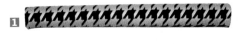

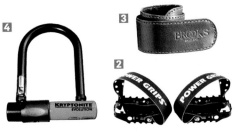

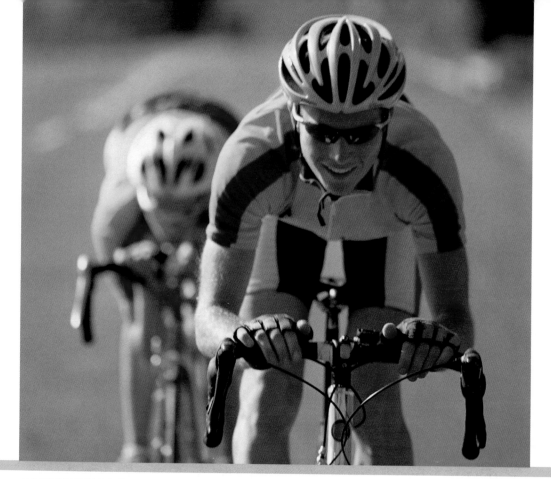

ANATOMY OF THE PERFECT PEDAL STROKE

Pros spend years perfecting their pedal strokes, says Chris Carmichael, the owner of Carmichael Training Systems and Lance Armstrong's longtime coach. "The vast majority of power comes from the downstroke, but with training you can increase power by programming muscles to engage earlier and finish later in the stroke." Carmichael tells his athletes to visualize each stroke in four parts.

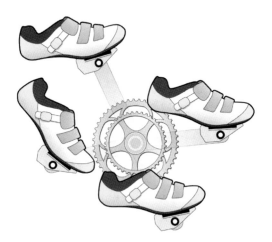

PUSH FORWARD. As you near the top of the stroke (at 11 o'clock), kick your foot forward to initiate an early push for the next revolution.

PUSH DOWN. Keep this part of the stroke simple: Push the pedal down. Most riders naturally keep their heel just above their toes. Adding ankle flexion and extension actually wastes energy and can lead to injuries.

LIGHTEN UP. Pulling your foot up is pointless; the downstroke of the other pedal is stronger. Just unweight your foot between the 8 o'clock and 10 o'clock points so it's not holding the other foot back.

PULL BACK. Once your foot approaches the bottom of the stroke, at about the 5 o'clock position, pull your foot backward with your hamstring, as if you're scraping mud off the bottom of your shoe.

Injury-Proof Your Workout

AVOID SIX SPORTS-RELATED SCRAPES AND SORES WITH THESE SIMPLE TWEAKS

Fitness should boost your body, not break it down. "Most nagging injuries are caused by pressure, friction, or tension," says Sean Collins, PT, ScD, physical therapy chairman at the University of Massachusetts at Lowell. Adjust your approach with this guide.

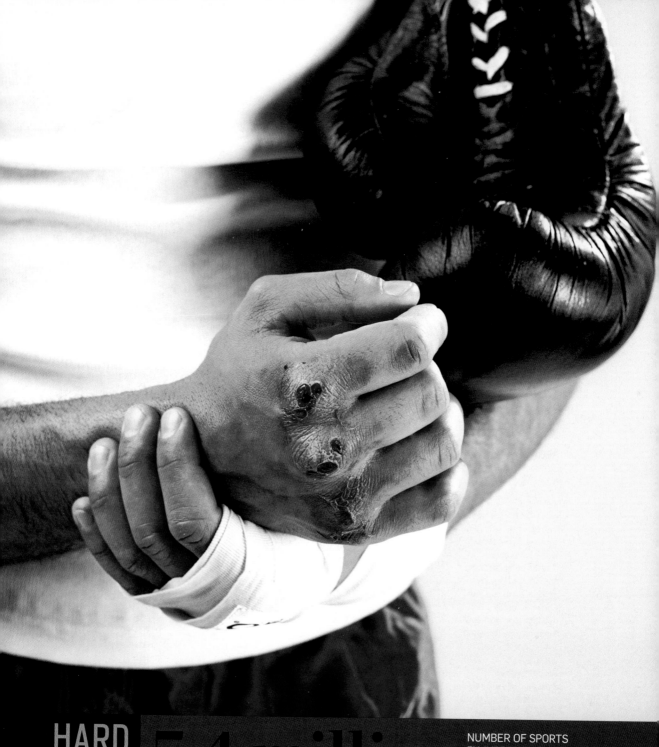

PROBLEM:
BURNING EYES FROM SWIMMING

Cause: Even if you suction-pumped your goggles to your eye sockets, chlorine-infused water could still infiltrate during your flip turns.
Fix: Before kicking off the wall, squeeze your outstretched arms against your ears and lead with the top of your head. "This creates a hole in the water that your body can flow through," says Richard Quick, head swimming and diving coach at Auburn University. You'll minimize drag and keep your goggles glued down.

PROBLEM:
DISCOMFORT FROM THE SQUAT BAR

Cause: The metal bar, combined with the pressure of the weight and insufficient cushioning, can rub the bony vertebra at the base of your neck.
Fix: Position the bar a half inch to an inch lower than you usually would, to take pressure off the bony protrusion, says Joseph M. Warpeha, director of the exercise physiology laboratories at the College of St. Scholastica. If the bar has no padding, wrap a gym towel around it or swap in a pair of dumbbells.

PROBLEM:
TENDER SKIN AFTER PULLUPS

Cause: The portion of thicker flesh just below your fingers jams beneath the pressure of the bar, pinching with every shift in weight.
Fix: To reduce impact, "slide your hand up to the bar to push the fleshy part down and out of the way," says Collins. Be sure to grip the bar at the crease where your fingers meet your palms, and then wrap your fingers around it.

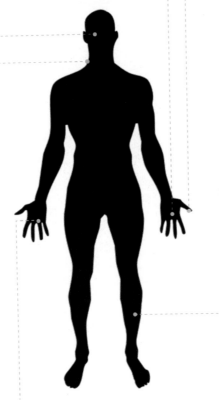

PROBLEM:
BLOODY BOXING KNUCKLES

Cause: Skilled boxers throw punches fast and frequently. But your skin doesn't always toughen as quickly as your muscles do.
Fix: Build tolerance by hitting the bag harder but less frequently and for shorter time frames, says Julien Baker, PhD, a professor of applied physiology at the University of Glamorgan. If you usually punch for 3 minutes at 50 percent strength, say, try 1 minute at full strength until your knuckles can last longer.

PROBLEM:
TENNIS THUMB BLISTERS

Cause: You have those nasty fluid bubbles because you're gripping your racket too hard, causing friction between your skin and the handle.
Fix: Relax your hand. You'll hit with surprisingly greater racket speed while reducing postmatch pain, says Kris Berg, EdD, a professor of exercise physiology at the University of Nebraska at Omaha. You can increase your sessions after your skin develops tolerance.

PROBLEM:
DEADLIFT SHIN SCRAPES

Cause: The rough gripping area of the bar (called the knurling) drags against your legs as you lift, grating your skin.
Fix: Before liftoff, "position your shoulders in front of the bar and your shoulder blades directly over the bar," says Alexander J. Koch, PhD, an associate professor of health and exercise sciences at Truman State University in Missouri. You'll avoid pulling the bar into your shins, resulting in a cleaner, safer lift.

EXERCISE SCIENCE

RUN FOR YOUR LIFE

It's official: Running increases your chances of living longer. Stanford researchers recently completed a 21-year study of 284 runners and 156 healthy nonrunners. They found that middle-aged and older runners cut their risk of disability and death from all major diseases by 40 percent. The scientists believe it's due to the sport's ability to increase cardiovascular fitness, improve aerobic capacity, expand organ reserve, boost skeletal and muscle mass, lower circulating inflammatory markers, and improve cognitive functions.

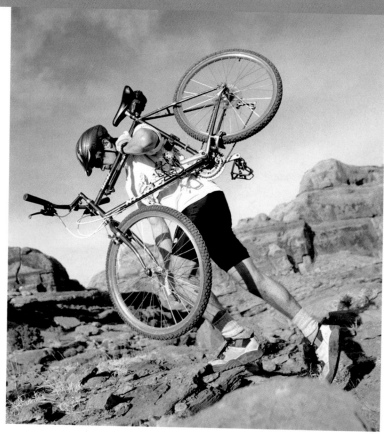

CLIMB HIGHER

A professor who studied stair running says it requires less flexing of the foot and ankle than hill running at the same incline does, so it's easier.

Alberto Minetti, MD, a physiology professor at the University of Milan, says running steep hills generally provides a harder workout for each vertical meter than running stairs does. A charity stairs race is still a fun workout. Find one with the American Lung Association (lungusa.org).

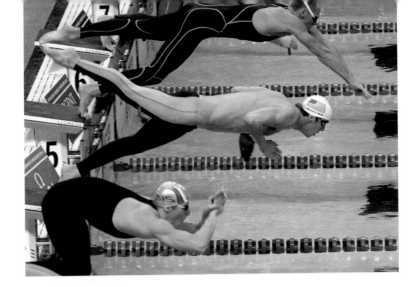

DON'T DREAD THE TREAD

If you're shopping for a treadmill, check out a motorless model. British scientists found that manually powered treadmills simulate over-ground running significantly better than motor-driven machines do. The mechanism: Conventional treadmills pull your feet back, causing you to run with straighter-than-normal legs, says study coauthor Phil Riches, PhD. A manual belt, on the other hand, forces you to push off with each foot as you would on hard ground. The powerless units do require se-rious torque to speed up, but once you're in full stride

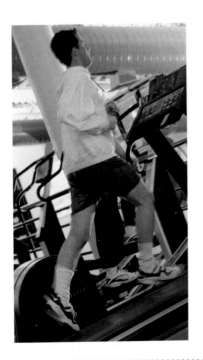

you won't miss the powered belt. Already own a motorized model? Run on an incline, which requires you to push off the belt with bent knees and added force.

But at the end of the day, a treadmill is no match for solid ground. When Wake Forest University scientists allowed exercisers to set their own pace on either a treadmill or a running track, the 'mill users preferred slower speeds and shorter stride lengths than those of the track athletes. And even when they were assigned a specific pace, the speed of the ground pounders remained higher. One reason: Treadmill users feel more negative about and derive less enjoyment from their training program than outdoor runners do, according to the study authors.

Running a 7-minute mile on the machine equals the effort of about a 7:30 pace on a track.

BE SLEEK; BE SPEEDY

Swimmers wearing full-body or waist-down suits expend about 5 percent less energy than when wearing conventional racing suits, tests found. Swimmers experienced less drag and lowered their times—by about 3 percent in full-body suits and almost 2 percent in legs-only suits.

Michael Phelps wears the Speedo LZR Racer, which has even less drag than the company's Fastskin, and goes for $290 and up at speedousa.com. Or use an old-style suit, work harder, and become fitter.

BE YOUR BEST

Want to score a personal best in that upcoming 10-K? Avoid new weight-training exercises, plyometric drills, and running downhill in the final few days before your big race. British researchers discovered that doing these types of activities within 48 hours of a timed event reduced the distance that runners could cover by as much as 7 percent.

"The exercises cause a high level of muscle damage, which seems to have an effect on the brain, significantly increasing an athlete's level of exertion even if he doesn't feel sore," says Samuele Marcora, PhD, the study's coauthor.

HIT YOUR STRIDE

The longer your stride, the more effective your workout, say University of Idaho researchers. They found that an extended stride length on cardio equipment can boost oxygen consumption by up to 12 percent and heart rate by 6 percent. At 44 inches, the stride length of the FreeMotion 5.8s is nearly twice that of a conventional elliptical machine, for a calorie thrashing that's easier on hip and knee joints. ($3,000, freemotionfitness.com)

WAKE UP TO WIN

It's not worth jumping out front during a triathlon's swim: You can save energy in the water by sticking close to the pack. After a series of lab tests, Portuguese scientists concluded that a swimmer who stays

2 feet behind another athlete's foot kicks experiences 44 percent less drag through the water. What's more, you can draft off another triathlete from as far back as 19 feet and still reduce your drag by 16 percent. "You'll maintain an overall

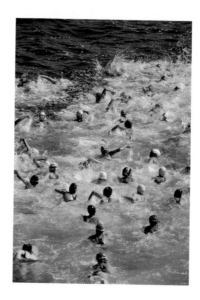

higher race pace, since you'll be sparing energy," says António José Silva, PhD, the study's lead author.

A tri tip: The sooner you drink water after the swim, the faster your closing run will be, say scientists at UNC-Chapel Hill.

PROTECT YOUR POWER

Can you stomach the demands of cycling? According to a new study from the University of

Pittsburgh, strong core muscles decrease your risk of lower-body cycling injuries. After analyzing riders, the researchers found that those with the weakest cores saw their mechanics fail during endurance rides.

"They began to flap their legs," says study author John Abt, PhD. In other words, the cyclists pedaled with a sideways motion instead of in proper up-and-down fashion. Although the riders were able to maintain their power, "this breakdown in technique could lead to a serious knee injury," Dr. Abt says.

BEAT THE SUMMERTIME BLUES

Think you slow down in the heat of the summer? You probably do. An Australian study charted differences in power output when elite cyclists completed 30-minute time trials in 73° and 90°F temperatures. But don't feel discouraged. Your performance will probably boost back up in the cooler weather.

GO GOLFING

Assuming the average golfer can dodge errant balls, he will live 5 years longer than a nonswinger, say Scandinavian scientists in the *Scandinavian Journal of Medicine &*

Science in Sports. They studied 300,000 golfers who regularly traversed 18 holes (sans golf cart). The researchers found that the death rate for golfers is 40 percent lower than that of other people of the same sex, age, and socioeconomic status. This corresponds to a 5-year increase in life expectancy, say the study authors, who credit this life-extending effect to the fact that golfers are outside for hours at a time, walk about 4 miles, and are engaged in a stress-reducing social activity.

HELP YOUR HANDICAP

Look out, Tiger. Phosphatidylserine (PS), a newcomer on the dietary-supplement scene, might help improve your golf game, report German researchers. When golfers with handicaps ranging from 15 to 40 took 200 milligrams of PS daily for 6 weeks, their combined accuracy levels increased nearly 25 percent.

That's because phosphatidylserine might help dampen stress hormones, allowing you to concentrate better, say the researchers, who will test a PS-infused snack bar on golfers later this year. In the meantime, a 200-milligram

dose of the supplement could make that next 8-foot birdie putt a bit easier to drain.

SAVE YOUR KNEES

Here's another instance where a rubber can save you: Neoprene sleeves help protect your knees from injury. That's because the braces significantly boost joint stability, say researchers in Belgium. According to Damien Van Tiggelen, PT, the study's lead author, injuries often occur when knee stability breaks down due to fatigue. He suggests reaching for the sleeves before the fourth quarter of a basketball game or any other period of high fatigue, such as a run that follows a weight-lifting session.

"The brace provides support but doesn't impair muscle function, so there's no detrimental effect," he says, adding that the increase in proprioception (sense of balance) can potentially smooth your movements. We like McDavid's Level 1 knee support ($13, mcdavidusa.com).

PLAY BALL

Don't let the goofy goggles stop you: Racquetball is a worthy cardio challenge, according to a new study in the *Journal of Sports Medicine*

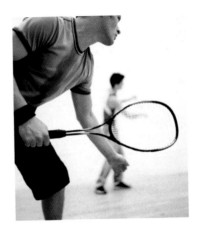

and Physical Fitness.

When the researchers had recreational players compete in 40-minute matches, they found that the exercise intensity of the court sport was on par with bicycling and jogging, which was a surprise because the action is intermittent.

What's more, racquetball builds explosive power due to its emphasis on quick stops, starts, and lunges.

To find a court, go to usra.org, click on "Lists & Links," and select your state's racquetball home page. ■

TRAINING TIPS

Q: I want to start running. How do I find the best shoe?

A: Measure the length of your foot both standing and sitting. If the difference is ¼ inch or less, you have a neutral foot, which rolls inward, or pronates, to absorb impact. If the difference is ¼ inch or more, your foot is flexible; your arch collapses as your foot lands, forcing your ankle muscles to work harder to keep you stable. If there's no change, you have a rigid foot—the impact force travels up your leg, possibly causing knee pain.

"The correct shoe reduces the muscle activity needed to run and makes your movement more efficient," says Benno M. Nigg, DrScNat, who studies biomechanics at the University of Calgary. Start shopping with our favorites that follow.

Motion Control
They're tanklike. These sturdy, durable shoes offer enough arch support to balance wobbly feet.

Good for: Flexible foot

Asics Gel-Foundation 8: Memory foam increases comfort by lining and cushioning your foot, and the wide base creates a solid foundation. ($90)

Brooks Trance 8: The segmented outsole (unlike a one-piece outsole) acts like a series of shock absorbers, smoothing your stride from heel to toe. ($140)

Stability
These shoes balance rigidity and cushioning with moderate arch support to stabilize foot roll.

Good for: Neutral foot

Asics Gel-Kayano 14: Its midsole is a lightweight foam that compresses just slightly as your foot rolls in. ($135)

Nike Air Zoom Structure Triax+ 11: Dense padding along the arch ensures a smooth heel-to-toe transition, while air pockets provide the cushioning. ($95)

Neutral Cushioned
Minimal arch support and softer midsoles encourage the foot to roll in to absorb the impact.

Good for: Rigid foot

Adidas Supernova Cushion 7: The lightweight foam midsole provides uniform cushioning along the length of the shoe. ($90)

Mizuno Wave Rider 11: Well-placed grooves in the sole increase the shoe's flexibility, and an elastic panel in the heel relieves stress and helps maintain the shoe's shape. ($95)

Q: Can you burn more fat by running in the sunshine?

A: Not enough to matter, says Alan Aragon, a nutritionist in Westlake Village, California, and the *Men's Health* Weight-Loss Coach.

This notion stems from the idea that light therapy can boost weight loss, a conclusion based on a 2007 study in the journal *Obesity*. The study found that people who exercised under bright lights lost about 2 percent body fat, while a control group's body fat stayed the same. But because these changes took place over 6 weeks, they're not terribly impressive. Also, the method used to assess body composition wasn't the most accurate one available.

If you burn the same amount of calories, sunshine won't offer any inherent fat-loss advantage over an indoor environment. Stick with the setting that motivates you best. It's far more important to have a regular routine of exercise, no matter where you're doing it.

Q: I take creatine before I lift weights. Should I also take it before I run?

A: It won't hurt, but it probably won't help either. Creatine increases the body's ability to produce energy rapidly. The more energy you produce, the harder you can train, and the faster your muscles will grow. At least that's what a handful of studies suggest for weight lifting and explosive activities such as football and baseball. The jury is still out on whether it can improve endurance or boost aerobic capacity. Besides, your kidneys and pancreas produce about 1 gram of the stuff on their own, which, when combined with the additional gram most people get from foods such as chicken and fish, is enough for cardio training.

Q: Will riding a bike affect my fertility?

A: Recent studies suggest there is a correlation between erectile dysfunction, sperm count, and time spent in the saddle, says Jordan D. Metzl, MD, a sports medicine specialist at the Hospital for Special Surgery, in New York City.

In fact, Austrian researchers found that the sperm production of cyclists who rode more than 3,000 miles a year was a third lower than that of noncyclers. That said, some experts warn to take such studies with a grain of salt, pointing to European nations with high numbers of male cyclists and normal rates of infertility and ED. Dr. Metzl's advice: Hedge your bets with a seat designed to ease the pressure on your privates—Specialized makes some great ones—and stand up for 60 seconds after every 30 minutes of riding.

Q: What can I do to make my back stop hurting after I play golf?

A: Start treating golf like a sport. Successful pro athletes don't hit the court or field without priming their bodies for action. Neither should you. Strengthen your back and torso with targeted exercises—we like back extensions and bicycle crunches—and do this stretch before you tee off: Standing in your address position, hold your five iron horizontally in front of you with your hands at each end and your elbows straight. Turn back and through, as if you were swinging. Pause for five seconds at the top of your backswing and again in the finish position. Repeat.

Q: **How can I prevent soreness after a day on the slopes?**

A: The single best way to ease next-day pain is to hydrate like mad, says Kevin Stone, MD, the founder of the Stone Clinic in San Francisco and a surgeon for the Jeep Ski Tour.

Water flushes lactic acid (a primary cause of soreness and stiffness) from muscle cells and lubricates joints. Drink two glasses with each meal and after every few runs. Also, jump into the hot tub for 15 minutes both before and after you hit the slopes, taking time to stretch your back and hamstrings by placing one leg at a time on the side of the tub and curling your head toward your knee. Warm muscles aid athletic performance; cold ones snap under the pressure.

Q: **If you break a bone, does it really grow back stronger than before?**

A: "It grows back as strong, sometimes stronger," says Andrew J. Feldman, MD, the director of sports medicine at St. Vincent's Medical Center in New York City, as well as a clinical instructor at New York Medical College in Valhalla, New York. "The body tells the broken bone to lay down new calcium, which may cause extra bone to form."

Q: **When I recover from one injury, another crops up. Could I be overtraining?**

A: An increased incidence of injuries is one sign of overtraining, but it's not the only one, says Dr. Metzl. Here's how to know for sure: Lie down and rest for 15 minutes, and then record your pulse rate. Stand up, wait 15 seconds, and record your pulse again. If the difference is greater than 15 beats per minute, you're overtraining. Ease up on your workout intensity and start cross-training. Overuse injuries usually occur in people who focus on one sport, which is why triathletes so rarely suffer them. ■

CREDITS

INDEX

Boldface page references indicate photographs. <u>Underscored</u> references indicate boxed text.

cholesterol-lowering drugs and,
306
failure of, pushing to, 182
mass, preserving, 100–101
soreness, managing, 100,
180–81, 351
strength test, 110–13, **111–13**
triceps, developing, 184
Mushrooms, 60
Music and weight lifting, 179
Myopathy, 306

N

Nasal congestion, 235
National Academy of Sports
Medicine (Calabasas,
California), 149
Nausea, 269
NEAT (non-exercise activity
thermogenesis), 306
Neck, stiff, 305
Neti pot, 263
Nexium, 262–63
Noise pollution, 247
Non-steroidal anti-inflammatory
drugs (NSAIDs), 262
NorCal Strength & Conditioning
(Chico, California), 142
Nori, 71, **71**
NSAIDs, 262
Nutrition. *See* Diet; *specific food*
Nuts, 20, **21**

O

Oatmeal, 20, **21**
OGTT, 273–74
Oily skin, 236
Olive oil, 309
Omega-3 fatty acids, 62
Omron Deluxe Blood Pressure
Monitor, 307
1,4 dioxane, 217
Oral glucose-tolerance test
(OGTT), 273–74
Orange juice, 26–27, 62
Orlando Barbell (Oviedo,
Florida), 146
Osteoarthritis, 305
Osteoporosis, 101–2
Overeating, 18–19
Overtraining, 351
Overweight

fitness and, 178
friends, 246–47
health risks of, 50
longevity and, 178
obesity epidemic and, 246
running and, 53

P

Pancreas, 280–82
Panera food, **4–5**, 4–5
Parabens, 217
Pasta, 63
Pastries, **7**, 7
Paullinia cupana, 269
Peanut oil, 309
Pedialyte, 106
PEG, 217
Performance Training Center
(Beaverton, Oregon), 149
Perspiration, 234–35
Phenylephrine, 263
Philippi Sports Institute (Las
Vegas, Nevada), 143,
146
Phosphatidylserine (PS), 348
Phthalates, 217
Phytoecdysteroids, 102
Pizza Hut food, 4, 4
Platelets, aspirin in unclogging,
275
Polit, Mario, 170, **171**, 173
Pollution, 247
Polyethylene glycol (PEG), 217
Pomegranate juice, 62
Portion sizes, 11, 36
Posture, 233
Potassium, 100–101, 101
Potato chips, 65
Potatoes, 61–62, 105
Prescription drugs, 260–63. *See
also specific type*
Prilosec, 262–63
Probiotics, 103
Propecia, 219
Prostate cancer, 274–75
Prostate-specific antigen (PSA),
275
Protein, 25, 30, 51, 104
Protein powder, 100, 104, 266
Protein shakes, 107
PS, 348
PSA, 275
Pseudoephedrine, 263

Pumpkin-seed oil, 219
Punctuality, 209

Q

Quinoa, 20, **21**, 63–64

R

Racquetball, 348, **348**
Raisins, 103, **103**
Red wine, 65
Resistance bands, 149, 159–61
Results Fitness (Santa Clarita,
California), 146, 148
Resveratrol, 65
Robiola cheese, 75
Rogaine, 219
Roncal cheese, 75
Rooibos tea, 69–70, **69**
Rosiglitazone, 261
Running. *See also* Marathons
adaptations of body for, 324
brain and, 324
creatine and, 350
hills, 345
injury prevention and, 322, 327
longevity and, 345
overweight and, 53
pain-free, 327
personal best and, reaching,
346–47
shoes for, 349
stride, 347
in sunshine, 350
treadmill, 346, **346**
in triathlons, 325, 347, **347**
R.W. Knudsen Family Tangerine
drink, 26, 26

S

Sainte-Maure cheese, 76
Salads, **5**, 5
Salmon, 20, **21**, 62–63
Sandbags for weight lifting, 142
Sandwiches, **3–6**, 3–6, **40**, 40
Saw palmetto, 219
Scalp, 233
Scents, 197–98, **198**
Secondhand smoke, 269
Selenium, 60
7-Eleven Double Big Gulp drink,
26, 26